Statistics for Biology and Health

Series Editors
Mitchell Gail
Jonathan M. Samet
B. Singer
Anastasios Tsiatis

More information about this series at http://www.springer.com/series/2848

George J. Knafl • Kai Ding

Adaptive Regression for Modeling Nonlinear Relationships

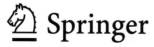 Springer

George J. Knafl
University of North Carolina
   at Chapel Hill
Chapel Hill, NC, USA

Kai Ding
University of Oklahoma Health Sciences Center
Oklahoma City, OK, USA

Additional material to this book can be downloaded from
http://www.unc.edu/~gknafl/AdaptReg.html

ISSN 1431-8776   ISSN 2197-5671   (electronic)
Statistics for Biology and Health
ISBN 978-3-319-81638-8   ISBN 978-3-319-33946-7   (eBook)
DOI 10.1007/978-3-319-33946-7

Printed on acid-free paper

This Springer imprint is published by Springer Nature
The registered company is Springer International Publishing AG Switzerland

Preface

This book addresses how to incorporate nonlinearity in one or more predictor (or explanatory or independent) variables in regression models for different types of outcome (or response or dependent) variables. Such nonlinear dependence is often not considered in applied research. While relationships can reasonably be treated as linear in some cases, it is not unusual for them to be distinctly nonlinear. A standard linear analysis in the latter cases can produce misleading conclusions, while a nonlinear analysis can provide novel insights into data not otherwise possible. A variety of examples of the benefits to the modeling of nonlinear relationships are presented throughout the book.

Methods are needed for deciding whether relationships are linear or nonlinear and for fitting appropriate models when they are nonlinear. Methods for these purposes are covered in this book using what are called fractional polynomials based on power transformations of primary predictor variables with real valued (and so possibly fractional) powers. An adaptive approach is used to construct fractional polynomial models based on heuristic (or rule-based) searches through power transforms of primary predictor variables. The book covers how to formulate and conduct such adaptive fractional polynomial modeling in a variety of contexts including adaptive regression of continuous outcomes, adaptive logistic regression of discrete outcomes with two or more values, and adaptive Poisson regression of count outcomes, possibly adjusted into rate outcomes with offsets. Power transformation of positive valued continuous outcomes is covered as well as modeling of variances/dispersions with fractional polynomials. The book also covers alternative approaches for modeling nonlinear relationships including standard polynomials, generalized additive models computed using local regression (loess) and spline smoothing approaches, and multivariate adaptive regression splines.

Part I covers modeling of nonlinear relationships for continuous outcomes using adaptive regression modeling. Adaptive models of this type are linear in the parameters for modeling the means, as are commonly used regression models based on untransformed primary predictor variables. However, adaptive models can depend on nonlinear transformations of available primary predictor variables.

Chapters 2 and 3 address nonlinear modeling of means and variances of univariate continuous outcomes using fractional polynomials. Chapters 4 and 5 extend this to modeling of means and variances of multivariate continuous outcomes, including marginal models based on either maximum likelihood estimation or generalized estimating equations (GEE) and conditional models with current outcome values depending on either prior outcome values (that is, transition models) or all other outcome values. Chapters 6 and 7 cover transformation of positive valued continuous outcomes as well as their predictors.

Part II extends fractional polynomial modeling to discrete outcomes, either dichotomous with two values or polytomous with more than two values, using adaptive logistic regression. Chapters 8 and 9 address modeling of means and dispersions of univariate dichotomous and polytomous outcomes. Polytomous outcomes are modeled both with adaptive ordinal regression using cumulative logits under the proportional odds assumption and with adaptive multinomial regression using generalized logits as needed for nominal outcomes. Chapters 10 and 11 extend this modeling to multivariate discrete outcomes.

Part III extends fractional polynomial modeling further to count outcomes using adaptive Poisson regression, possibly adjusted to models of rate outcomes using offsets. Chapters 12 and 13 address modeling of means and dispersions of univariate count/rate outcomes. Chapters 14 and 15 extend this modeling to multivariate count/rate outcomes.

Part IV covers modeling of nonlinear relationships for univariate continuous and dichotomous outcomes using generalized additive models (GAMs) and multivariate adaptive regression splines (MARS) models. It also compares GAMs as generated by SAS® PROC GAM and MARS models as generated by PROC ADAPTIVEREG to associated adaptive regression models. Chapters 16 and 17 address modeling of nonlinear relationships using GAMs for means of univariate continuous and dichotomous outcomes. Chapters 18 and 19 address modeling of nonlinear relationships using MARS models for means of these two types of outcomes. Modeling of variances/dispersions, correlated multivariate outcomes, and polytomous discrete outcomes are not covered since PROC GAM and PROC ADAPTIVEREG do not currently support such modeling. Modeling of count/rate outcomes is also not considered for brevity.

Chapters 2–19 present a series of analyses of selected data sets. These analyses demonstrate how to conduct adaptive regression modeling, generalized additive modeling, and MARS modeling in the regression, logistic regression, and Poisson regression contexts as well as the need for such nonlinear modeling. Overviews of analysis results are provided in even-numbered chapters. Statistical formulations for associated regression models are also provided in some of these chapters. Part V (Chap. 20) provides a summary of these formulations and their extensions to distributions in the exponential family. It also covers the heuristics underlying the adaptive modeling process. Familiarity with vector and matrix notation and calculus is needed to understand the formulations, but not the analyses and the example code. An informal overview of the adaptive modeling process is provided in Sect. 1.3.

Direct support for adaptive regression modeling based on fractional polynomials is not currently available in standard statistical software tools like SAS version 9.4 (SAS Institute Inc., Cary, NC). Consequently, SAS macros have been developed for these purposes. Detailed descriptions of how to use these macros and of their output are provided in odd-numbered chapters (except for Chap. 1). A working knowledge of SAS is assumed, so the book does not provide an introduction to the use of SAS.

The intended audience includes data analysts, both applied researchers conducting analyses of their own data and statisticians conducting analyses for applied researchers. Readers can choose to focus on a specific type of regression analysis (for example, logistic regression of univariate dichotomous outcomes as covered in Chaps. 8 and 9) but should review Chaps. 2 and 3 first for an introduction to adaptive regression modeling and Sects. 4.5.3 and 4.5.4 on moderation analyses using geometric combinations. Practice exercises are provided at the end of odd-numbered chapters (except for Chap. 1) for readers to practice conducting analyses like those in the related even-numbered chapters, and so the book can be used as a text for a course or workshop on adaptive regression modeling. The lectures can present the analyses in the text along with underlying formulations and students can use the exercises to practice conducting adaptive regression analyses. The data sets are primarily taken from the health sciences, but the methods apply generally to all application areas.

References are provided at the end of each chapter. Supplementary materials are available on the Internet (http://www.unc.edu/~gknafl/AdaptReg.html) including Internet sources for data sets used in Chaps. 2–19, the SAS macros used in analyses reported in Chaps. 2–19, detailed descriptions of those macros, and code for conducting the analyses reported in Chaps. 2–19.

Chapel Hill, NC, USA   George J. Knafl
Oklahoma City, OK, USA   Kai Ding

Acknowledgments

We thank Hannah Bracken of Springer for her support and our families for all their encouragement. The development of the genreg macro used in reported analyses was partially supported by grants R01 AI57043 from the National Institute of Allergy and Infectious Diseases and R03 MH086132 from the National Institute of Mental Health.

Contents

Abbreviations

AIC	Akaike information criterion
AIC′	Akaike information criterion adjusted so that larger scores indicate better models
AIC$^+$	Extended Akaike information criterion adjusted so that larger scores indicate better models
AR1	Order 1 autoregressive
BIC	Bayesian information criterion
BIC′	Bayesian information criterion adjusted so that larger scores indicate better models
BIC$^+$	Extended Bayesian information criterion adjusted so that larger scores indicate better models
CV	Cross-validation
DF	Degrees of freedom
EC	Exchangeable correlations
GAM	Generalized additive model
GC	Geometric combination
GCV	Generalized cross-validation
GEE	Generalized estimating equations
LCV	Likelihood cross-validation
LCV(λ)	Power-adjusted likelihood cross-validation (for an outcome raised to the power λ)
LCV$^+$	Extended likelihood cross-validation
loess	Local regression
log	Natural logarithm
LOO	Leave-one-out
LSCV	Least squares cross-validation
MARS	multivariate adaptive regression splines
ML	Maximum likelihood
ODS	Output delivery system
OR	Odds ratio

PCDP	Proportion of correct deleted predictions
PD	Percent decrease
PI	Percent increase
PLC	Penalized likelihood criterion
PLC$'$	Penalized likelihood criterion adjusted so that larger scores indicate better models
PLCV	Pseudolikelihood cross-validation
PLCV$^+$	Extended pseudolikelihood cross-validation
PRESS	Prediction sums of squares
QIC	Quasi-likelihood information criterion
QIC$'$	Quasi-likelihood information criterion adjusted so that larger scores indicate better models
QLCV$^+$	Extended quasi-likelihood cross-validation
UN	Unstructured

About the Authors

George J. Knafl is Professor and Biostatistician in the School of Nursing of the University of North Carolina at Chapel Hill where he teaches statistics courses to doctoral nursing students, consults with graduate students and faculty on their research, and conducts his own research. He has over 35 years of experience in teaching, consulting, and research in statistics. His research involves development of methods for searching through alternative models for data to identify an effective choice for modeling those data and the application of those methods to the analysis of health science data sets. He is also Professor Emeritus in the College of Computing and Digital Media at DePaul University and has also taught in Schools of Nursing at Yale University and the Oregon Health and Sciences University.

Kai Ding is Assistant Professor, Department of Biostatistics and Epidemiology at the University of Oklahoma (OU) Health Sciences Center. He is also Associated Member of the Peggy and Charles Stephenson Cancer Center (SCC) of OU Medicine. Dr. Ding received his Ph.D. in Biostatistics from the University of North Carolina at Chapel Hill in 2010. His research focuses on survival analysis and semiparametric inference. He has been involved in the design and analysis of numerous research studies in cancer and ophthalmology and currently serves on the Scientific Review Committee and the Protocol Monitoring Committee of the SCC.

Chapter 1
Introduction

1.1 Purpose

Nonlinearity in one or more predictor (or explanatory or independent) variables in regression models for different types of outcome (or response or dependent) variables is often not considered in applied research. While relationships can reasonably be treated as linear in some cases, it is not unusual for them to be distinctly nonlinear. A standard linear analysis in the latter cases can produce misleading conclusions while a nonlinear analysis can provide novel insights into data not otherwise possible.

Methods are needed for deciding whether relationships are linear or nonlinear and for fitting appropriate models when they are nonlinear. Methods for these purposes are covered in this book using what are called fractional polynomials (Royston and Altman 1994) based on power transformations of primary predictor variables with real valued (and so possibly fractional) powers. An adaptive approach is used to construct fractional polynomial models based on heuristic (or rule-based) searches through power transforms of primary predictor variables (see Sect. 1.3 for an overview and Chap. 20 for details).

As an example, analyses are presented in Chap. 2 of death rates in 60 metropolitan statistical areas. Figure 1.1 displays a portion of these data along with a fitted nonlinear curve. The regression model for the death rates as a linear function of associated nitric oxide pollution index values suggests that the mean death rate does not depend on the nitric oxide pollution index ($P = 0.557$) as do the associated quadratic and cubic polynomial models. Consideration of fractional polynomials is required to identify that the mean death rate does distinctly nonlinearly depend on the nitric oxide pollution index (the power used in Fig. 1.1 is -0.8). See Sect. 2.20 for a summary of analyses conducted in Chap. 2 of the death rate data.

As a second example, analyses are conducted in Chap. 4 of dental measurements at 8, 10, 12, and 14 years old for 27 children, including 16 boys and 11 girls, as a function of their age, gender, and the interaction (that is, the product) of age and

© Springer International Publishing Switzerland 2016
G.J. Knafl, K. Ding, *Adaptive Regression for Modeling Nonlinear Relationships*,
Statistics for Biology and Health, DOI 10.1007/978-3-319-33946-7_1

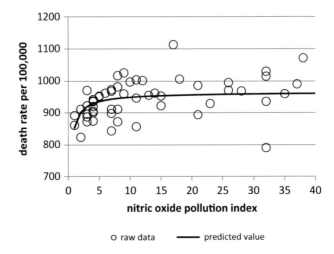

Fig. 1.1 The death rate per 100,000 as a function of the nitric oxide pollution index

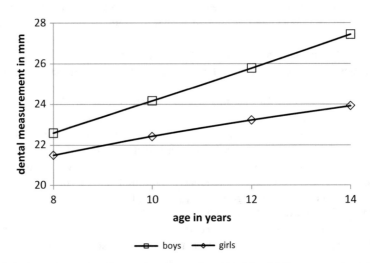

Fig. 1.2 Estimated mean dental measurements as a function of the child's age as moderated by the child's gender

gender, an issue called moderation or modification (see Sect. 4.5.3). The model linear in these three terms under autoregressive correlations with constant variances suggests that the dependence on age is reasonably treated as the same for boys and girls ($P = 0.116$ for the interaction). Consideration of fractional polynomials is required to identify that in fact the dependence on age is different for boys than it is for girls. The estimated moderation relationship is displayed in Fig. 1.2. Mean dental measurements increase for both girls and boys at lower levels for girls than for boys, at slower rates for girls as they age (the associated power for girl's ages is 0.19), and nearly linearly for boys as they age. See Sect. 4.16 for a summary of analyses conducted in Chap. 4 of the dental measurement data. Other examples of benefits to consideration of nonlinear relationships are presented throughout the book.

The book covers how to formulate and conduct adaptive fractional polynomial modeling in a variety of contexts including adaptive regression of continuous outcomes, adaptive logistic regression of dichotomous and polytomous outcomes with two or more values, and adaptive Poisson regression of count outcomes, possibly adjusted to rate outcomes using offsets. Power transformation of positive valued continuous outcomes is covered as well as modeling of variances/dispersions with fractional polynomials. The book also covers alternative approaches for modeling nonlinear relationships, including standard polynomials, generalized additive models (GAMs) (Hastie and Tibshirani 1999) computed using local regression (loess) (Cleveland et al. 1988) and spline (Ahlberg et al. 1967) smoothing approaches (through SAS PROC GAM), and multivariate adaptive regression splines (MARS) (Friedman 1991) models (through SAS PROC ADAPTIVEREG).

Direct support for adaptive regression modeling based on fractional polynomials is not currently available in standard statistical software tools like SAS (version 9.4). Consequently, SAS macros have been developed for these purposes. These macros are available on the Internet (http://www.unc.edu/~gknafl/AdaptReg.html) as is code for loading in the data and for conducting the analyses reported in the book. Base SAS is required as well as SAS/STAT and PROC IML. Detailed descriptions of how to use these macros and of their output are provided, assuming a working knowledge of SAS. See, for example, Der and Everitt (2006) for a thorough description of SAS. SAS output displays are generated in listing format, not in the default HTML format of SAS version 9.4. All reported analyses have been generated with SAS version 9.4 under Windows 7 using an Intel Core 2 Duo CPU.

A series of analyses of selected data sets are presented to demonstrate how to conduct adaptive regression modeling in a variety of contexts as well as the need for consideration of nonlinear relationships. This includes the regression context (see Part I) with continuous outcomes and models for their means linear in the coefficient parameters, the logistic regression context (see Part II) with either dichotomous outcomes with two values or polytomous outcomes with more than two values, and the Poisson regression context (see Part III) with count/rate outcomes. In the special case of polytomous outcomes, the analyses address both ordinal regression models using cumulative logits under the proportional odds assumption as well as multinomial regression models using generalized logits as needed for nominal outcomes. The analyses address both univariate and multivariate outcomes of these three types. The analyses also include a comparison of generalized additive modeling (Hastie and Tibshirani 1999) and MARS modeling (Friedman 1991), well-established nonparametric regression methods, to adaptive modeling (see Part IV). Statistical formulations for regression models of these types are provided. A separate summary of these formulations and their extensions to distributions in the exponential family along with the heuristics underlying the adaptive modeling process are also provided (see Part V). Familiarity with vector and matrix notation and calculus is needed to understand the formulations, but not the analyses and the example code.

1.2   Background

Regression models commonly assume that the mean of an outcome variable y, or some transform of that mean, is linear in available predictor variables. Nonlinearity of y in a primary predictor x can be addressed by inclusion of one or more transforms of x as predictors. Most commonly, this is achieved through standard polynomial models with powers limited to nonnegative integers. Usually, all nonnegative integer powers less than a fixed value are included in the polynomial model, for example, the fully specified cubic polynomial model with constant term x^0, linear term x^1, quadratic term x^2, and cubic term x^3. Standard polynomials can effectively model nonlinearity in x in some cases, but not in general (see Sect. 2.9). Moreover, fully specified polynomial models can overfit the data, and fully specified polynomial models of higher degree than the cubic model are infrequently used.

Royston and Altman (1994) proposed an alternative they called fractional polynomial modeling allowing powers to be real valued. Their work has been extended by Royston and Sauerbrei (2008). They recommended consideration of only a few selected powers, for example, -2, -1, -0.5, 0.5, 1, 2, 3 and the natural log transform as the 0 power case for degree 1 fractional polynomials with only one power transform. One choice within the fixed set is used, not the complete set as in fully specified standard polynomial models. Considering only powers from a fixed set can effectively model nonlinearity in a predictor x in many cases and can outperform standard polynomial modeling since that fixed set usually contains all the powers of linear, quadratic, and cubic polynomials. However, a fixed set of powers cannot address general nonlinearity in x (see Sects. 2.12 and 2.13 for an example based on a simulated data set and Sect. 13.3 for an example based on a real, non-simulated data set), and so unrestricted real valued powers are considered in the analyses reported in this book. Royston and Sauerbrei (2008) only addressed fractional polynomial modeling of means while fractional polynomials are also used in this book to model variances/dispersions as well as means. They also only considered modeling of univariate outcomes (except for a brief treatment of multi-level models in their Sect. 12.3.3) while both univariate and multivariate outcomes are addressed in this book.

Knafl et al. (2004) developed methods for adaptively selecting powers with arbitrary real values, not limited to a fixed set. These methods use a heuristic (that is, rule-based) approach to search through integer powers, then through single decimal digit powers, followed by two decimal digit powers, and continuing until there is no distinct benefit to changing the power (as defined in Sect. 20.4.3). Models are evaluated and compared using cross-validation (see Sect. 2.5 for an introduction to cross-validation) with the data randomly partitioned into k subsets called folds (Burman 1989). Cross-validation scores are adapted to the type of data by basing them on an appropriate likelihood for those data or in general on some kind of extended likelihood, for example, an extended quasi-likelihood (McCullagh and Nelder 1999). These possibly extended likelihood cross-validation (LCV) scores are used to control the adaptive modeling process. Penalized likelihood criteria (PLCs) can also be used for that purpose (see Sect. 2.10).

Knafl et al. (2004) only addressed adaptive Poisson regression modeling of univariate count/rate outcomes, but their approach extends to modeling means of univariate outcomes under generalized linear models (McCullagh and Nelder 1999). Knafl et al. (2010) extended this work further to adaptive modeling of variances/dispersions of univariate outcomes along with their means using extended quasi-likelihood methods. Knafl et al. (2006) extended adaptive methods to modeling of multivariate outcomes under the standard repeated measures approach based on exchangeable correlations. Their approach generalizes to other correlation structures for multivariate normal data. These are called marginal models (Fitzmaurice et al. 2011).

Likelihoods for marginal models for correlated categorical outcomes are usually difficult to compute, and so generalized estimating equations (GEE) methods (Liang and Zeger 1986) are often used to model such outcomes that avoid computation of likelihoods, complicating the generalization of adaptive modeling based on LCV to this context. However, it is possible to formulate appropriate extended likelihoods for GEE-based models (see Sect. 10.7), with which to compute extended LCV scores for adaptive GEE-based modeling. Conditional modeling (Diggle et al. 2002), on the other hand, is based on pseudolikelihoods, which can be used to compute pseudolikelihood cross-validation (PLCV) scores. Pseudolikelihoods can also be combined with extended quasi-likelihood methods to model variances/dispersions as well as means for conditional models. Moreover, since dependence is addressed in conditional models by modeling individual outcome measurements in terms of subsets of the other outcome measurements for subjects, adaptive methods can be used to generate fractional polynomial models based on primary predictors including averages of those subsets of other outcome measurements as well as other available variables. Transition (or autoregressive or Markov) models with dependence based on subsets of prior outcome measurements are important special cases of conditional models. Both transition models and general conditional models are considered in the example analyses (see Chaps. 4 and 5 for multivariate continuous outcomes, Chaps. 10 and 11 for multivariate dichotomous/polytomous outcomes, and Chaps. 14 and 15 for multivariate count/rate outcomes).

1.3 Overview of the Adaptive Modeling Process

The adaptive modeling process (as formalized in Sect. 20.4) is controlled by LCV scores and by tolerance parameters, changing with the sample size and indicating how much of a percent decrease in the LCV score can be tolerated at given stages of the process. LCV scores can be replaced by some kind of extended LCV scores, for example, scores based on extended quasi-likelihoods rather than on likelihoods, or by PLC scores adjusted so that larger scores indicate better models. The process starts with an expansion phase analogous to the usual forward selection procedure, systematically adding in transforms of primary predictors to a base model (usually the constant model). The next transform to add to the model is the one generating the best LCV score among transforms of primary predictors currently under consideration for expanding the model. Primary predictors generating distinctly inferior LCV scores (as determined by the associated tolerance parameter) at some stage of the expansion are dropped from further consideration. The expansion stops when the next transform to add to the model would reduce the LCV score by more than a tolerable amount (as determined by the expansion stopping tolerance parameter) or when all primary predictors have been dropped from consideration for expanding the model. The expansion can optionally also generate geometric combinations consisting of products of powers of primary predictors generalizing standard interactions (see Sect. 4.5.4).

Expanded models often need simplification to be effective. This is addressed through a contraction phase analogous to the usual backward elimination procedure, removing extraneous transforms from the expanded model and retransforming the remaining transforms in the model. The next transform to remove from the model is the one whose removal, along with retransformation of the remaining transforms, generates the best LCV score among transforms currently under consideration for contracting the model. Transforms are removed from consideration for contracting the model, and so included in the final model possibly retransformed, when removing them at some stage of the contraction generates distinctly inferior LCV scores (as determined by the associated tolerance parameter). The contraction stops when the next transform to remove from the model would reduce the LCV score by more than a tolerable amount (as determined by the contraction stopping tolerance parameter) or when all model transforms have been dropped from consideration for contracting the model.

When the contraction removes any transforms from the expanded model, all the other transforms will be adjusted to improve the LCV score. However, when the contraction leaves the expanded model unchanged, the expanded model might be improved by transforming it. This is only needed for models with at least one non-indicator transform (i.e., not a transform with just the two values 0 and 1) that was added prior to the last step of the expansion. Under such conditions, the expanded, uncontracted model is transformed. Section 10.4.1 provides an example where such a conditional transformation distinctly improves an expanded, uncontracted model.

The adaptive modeling process can be applied to only the expectation (or mean) component of the model, to only the variance/dispersion component, or to both of these components in combination. For example, it is possible to generate an adaptive model for the means assuming constant variances/dispersions. Alternately, it is possible to start with a theory-based model for the means and generate an adaptive model for the variances/dispersions to test the theory-based model for the means under an appropriate model for the variances/dispersions. Finally, it is possible to generate an adaptive model for the variances/dispersions together with the means.

The transforms of an adaptively generated model typically have significantly nonzero slopes. For example, the adaptive model described in Tables 3.4 and 3.6 has two transforms, both of which have highly significant slopes at $P < 0.001$. These results support the effectiveness of the adaptive modeling process. However, they also indicate that it is usually inappropriate to make inferences based on tests for zero coefficients of adaptive models. An exception is a model with some of its terms included on the basis of theoretical considerations and only the other terms of the model adaptively generated. For example, in a study with an intervention group and a control group, the indicator variable for being in the intervention group can be included along with an intercept in the base model, expanded with transforms of available covariates, and contracted with the restriction that the base model should remain unchanged. The test for a zero slope for the intervention group indicator can then be used to assess whether there is an intervention effect on the outcome after controlling for an appropriate set of transformed covariates. Analyses like this could be considered semi-adaptive modeling.

Alternative adaptive models are usually more appropriately compared using χ^2-based LCV ratio tests (Sects. 2.7 and 4.4.2) analogous to likelihood ratio tests. Rather than use a P-value or a cutoff for a significant LCV ratio, LCV ratio tests are expressed in this book in terms of a cutoff for a substantial percent decrease in the LCV score. The value for this cutoff depends on the sample size (see Sect. 4.4.2 for the formula) and is reported in the output of the SAS macros developed to support adaptive modeling. A LCV ratio test is used in determining the contraction stopping tolerance, thereby adjusting its value for the sample size as are all of the tolerance parameters controlling the adaptive modeling process (see Sect. 20.4.8). LCV ratio tests can be used in place of tests for zero coefficients. For example, the adaptive modeling process can be applied first with a set of covariates as the primary predictors and then to those primary predictors together with the intervention group indicator. If the latter model does not include the intervention group indicator, then the covariates explain away its effect on the outcome. If the intervention group indicator is included in the latter model, whether that effect is of substance can be assessed by the LCV ratio test comparing the latter model to the former one computed from only the covariates.

LCV ratio tests are more conservative than tests of zero coefficients, and so similar in effect to multiple comparisons adjustments (Sect. 4.4.2 provides a partial justification for why this holds). For example, Riegel and Knafl (2014) identified 21 baseline risk factors for heart failure patients that individually were significantly ($P < 0.05$) related to hospitalization in the next 6 months. The associated LCV ratio tests comparing the individual risk factor models to the constant model were significant for only 16 (or 76.2 %) of these risk factors. As another example, Knafl and Riegel (2014) identified 12 baseline risk factors for heart failure patients that individually were significantly ($P < 0.05$) related to poor adherence in the next

6 months. The associated LCV ratio tests comparing the individual risk factor models to the constant model were significant only for 2 (or 16.7 %) of these risk factors.

References

Ahlberg, J. H., Nilson, E. N., & Walsh, J. L. (1967). *The theory of splines and their applications.* New York: Academic Press.

Burman, P. (1989). A comparative study of ordinary cross-validation, v-fold cross-validation and the repeated learning-testing methods. *Biometrika, 76*, 503–514.

Cleveland, W. S., Devlin, S. J., & Gross, E. (1988). Regression by local fitting. *Journal of Econometrics, 37*, 87–114.

Der, G., & Everitt, B. S. (2006). *Statistical analysis of medical data using SAS.* Boca Raton, FL: Chapman & Hall/CRC.

Diggle, P. J., Heagarty, P., Liang, K.-Y., & Zeger, S. L. (2002). *Analysis of longitudinal data* (2nd ed.). Oxford: Oxford University Press.

Fitzmaurice, G. M., Laird, N. M., & Ware, J. H. (2011). *Applied longitudinal analysis* (2nd ed.). Hoboken, NJ: John Wiley & Sons.

Friedman, J. H. (1991). Multivariate adaptive regression splines. *Annals of Statistics, 19*, 1–67.

Hastie, T. J., & Tibshirani, R. J. (1999). *Generalized additive models.* Boca Raton, FL: Chapman & Hall/CRC.

Knafl, G. J., Delucchi, K. L., Bova, C. A., Fennie, K. P., & Williams, A. B. (2010). A systematic approach for analyzing electronically monitored adherence data. In B. Ekwall & M. Cronquist (Eds.), *Micro electro mechanical systems (MEMS) technology, fabrication processes and applications, Chapter 1* (pp. 1–66). Hauppauge, NY: Nova. Retrieved from https://www.novapublishers.com/catalog/product_info.php?products_id=19133

Knafl, G. J., Fennie, K. P., Bova, C., Dieckhaus, K., & Williams, A. B. (2004). Electronic monitoring device event modeling on an individual-subject basis using adaptive Poisson regression. *Statistics in Medicine, 23*, 783–801.

Knafl, G. J., Fennie, K. P., & O'Malley, J. P. (2006). Adaptive repeated measures modeling using likelihood cross-validation. In B. Bovaruchuk (Ed.), *Proceedings of the second IASTED international conference on computational intelligence 2006* (pp. 422–427). Anaheim: ACTA Press.

Knafl, G. J., & Riegel, B. (2014). What puts heart failure patients at risk for poor medication adherence? *Patient Preference and Adherence, 8*, 1007–1018.

Liang, K.-Y., & Zeger, S. L. (1986). Longitudinal data analysis using generalized linear models. *Biometrika, 73*, 13–22.

McCullagh, P., & Nelder, J. A. (1999). *Generalized linear models* (2nd ed.). Boca Raton, FL: Chapman & Hall/CRC.

Riegel, B., & Knafl, G. J. (2014). Electronically monitored medication adherence predicts hospitalization in heart failure patients. *Patient Preference and Adherence, 8*, 1–13.

Royston, P., & Altman, D. G. (1994). Regression using fractional polynomials of continuous covariates: Parsimonious parametric modeling. *Applied Statistics, 43*, 429–467.

Royston, P., & Sauerbrei, W. (2008). *Multivariable model-building: A practical approach to regression analysis based on fractional polynomials for modelling continuous variables.* Hoboken, NJ: John Wiley & Sons.

Part I
Adaptive Regression Modeling

Chapter 2
Adaptive Regression Modeling of Univariate Continuous Outcomes

2.1 Chapter Overview

This chapter formulates and demonstrates adaptive regression modeling of univariate continuous outcomes treated as independent and normally distributed either with constant variances, as is common for regression modeling, or with non-constant variances. This type of regression is also called "linear" regression because models for the means are linear in their intercept and slope parameters. Adaptive regression models for means are linear in their intercept and slope parameters as well, but can also be nonlinear in the primary predictors determining those models due to the inclusion in the model of power transforms of those primary predictors. Thus, they could be called adaptive "linear" regression models, but since their purpose is to address nonlinear relationships, the "linear" part is dropped to avoid confusion. Hence, this book refers to adaptive models for continuous outcomes as adaptive regression models to distinguish them from adaptive logistic regression models for discrete outcomes and from adaptive Poisson regression models for count/rate outcomes. A description of how to generate adaptive regression models in SAS is provided in Chap. 3.

Section 2.2 describes the death rate data to be analyzed in this chapter. Section 2.3 provides a formulation of the bivariate regression model to be used in initial analyses and Sect. 2.17 extends this formulation to general multiple regression models. Section 2.4 introduces fractional polynomial models based on power transforms of primary predictor variables. Section 2.5 formulates cross-validation (CV) scores for model selection including likelihood CV (LCV) scores computed from likelihoods (in this case the normal density) with larger scores indicating better models for the data. Section 2.10 addresses the use of penalized likelihood criteria (PLCs) as alternatives to LCV for model selection, and Sect. 2.19 modeling of variances along with means. Sections 2.6–2.16 and 2.18–2.19 provide a series of adaptive regression analysis examples including model comparisons using LCV ratio tests analogous to likelihood ratio tests in Sect. 2.7, choosing the number of

© Springer International Publishing Switzerland 2016
G.J. Knafl, K. Ding, *Adaptive Regression for Modeling Nonlinear Relationships*,
Statistics for Biology and Health, DOI 10.1007/978-3-319-33946-7_2

folds in Sect. 2.8, and comparison of adaptive modeling to standard polynomial modeling in Sect. 2.9 and to standard fractional polynomial modeling in Sect. 2.12. Sections 2.20 and 2.21 provide overviews of the results of the analyses. Formulation sections are not needed to understand analysis sections.

2.2   The Death Rate Data

A data set on death rates per 100,000 for 60 metropolitan statistical areas in the US is available on the Internet (see Supplementary Materials). These data were analyzed by McDonald and Schwing (1973) and were published by McDonald and Ayers (1978) and by Gunst and Mason (1980, pp. 368–371). They are reanalyzed here to demonstrate how to conduct regression analyses that account for nonlinearity in predictor variables. The variable deathrate (deaths per 100,000) is the outcome for these analyses. The possible predictor variables are NOindex (the nitric oxide pollution index), SO2index (the sulfur dioxide pollution index), and rain (average annual precipitation in inches). There are 12 other predictors in the original data set (see Table 16.5), but they are not considered here.

The predictor NOindex is considered first. The standard linear polynomial regression model for deathrate as a function of NOindex produces a nonsignificant ($P = 0.557$) t test for zero slope for NOindex, suggesting that deathrate is constant in NOindex. However, a regression analysis of deathrate as a function of the natural logarithm log(NOindex) of NOindex produces a significant ($P = 0.024$) t test. Consequently, using a standard linear polynomial regression model in NOindex provides misleading information about the relationship between deathrate and NOindex. It suggests that deathrate does not depend on NOindex, when in fact it does if nonlinear relationships are considered.

2.3   The Bivariate Regression Model and Its Parameter Estimates

This section provides a formulation (which can be skipped) of the standard bivariate regression model for an outcome variable y as a function of a single predictor variable x. As is standard, y is assumed to be normally distributed with variances constant in x.

The observed data for the regression models of Sect. 2.2 consist of pairs of values (y_s, x_s) for subjects (or observations) $s \in S = \{s : 1 \leq s \leq n\}$ where the outcome variable $y = $ deathrate, the predictor variable $x = $ NOindex or $x = $ log(NOindex), and the sample size $n = 60$. The associated statistical model assumes that

$$y_s = \beta_1 + \beta_2 \cdot x_s + e_s$$

for $s \in S$ where the errors e_s are independent, normally distributed with means 0 and variances having constant value σ^2. The likelihood term L_s for the sth subject satisfies

$$\ell_s = \log(L_s) = -\frac{1}{2} \cdot e_s^2/\sigma^2 - \frac{1}{2} \cdot \log(\sigma^2) - \frac{1}{2} \cdot \log(2 \cdot \pi)$$

where π is the usual constant. Let $\boldsymbol{\beta}$ denote the 2×1 column vector of coefficients, that is, $\boldsymbol{\beta} = (\beta_1, \beta_2)^T$ where $\mathbf{v}^T$ denotes the transpose of an arbitrary vector $\mathbf{v}$. Let $\boldsymbol{\theta} = (\boldsymbol{\beta}^T, \sigma^2)^T$ denote the 3×1 column vector of all model parameters. The likelihood $L(S; \boldsymbol{\theta})$ is the product of the likelihood terms L_s over $s \in S$ satisfying

$$\ell(S; \boldsymbol{\theta}) = \log(L(S; \boldsymbol{\theta})) = \sum_{s \in S} \ell_s.$$

The maximum likelihood estimate $\boldsymbol{\theta}(S) = (\boldsymbol{\beta}(S)^T, \sigma^2(S))^T$ of $\boldsymbol{\theta}$ is computed by solving the estimating equations $\partial \ell(S; \boldsymbol{\theta})/\partial \boldsymbol{\theta} = \mathbf{0}$ obtained by differentiating $\ell(S; \boldsymbol{\theta})$ with respect to $\boldsymbol{\theta}$, where $\mathbf{0}$ denotes the zero vector, in this case a 3×1 vector. For simplicity of notation, parameter estimates $\boldsymbol{\theta}(S)$ are denoted as functions of the index set S for the data used in their computation without hat (^) symbols. With

$$e_s(S) = y_s - \beta_1(S) - \beta_2(S) \cdot x_s$$

denoting the residuals estimating the errors e_s for $s \in S$, the maximum likelihood estimate $\sigma^2(S)$ of σ^2 is given by

$$\sigma^2(S) = \frac{1}{n} \sum_{s \in S} e_s(S)^2.$$

Since this is a biased estimate of σ^2, standard regression procedures use instead the unbiased estimate (that is, on the average it equals σ^2) obtained by replacing n in the denominator by the degrees of freedom (DF), in this case, $DF = n - 2$. The above formulation also holds for any subset S' of S.

2.4   Power Transformed Predictors

The predictor $x = $ NOindex is positive valued (with values ranging from 1 to 319), and so power transforms x^p are well-defined for all real valued powers p. These power transforms can be used to account for nonlinear (or curvilinear) dependence of deathrate on $x = $ NOindex. Standard polynomial models include only power transforms with nonnegative integer powers and are usually fully specified including all nonnegative integer powers less than or equal to a fixed integer power. For example, the fully specified quadratic polynomial in x includes the predictors x^0 (the intercept or constant term), x^1 (the linear term), and x^2 (the quadratic term). More general polynomial models allowing real valued powers are called fractional polynomials (Royston and Altman 1994). Degree 1 fractional polynomials in x include only one real valued power transform x^p of the predictor x.

The zero power requires special treatment. Since x^0 is identically equal to 1, using it as a predictor would be redundant when the model already has an intercept. When the model has an intercept and a slope for the power transform x^p, it converges, as the power p converges to 0, to the model based on $\log(x)$ (see Sect. 2.13.2).

2.5   Cross-Validation

Alternate fractional power transform models for deathrate as a function of NOindex have been considered so far, but not how to evaluate and compare those models, and so make an informed choice between them. One way to accomplish this is through cross-validation (CV). In CV, data are partitioned into disjoint subsets called folds, the data in each fold are predicted using parameter estimates computed from the rest of the data in the complement of the fold, and these deleted predictions are combined over all folds into CV scores. Depending on the type of CV, either smaller or larger scores indicate better models for the data. Formulations are provided for several CV approaches in this section. The approach called likelihood CV (LCV), with scores based on deleted likelihoods for folds, is used in analyses of deathrate reported in this chapter. Larger LCV scores indicate better models. The k-fold version uses k randomly selected folds to compute LCV scores. The leave-one-out (LOO) version assigns each data point to its own fold. Details are provided in Sects. 2.5.1 and 2.5.3, but can be skipped. Section 2.5.2 provides an example analysis using the LOO type of CV called the prediction sum of squares (PRESS) (Allen 1974). As formalized in Sect. 2.5.1, PRESS is the sum of squared deleted residuals, each computed from the observed data values for an observation along with parameter values estimated using data values for all the other observations. Smaller PRESS scores indicate better models.

General LCV is not directly supported in SAS (using version 9.4). Also, searching over the many alternative power transformations can be challenging. For those reasons, a SAS macro called genreg (for general regression) has been implemented for conducting such searches based on LCV. This macro uses heuristic (that is, rule-based) search techniques to adaptively identify appropriate power transforms of available predictors for outcomes (see Sect. 1.3 for an overview and Chap. 20 for details). The searches use scores based on either k-fold LCV or penalized likelihood criteria (PLCs) to evaluate and compare models. The genreg macro is available on the Internet (see the Supplementary Materials). Reported analyses are generated using this macro. See Chap. 3 for a description of its use in generating results reported in this chapter.

2.5.1   PRESS Formulation

One basic type of CV can be conducted using the PRESS score (Allen 1974; called "predicted residual SS" in the SAS PROC REG output). Let $S\backslash\{s\}$ denote the subset of the subject index set S consisting of indexes other than s. PRESS is defined as

$$\text{PRESS} = \sum_{s \in S} e_s(S\backslash\{s\})^2.$$

In other words, it is the sum of squares of the deleted residuals computed for each subject s with that subject's data (y_s, x_s) and with coefficients $\beta(S\backslash\{s\})$ estimated from the data for the other subjects with indexes in $S\backslash\{s\}$. Smaller PRESS scores indicate better models.

2.5.2   PRESS Assessment of the Death Rate as a Function of the Nitric Oxide Pollution Index

Table 2.1 contains PRESS scores for a selection of integer powers for modeling deathrate as a function of NOindex. The best (lowest) PRESS score of Table 2.1 is generated by the power -1. Consequently, a PRESS assessment indicates that $NOindex^{-1}$ is an effective predictor among integer power transforms. Improvements may be possible by searching through fractional powers around -1, but that issue is addressed later. In any case, these results suggest that the relationship between deathrate and NOindex is nonlinear. This is further supported by a significant ($P = 0.001$) slope for $NOindex^{-1}$ in the selected nonlinear model.

2.5.3   Formulation for Other Types of Cross-Validation

PRESS provides for a leave-one-out (LOO) type of CV, deleting one subject at a time to compute deleted parameter estimates. Other types of CV approaches are

Table 2.1 Selection of an integer power transform of the nitric oxide pollution index for predicting the death rate per 100,000

Power	PRESS
−3	217,602
−2	212,477
−1	201,887
0	229,515
1	260,762
2	230,940
3	238,679

PRESS: prediction sums of squares

possible. Splitting (or holdout or learning-testing) (Burman 1989) is the simplest type of CV. The data are partitioned into two subsets: the training (or calibration or learning) set with indexes S' and the holdout (or validation or test) set with indexes in the complement $S\backslash S'$ of S'. The training set is used to estimate model parameters and the holdout set to evaluate those estimates. In the regression context of Sect. 2.3, the splitting CV score can be computed as

$$\text{SPLIT} = \sum_{s \in S\backslash S'} e_s(S')^2.$$

A k-fold CV (Burman 1989) is intermediate between the splitting and LOO cases. The index set S is partitioned into $k > 1$ disjoint sets F(h), called folds, for $h \in H = \{h : 1 \leq h \leq k\}$. The CV score is then based on contributions for each subject computed with the data for that subject and with parameter estimates based on the data in the complement of the fold for the subject. In the regression context of Sect. 2.3, the k-fold CV score can be computed as

$$\text{CV} = \sum_{h \in H} \sum_{s \in F(h)} e_s(S\backslash F(h))^2.$$

So far, CV scores have been computed as sums, but they could have been computed as averages without affecting the conclusions. Also, scores have been based on a least squares CV (LSCV) approach. This is a natural choice for regression models based on normally distributed data. For general distributions, on the other hand, it seems more appropriate to base CV scores on those distributions. This can be accomplished with likelihood CV (LCV), an idea that goes back to Stone (1977) and Geisser and Eddy (1979). LCV scores are defined as

$$\text{LCV} = \prod_{h \in H} L(F(h); \boldsymbol{\theta}(S\backslash F(h)))^{1/n},$$

where the likelihood function $L(\cdot; \boldsymbol{\theta})$ varies with the distribution for the data and includes as a special case the normal likelihood for the regression problem considered in Sect. 2.3. In other words, deleted likelihoods are computed for each fold F(h) using the data in that fold and deleted parameter estimates based on all the other data (that is, the data in the fold complement $S\backslash F(h)$). These deleted fold likelihoods are normalized by the sample size n and multiplied up to generate the LCV score. LCV scores are geometric averages of deleted fold likelihoods with larger scores indicating better models for the data. Also, all model parameters are used in computing LCV scores, including for regression models the variance parameter σ^2 and not just the vector $\boldsymbol{\beta}$ of parameters for the means as in the LSCV formulation.

LOO LCV is the special case of k-fold LCV with $k = n$ folds, each consisting of an index for a single subject. In that case, maximizing LOO LCV scores for regression models is equivalent to minimizing

$$-2 \cdot \log(\text{LCV}) - \log(2 \cdot \pi) = \frac{1}{n}\text{PRESS} + \frac{1}{n}\sum_{s \in S} \log\left(\sigma^2(S \setminus \{s\})\right).$$

Hence, LCV in the regression context generalizes PRESS, a type of LSCV, to account for deleted estimates of the variances as well as deleted estimates of the parameters for the means. Moreover, LOO LCV for regression models under the normal distribution with known value for the variance parameter is equivalent to CV using PRESS.

LCV scores are based on likelihoods, and so for consistency they are computed in reported analyses with maximum likelihood estimates of all model parameters including the variance parameter, even though that estimate is biased. Subjects are randomly assigned to folds. Specifically, independent uniform random values u_s in (0,1) are used to generate fold assignments with subjects s assigned to folds $F(h(s))$ where $h(s) = \text{int}(k \cdot u_s) + 1$ for $s \in S$, with $\text{int}(k \cdot u_s)$ denoting the integer part of the positive real number $k \cdot u_s$. This means that subjects are equally likely to be assigned to each of the folds $F(h)$ but that those folds can vary in size and can even be empty (in which case they are not used in computing the LCV score). The same initial seed is used to generate the random values u_s determining the folds with all models for the same outcome so that LCV scores for different models for that outcome are comparable to each other. The data should also always be in the same order since otherwise observations would be assigned to different folds and then LCV scores are different (but parameter estimates are not affected).

2.6   Death Rate as a Function of the Nitric Oxide Pollution Index

As a starting point, set the number k of folds to 10 (and so the average fold size is $60/10 = 6$). The adaptively chosen model (using the genreg macro; see Chap. 3) for deathrate constrained to have an intercept and a single power transform of NOindex includes the transform $\text{NOindex}^{-0.8}$ with 10-fold LCV score 0.0041051. When multiple transforms of NOindex are allowed, the associated expanded model is based on the three transforms: $\text{NOindex}^{-0.8}$, $\text{NOindex}^{1.1}$, and NOindex^{-6}, together with an intercept, and the LCV score improves to 0.0042534.

It is likely that some of the transforms of the above expanded model are extraneous. Expanded models can often be improved further by contracting them, removing extraneous transforms possibly including the unit transform corresponding to the intercept, and adjusting the powers of the remaining transforms. Removing transforms produces more parsimonious models, but not necessarily always better LCV scores. However, if these scores are not too much smaller, then the contracted model is preferable as a parsimonious, competitive alternative. For the analysis of deathrate as a function of NOindex, the expanded model can be contracted to the model with the two transforms $\text{NOindex}^{-0.04}$ and $\text{NOindex}^{-0.39}$

(in that order) without an intercept and with reduced 10-fold LCV score 0.0042256. An approach is needed to be able to decide whether this is a tolerable reduction in the LCV score or not.

2.7 Model Comparisons

A larger LCV score does not always indicate a distinctly better model. A model with a smaller score is a competitive alternative to a model with a larger score if that smaller score is not too much smaller. If it is also simpler, as for the contracted model in NOindex compared to the associated uncontracted model, then it is a parsimonious, competitive alternative and so preferable. On the other hand, if the smaller score is substantially smaller, then the model with the larger score provides a distinct improvement over the model with the smaller score. A formal approach is needed for making such assessments.

This is possible with LCV ratio tests analogous to likelihood ratio tests. Rather than use a P-value or a cutoff for a significant LCV ratio, a LCV ratio test is expressed as a function of a cutoff for a substantial percent decrease (PD) in the LCV scores (see Sect. 4.4.2 for the formula for computing the cutoff). A PD is treated as substantial when it is larger than the value at the cutoff given by the 95th percentile 3.84146 of the χ^2 distribution with $DF = 1$ (but see Sect. 9.8 for an exception when the cutoff is based on $DF = 2$). Thus, a substantive PD exceeds what would be a significant amount for nested models (that is, models with predictors a subset of another model's predictors) differing by the smallest possible nonzero integer number of parameters. This is called substantial (or distinct) rather than significant since it might not involve nested models. The value for this cutoff depends on the sample size n.

For example, the cutoff for a substantial PD for the death rate data with $n = 60$ is 3.15 % (as reported in the genreg output). The PD for the contracted model in NOindex compared to the uncontracted model using their 10-fold LCV scores and rounded to two decimal digits is

$$100 \% \cdot (0.0042534 - 0.0042256)/0.0042534 = 0.67 \%.$$

Since 0.67 % is smaller than the cutoff of 3.15 % for the data, the contracted model is a competitive alternative to the uncontracted model with the larger LCV score, and so preferable since it is also simpler. Had the PD been greater than 3.15 %, the uncontracted model would have provided a distinct improvement (and so the genreg macro would have produced a different contracted model). Figure 2.1 displays the predicted value curve generated by the preferable, contracted model for deathrate as a function of NOindex and the raw data used to compute those estimates. The estimated mean deathrate increases at a relatively fast rate for relatively low NOindex values and then decreases gradually for higher NOindex values.

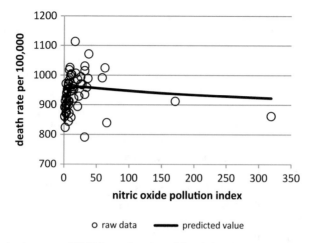

Fig. 2.1 The death rate per 100,000 as a function of the nitric oxide pollution index

Table 2.2 Impact of the number of folds on the adaptive model for the death rate per 100,000 as a function of the nitric oxide pollution index

Fold count k	Selected transforms	k-Fold LCV score	Percent decrease in k-fold LCV scores	5-fold LCV score	Percent decrease in 5-fold LCV scores (%)
5	NOindex$^{-0.32}$, NOindex$^{-0.05}$	0.0042303	0.00	0.0042303	0.00
10	NOindex$^{-0.04}$, NOindex$^{-0.39}$	0.0042256	0.11	0.0042193	0.26
15	NOindex$^{-0.04}$, NOindex$^{-0.4}$	0.0041872	1.02	0.0042186	0.28

LCV: likelihood cross-validation

2.8 Choosing the Number of Cross-Validation Folds

A fixed value for the number of folds, like 10 folds as used so far, is unlikely to be appropriate for all data sets. An assessment of the impact of the choice of the number of folds on conclusions can be conducted by comparing results over alternative fold counts for an important benchmark analysis for the data. For example, for the deathrate data, generating an adaptive model for how deathrate depends on NOindex is a reasonable choice for a benchmark analysis. If the number of folds is set appropriately for this analysis, that choice can be expected to work well for other analyses of deathrate.

This issue is addressed in Table 2.2. For numbers k of folds varying from 5 to 15 over multiples of 5, the associated adaptive models for deathrate as a function of NOindex include two transforms of NOindex all without an intercept. The choice of k = 5 folds generates the largest Table 2.2 k-fold LCV score, and PDs for scores generated for the other choices of k are smaller than the cutoff of 3.15 % for the data. However, that does not necessarily mean that the models generated using those other values of k are reasonably close to each other. LCV ratio tests are best conducted using scores computed with the same number of folds. Table 2.2 uses the value of $k = 5$ with the largest of the Table 2.2 k-fold LCV scores for this comparison. The adaptive models based on values of k other than $k = 5$ generate the smaller 5-fold scores with PD at most the insubstantial value 0.28 %, indicating that these models are competitive alternatives. These results suggest that adaptive modeling is reasonably robust to the choice for k, at least for these data and most likely more generally. Other regression modeling examples are provided in this book where selected power transforms are not too different for alternative numbers k of folds. Knafl and Grey (2007) and Knafl et al. (2012) provide further examples in the factor analysis context. Also, Hastie et al. (2009, p. 243) recommend using either $k = 5$ or $k = 10$ for non-likelihood CV in the statistical learning context.

For these data, fold sizes (as reported in the genreg output) for $k = 5$ folds range from 8 to 15 subjects with average 12, for $k = 10$ from 3 to 10 subjects with average 6, and for $k = 15$ from 1 to 8 subjects with average of 4. Larger values of k produce relatively small fold sizes for data sets like this with $n = 60$ subjects. The impact of larger numbers of folds can be assessed by consideration of a leave-one-out (LOO) LCV with each observation in its own fold. The adaptively generated model for that case has the two transforms $NOindex^{0.032}$ and $NOindex^{0.9}$ without an intercept and LOO LCV score 0.0042287. The 5-fold LCV score for this model is 0.0042634, and so the LCV score for the adaptive 5-fold model generates an insubstantial PD of 0.78 % compared to the LCV score for the model selected with LOO LCV. This suggests that large numbers k of folds relative to the sample size (for example, with average fold size less than 4 as in this example) might generate somewhat better models, but not distinctly better models than those generated by smaller k, and so the extra computation they require does not seem warranted.

The recommended approach for setting the number k of folds in general is as follows. First, select an important benchmark adaptive analysis for a data set. Then vary the value of k starting at 5 folds over multiples of 5 folds until a local maximum in the LCV score occurs (see Sect. 2.12 for an example where the first local maximum is at $k = 10$). Use that first local maximum in k for all subsequent analyses of the data set. When the LCV score decreases from the first value at $k = 5$ to the second one at $k = 10$ as for the deathrate data, $k = 5$ can be used, but it is not necessarily a local maximum. In that case, it seems important to also consider values of k larger than 10. If the LCV score is also smaller for $k = 15$ as for the deathrate data, it seems reasonable to use $k = 5$ in subsequent analyses, and so all subsequent analyses of deathrate use 5-fold LCV scores. However, if the LCV score for $k = 15$ is larger than the score for $k = 5$, it seems reasonable to continue searching and use the next local maximum (see Sect. 4.12 for an example). When sample sizes are small (for example, the data set used in Chap. 12 with 15 observations), the k-fold approach can generate folds whose complements are relatively small, and so estimates based on those complements might not be reliable. In such cases, the LOO LCV approach seems more reliable since it maximizes the sizes of the fold complements.

Table 2.3 Comparison of standard polynomial models to the adaptive model for the death rate per 100,000 as a function of the nitric oxide pollution index

Model	Transforms[a]	5-fold LCV score	Percent decrease (%)
Constant	1	0.0038136	9.85
Linear polynomial	1, NOindex	0.0036979	12.59
Quadratic polynomial	1, NOindex, NOindex^2	0.0019677	53.49
Cubic polynomial	1, NOindex, NOindex^2, NOindex^3	2.253e−55	100.00
Adaptive	NOindex$^{-0.32}$, NOindex$^{-0.05}$	0.0042303	0.00

LCV: likelihood cross-validation, NOindex: nitric oxide pollution index
[a]The predictor 1 corresponds to including an intercept in the model

2.9   Comparison to Standard Polynomial Models

Standard polynomials are often used to account for nonlinearity in predictors. These are usually fully-specified, including terms for all nonnegative integer powers less than or equal to a given integer power. Table 2.3 provides a comparison of fully-specified standard polynomial models to the adaptive model for predicting deathrate from NOindex. The most commonly used standard polynomial models are considered, including the constant, linear, quadratic, and cubic polynomial models of degrees 0–3. The constant polynomial model of degree 0 generates the best LCV score for these polynomial models, but with a PD compared to the adaptive model of 9.85 %, well above the cutoff of 3.15 % for the data. Consequently, standard polynomial models are ineffective for identifying the form for the nonlinearity of the relationship between deathrate and NOindex. Moreover, since the constant model generates the best score for the standard polynomial models, consideration of only those models suggests that deathrate does not depend on NOindex when in fact it does. A nonlinear, fractional polynomial model is needed to identify that deathrate does in fact distinctly depend on NOindex.

2.10   Penalized Likelihood Criteria for Model Selection

Section 2.10.1 provides a formulation (which can be skipped) for the two most commonly used penalized likelihood criteria (PLCs): the Akaike information criterion (AIC) with penalty based on the number of parameters and the Bayesian information criterion (BIC) with penalty based on the sample size as well as the number of parameters. The less commonly used Takeuchi information criterion (TIC), also called the robust AIC, is also formulated. PLCs are usually formulated so that smaller scores indicate better models, but they can be adjusted so that larger scores indicate better models. These adjusted scores are denoted by adding a prime

($'$) to the name, for example, the adjusted AIC score is denoted AIC$'$. Adjusted PLC scores can be used in place of LCV scores to generate adaptive models. Section 2.10.2 provides examples of such analyses.

2.10.1   Formulation

PLCs are commonly used in model selection (Sclove 1987). The AIC with penalty based on the number of model parameters is the best known PLC. Formally,

$$\text{AIC} = -2 \cdot \log(L(S; \boldsymbol{\theta}(S))) + 2 \cdot \dim(\boldsymbol{\theta}),$$

where $L(S; \boldsymbol{\theta}(S))$ is the likelihood for observations with indexes in S and model based on the estimate $\boldsymbol{\theta}(S)$ of the parameter vector $\boldsymbol{\theta}$ of dimension $\dim(\boldsymbol{\theta}(S)) = \dim(\boldsymbol{\theta})$. Smaller scores indicate better models. BIC is another commonly used PLC and is also called the Schwarz criterion. It adjusts the weight 2 for the number $\dim(\boldsymbol{\theta})$ of parameters in the AIC penalty to a function of the sample size n, that is,

$$\text{BIC} = -2 \cdot \log(L(S; \boldsymbol{\theta}(S))) + \log(n) \cdot \dim(\boldsymbol{\theta}),$$

also with smaller scores indicating better models. AIC and BIC scores are generated for a variety of modeling situations in SAS.

The Takeuchi information criterion (TIC) is a third PLC (Takeuchi 1976), but is not as widely used as AIC and BIC, nor is it directly supported in SAS. The number of parameters $\dim(\boldsymbol{\theta})$ of the AIC score is replaced by an estimate, that is,

$$\text{TIC} = -2 \cdot \log(L(S; \boldsymbol{\theta}(S))) + 2 \cdot \text{tr}\Big(J(\boldsymbol{\theta}(S))^{-1} \cdot K(\boldsymbol{\theta}(S))\Big),$$

where

$$J(\boldsymbol{\theta}) = -\frac{1}{n} \sum_{s \in S} \frac{\partial \ell_s^{\,2}}{\partial \boldsymbol{\theta} \partial \boldsymbol{\theta}^{\mathrm{T}}}$$

is computed from the second derivatives of the log likelihood terms ℓ_s (as defined in Sect. 2.3),

$$K(\boldsymbol{\theta}) = \frac{1}{n} \sum_{s \in S} \partial \ell_s / \partial \boldsymbol{\theta} \cdot (\partial \ell_s / \partial \boldsymbol{\theta})^{\mathrm{T}}$$

is computed from the first derivatives of the log likelihood terms ℓ_s, and tr($\mathbf{A}$) denotes the trace of an arbitrary square matrix $\mathbf{A}$, that is, the sum of its main diagonal entries. Once again, smaller scores indicate better models. TIC is also called the robust AIC since it allows for the true likelihood to be different from the assumed likelihood L used to generate estimates of $\boldsymbol{\theta}$. Moreover, when the true likelihood is same as the assumed likelihood, TIC and AIC are asymptotically equivalent. This holds since, in that case, $J(\boldsymbol{\theta}(S))$ and $K(\boldsymbol{\theta}(S))$ are asymptotically equal (Claeskens and Hjort 2009) so that $J(\boldsymbol{\theta}(S))^{-1} \cdot K(\boldsymbol{\theta}(S))$ is asymptotically an identity matrix of dimension $\dim(\boldsymbol{\theta})$ with trace equal to $\dim(\boldsymbol{\theta})$, and so the TIC penalty term $2 \cdot \text{tr}(J(\boldsymbol{\theta}(S))^{-1} \cdot K(\boldsymbol{\theta}(S)))$ is asymptotically equal to the penalty term $2 \cdot \dim(\boldsymbol{\theta})$ of AIC. TIC is also asymptotically equivalent to LOO LCV (Eq. 2.30, Claeskens and Hjort 2009).

PLCs can be used instead of LCV to select models using the adaptive modeling process, but they need to be adjusted first. Specifically, a PLC score is adjusted to

$$PLC' = \exp\left(-\frac{1}{2n} \cdot PLC\right)$$

so that it represents a geometric average with larger scores indicating better models. The advantage of using adjusted PLCs over LCV is the reduced computational times, which is especially important for large sample sizes. However, competitive models might not always be generated (see Sect. 4.8.4 for examples).

2.10.2 Adaptive Analyses Using Penalized Likelihood Criteria

Table 2.4 describes models adaptively generated using AIC, BIC, and TIC scores (as defined in Sect. 2.10.1) and the adaptive model based on 5-fold LCV scores. The models are all based on two transforms of NOindex without an intercept. Table 2.4 also provides a comparison of 5-fold LCV scores. LCV scores for these three models. BIC generates the model with BIC' score 0.0040727 (not in Table 2.4) and the best LCV score 0.0042503 of Table 2.4. LCV generates the next best LCV

Table 2.4 Comparison of penalized likelihood criteria to likelihood cross-validation for generating adaptive models for the death rate per 100,000 as a function of the nitric oxide pollution index

Model selection criterion	Model transforms	5-fold LCV score	Percent decrease (%)
AIC	NOindex$^{-0.38}$, NOindex$^{-0.04}$	0.0042195	0.72
BIC	NOindex$^{0.037}$, NOindex$^{0.9}$	0.0042503	0.00
TIC	NOindex$^{1.1}$, NOindex$^{0.032}$	0.0041874	1.48
5-fold LCV	NOindex$^{-0.39}$, NOindex$^{-0.04}$	0.0042303	0.47

AIC: Akaike information criterion, BIC: Bayesian information criterion
LCV: likelihood cross-validation, TIC: Takeuchi information criterion
NOindex: nitric oxide pollution index

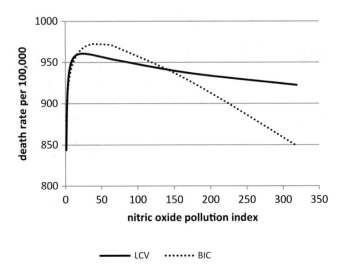

Fig. 2.2 Comparison of estimated mean death rate per 100,000 as a function of the nitric oxide pollution index for the adaptive fractional polynomial models based on LCV and on BIC

score 0.0042303 and insubstantial PD of 0.47 %. AIC generates a model with AIC$'$ score 0.0042009 (not in Table 2.4) and competitive LCV score 0.0042195 with PD 0.72 %. TIC generates a model with TIC$'$ score 0.0042607 (not in Table 2.4) and the smallest LCV score 0.0041874 but with insubstantial PD 1.48 %. In this case, all the PLC-based models and the LCV-based model are competitive alternatives.

Figure 2.2 displays estimated mean curves for adaptive models generated with LCV and BIC. The AIC plot is almost the same as for LCV and the TIC plot almost the same as for BIC. Compared to the estimated mean curves generated with LCV and AIC, the estimated mean curves generated with BIC and TIC are more highly influenced by the few extreme observations with very large NOindex values (see Fig. 2.1). Thus, model selection based on some PLCs can be more highly influenced by chance variation (like outliers) in the data than when based on k-fold LCV or on other PLCs, and so it seems best to use LCV for model selection, as is further supported by the analyses presented in Sect. 4.8.4, for which the LCV-based model distinctly outperforms models based on AIC, BIC, and TIC.

2.11 Monotonic Models

The relationship depicted in Fig. 2.1 is counterintuitive, suggesting that death rates per 100,000 decrease somewhat for very high levels of nitric oxide pollution levels. A strictly increasing, monotonic relationship would have been expected instead. An adaptive monotonic relationship can be generated by restricting the search to a single transform of NOindex, possibly with or without an intercept. The associated monotonic model includes the single transform NOindex$^{-0.8}$ with an intercept (and the estimated slope is negative so that the estimated mean deathrate increases with NOindex). The LCV score is smaller at 0.0041005, but the associated PD compared to the fully adaptive, non-monotonic model is 3.07 %. Since this is smaller than the cutoff of 3.15 % for the data, the monotonic model is a competitive alternative to the non-monotonic model with the larger LCV score.

LCV ratio tests, like likelihood ratio tests, are based on χ^2 distributions, and so formally they only apply when the two models are nested. However, non-nested models often need to be compared, as is the case for the above comparison of the monotonic model with a single transform of NOindex with an intercept to the non-monotonic, contracted model also with two terms, both transforms of NOindex. To cover such cases, the cutoff for a substantial PD is computed from the χ^2 distribution with DF = 1 set to its smallest possible nonzero integer value (but see Sect. 9.8 for an exception). This is a conservative choice in the sense that if the appropriate DF should be larger than 1, the cutoff for a substantial PD should be smaller, and so the more complex model might be considered not to provide a substantial improvement in cases where it has.

There are two distinctly outlying data points in Fig. 2.1 corresponding to the two very large NOindex values of 171 and 319. In contrast, the other NOindex values range from 1 to 66. These outlying values appear to have highly influenced the results of the non-monotonic analysis of deathrate as a function of NOindex (an assessment of this issue is left as an exercise; see Practice Exercise 3.4). Their effect is to counterintuitively lower the estimated mean deathrate for very high NOindex values. When such counterintuitive results occur, it is important to assess whether or not they are distinct by comparing them to associated monotonic models. In this case, a monotonic relationship, as would be expected for the relationship of the death rate per 100,000 with a pollution index, provides a competitive alternative. Predicted values for this monotonic relationship along with the raw data are plotted in Fig. 2.3. These results suggest the intuitive conclusion that the mean death rate increases at a very fast rate for low nitric oxide pollution values and then levels off to a relatively constant level.

2.12 Comparison to Standard Fractional Polynomial Modeling

Fractional polynomials, as considered in adaptive modeling, are commonly used with powers limited to specific choices (Royston and Altman 1994). The recommended set for first degree fractional polynomial models consists of the eight powers -2, -1, -0.5, 0, 0.5, 1, 2, and 3, where the zero power corresponds to the log transform (see Sect. 2.13.2 for the justification). These models also always include intercepts. Results are given in Table 2.5 for the constant model, the recommended degree 1 fractional polynomial models, and the adaptive

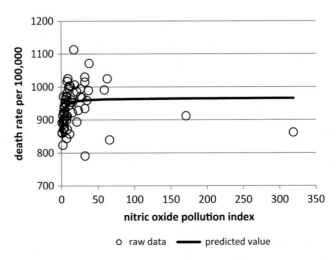

Fig. 2.3 The death rate per 100,000 as a monotonic function of the nitric oxide pollution index

Table 2.5 Comparison of recommended degree 1 fractional polynomial models to the adaptive monotonic model for the death rate per 100,000 as a function of the nitric oxide pollution index

Model	Transforms[a]	5-fold LCV score	Percent decrease (%)
Constant model	1	0.0038136	7.00
Power $= -2$	1, NOindex^{-2}	0.0039949	2.58
Power $= -1$	1, NOindex^{-1}	0.0040929	0.19
Power $= -0.5$	1, NOindex$^{-0.5}$	0.0040684	0.78
Power $= 0$	1, log(NOindex)	0.0038741	5.52
Power $= 0.5$	1, NOindex$^{0.5}$	0.0036775	10.32
Power $= 1$	1, NOindex^{1}	0.0036979	9.82
Power $= 2$	1, NOindex^{2}	0.0038597	5.87
Power $= 3$	1, NOindex^{3}	0.0037732	7.98
Adaptive monotonic	1, NOindex$^{-0.8}$	0.0041005	0.00

LCV: likelihood cross-validation, NOindex: nitric oxide pollution index
[a]The predictor 1 corresponds to including an intercept in the model

monotonic model since it has degree 1 like the recommended models. The adaptive model generates the best LCV score of Table 2.5. The recommended model based on the -1 power transform generates the best LCV score of the recommended degree 1 models with an insubstantial PD of 0.19 % compared to the adaptive monotone model. Royston and Altman (1994) also recommend choices for pairs of powers for degree 2 fractional polynomial models, but those are not considered here (they are addressed in Sect. 2.13). They also recommend choosing the power from the recommended set by maximizing the likelihood and not with LCV scores. This approach is equivalent to using either AIC or BIC scores since all recommended powers of a fixed degree generate models with the same number of parameters and so with the same AIC and BIC penalties.

The expansion process used to generate adaptive models starts with a grid search over a range of powers. The power generating the largest LCV score over these powers is then used as the initial power for further heuristic search adjustments (see Chap. 20). By default, the grid search uses the powers $-3, -2.5, \cdots, -0.5, 0.5, 1, \cdots, 3$. This includes all the recommended degree 1 fractional powers except the log transform corresponding to the 0 power, and so adaptive modeling is likely to generate an improved model compared to that recommended set, but not necessarily a distinctly better model. When the grid search selects the lowest (highest) value, -3 (3) in the default set, the adaptive search continues through smaller (larger) integer values before searching over single decimal powers.

The results of Table 2.5 suggest that consideration of powers outside the recommended set can provide improvements, but that the recommended set should often provide a competitive alternative. Whether the adaptive model ever outperforms the recommended set is investigated using a simulated data set with 1,001 observations, an outcome variable ysim, and a predictor variable xsim. Equally-spaced values are generated for xsim ranging from 0.5 to 1 over multiples of 0.0005 with associated ysim values satisfying $ysim = 25 + xsim^{-7} + e$ where the errors e are independent normal with mean 0 and standard deviation 5. The intercept was set to 5 times the standard deviation so that ysim values would be positive with probability essentially 1. The data are plotted in Fig. 2.4. The cutoff for a substantial PD is 0.19 %.

The adaptive model for ysim as a function of xsim using 5-fold LCV has the single power transform $xsim^{-6.89}$ with an intercept and LCV score 0.047781. For 10 folds, the generated model has one power transform $xsim^{-6.9}$ with an intercept and increased LCV score 0.047782. For 15 folds, the generated model has the single power transform $xsim^{-6.89}$ with an intercept and decreased LCV score 0.047779. So, $k = 10$ is the first local maximum for this analysis, but there is little difference in the scores with the largest PD of 0.01 % for $k = 15$. The adaptively generated model for $k = 10$ has estimated intercept 25.02 and estimated slope 1.06 for the transform with power -6.9, and so is quite close to the true function with intercept

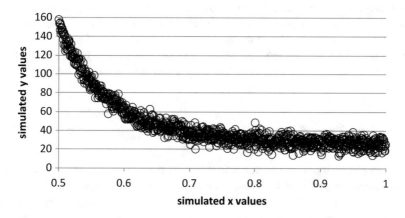

Fig. 2.4 Simulated fractional polynomial data

Table 2.6 Comparison of recommended degree 1 fractional polynomial models to the adaptive monotonic model for the simulated data

Model	Transforms[*]	10-fold LCV score	Percent decrease (%)
Constant model	1	0.008297	82.6
Power $= -2$	1, xsim^{-2}	0.021106	55.8
Power $= -1$	1, xsim^{-1}	0.017911	62.5
Power $= -0.5$	1, $\text{xsim}^{-0.5}$	0.016663	65.1
Power $= 0$	1, $\log(\text{xsim})$	0.015601	67.3
Power $= 0.5$	1, $\text{xsim}^{0.5}$	0.014695	69.2
Power $= 1$	1, xsim^{1}	0.013922	70.9
Power $= 2$	1, xsim^{2}	0.012694	73.4
Power $= 3$	1, xsim^{3}	0.011789	75.3
Adaptive monotonic	1, $\text{xsim}^{-6.9}$	0.047782	0.0

LCV: likelihood cross-validation, xsim: simulated x value
[a]The predictor 1 corresponds to including an intercept in the model

25, slope 1, and power -7. Also, the estimated standard deviation is 5.05, close to the true value of 5. The true model with an intercept and power transform xsim^{-7} has estimated intercept 25.28, slope 0.99, and standard deviation 5.05, also all close to the true values. Moreover, its 10-fold LCV score is 0.047746 with insubstantial PD of 0.08 % compared to the adaptively generated model, and so the true model is a competitive alternative for these data. Also, the adaptive monotonic model is the same as the unrestricted adaptive model. These results support the validity of the adaptive model selection process.

Table 2.6 contains a comparison of the recommended set of power transforms to the adaptive monotonic model, also with an intercept and a single power transform of xsim. For these data, the adaptive monotonic model distinctly outperforms all the recommended degree 1 power transforms with best PD of 55.8 %, very much larger than the cutoff of 0.19 % for a substantial PD. These results indicate that the recommended set of degree 1 powers can be very ineffective in cases like this with the true power outside the range of that set. Consequently, adaptive selection of powers is needed to generate effective models in general modeling situations. If only recommended degree 1 powers are considered in an analysis and the selected power is -2 (3), then it would be best to consider integer powers less (more) than -2 (3). See Sect. 13.3 for another example where adaptive modeling distinctly outperforms the recommended degree 1 powers, but using a real, non-simulated data set.

2.13   Log Transforms

The zero power transform is not considered in the adaptive modeling process to avoid having to decide if it corresponds to the unit or log transform. Since small powers are considered and these approximate the log transform when the model contains an intercept, models generated using only nonzero power transforms without considering the log transform are likely to be competitive alternatives to models generated from both nonzero power transforms and the log transform. As an example, the adaptively generated model (that is, expanded and then contracted) for deathrate as a function of NOindex and its log contains the transforms $NOindex^{0.042}$ and $(\log(NOindex))^{3.6}$ without an intercept. Its LCV score is 0.0043239. The adaptive model based on only nonzero power transforms of NOindex generates an insubstantial PD of 2.18 %, suggesting that log transforms might not be needed to generate effective adaptive models. Consideration of log transforms along with power transforms can generate larger LCV scores but the improvements may not justify the extra processing time.

2.13.1 Recommended Degree 2 Fractional Polynomials

Royston and Altman (1994) also recommend a finite set of degree 2 fractional polynomial models in a predictor x to consider, all with intercepts and possibly involving log transforms. These models are based on two powers p and p' with $p \leq p'$ for p and p' one of the eight recommended degree 1 powers (and so $8 \cdot 9/2 = 36$ pairs of powers). When $0 < p < p'$, the two transforms of the model are x^p and $x^{p'}$. When $0 = p < p'$, the two transforms of the model are $\log(x)$ and $x^{p'}$. When $p = p' \neq 0$, the two transforms are x^p and $x^p \cdot \log(x)$ and when $p = p' = 0$, the two transforms are $\log(x)$ and $(\log(x))^2$. The $p' = p$ models are limits of models based on x^p and $x^{p'}$ for $p' > p$ as p' converges to p (see Sect. 2.13.2).

The model for deathrate as a function of NOindex with two powers $p' = p = 0$ plus an intercept generates the best LCV score of 0.0043085 among all degree 2 recommended models. The comparable adaptive model based on NOindex and log(NOindex) has larger LCV score 0.0043239 and is simpler with two transforms and no intercept. The best recommended degree 2 model is competitive with insubstantial PD of 0.36 %. These results suggest that recommended sets of power transforms will often be competitive alternatives to adaptive models but can also be more complex.

For the simulated data of Sect. 2.12, the model with powers $p' = p = -2$ generates the best LCV score of 0.041544 among all recommended degree 2 models. This is a substantial improvement over the best degree 1 recommended model with power $p = -2$ and LCV score 0.021106 (see Table 2.6), and so a PD of 49.2 %. However, this best recommended degree 2 model generates a substantial PD in the LCV scores of 13.1 % compared to the adaptive model in xsim, much larger than the cutoff of 0.19 % for the data. These results indicate that, while recommended degree 2 models can provide distinct improvements over degree 1 recommended models, they can still have substantially lower LCV scores than adaptively generated models when true powers are outside the range of recommended powers. See Sect. 13.3 for an example where adaptive modeling distinctly outperforms the recommended degree 2 powers using a real, non-simulated data set (and the recommended degree 1 powers too).

2.13.2 Limits of Fractional Polynomials

This section provides a justification of the use of the natural log transform in the recommended degree 1 and degree 2 fractional polynomials. It can be skipped to focus on analyses.

For positive valued predictors x, power transforms x^p are well-defined for all real valued powers p. The zero power requires special treatment. Since x^0 is identically equal to 1, using it as a predictor would be redundant when the model already has an intercept. When the model has an intercept β_1 and a slope β_2 for the power transform x^p, it converges, as the power p converges to 0, to the model based on log(x). To see this in the simple case of a degree 1 fractional polynomial, let $\beta_1' = \beta_1 + \beta_2$ and $\beta_2' = \beta_2 \cdot p$ so that

$$y = \beta_1 + \beta_2 \cdot x^p + e = \beta_1' + \beta_2' \cdot \frac{x^p - 1}{p} + e,$$

which converges, for arbitrary fixed values of β_1' and β_2', as p converges to 0 to $y = \beta_1' + \beta_2' \cdot \log(x) + e$ by L'Hôpital's rule so that the maximum likelihood estimates of β_1' and β_2' for the model with the predictor $(x^p - 1)/p$ converge to the maximum likelihood estimates of β_1' and β_2' for the model with the predictor log(x). The case with two power transforms x^p and $x^{p'}$ with $p' > p$ can be expressed as

$$y = \beta_1 + \beta_2 \cdot x^p + \beta_3 \cdot x^{p'} + e = \beta_1 + \beta_2' \cdot x^p + \beta_3' \cdot x^p \cdot \frac{x^{p'-p} - 1}{p' - p} + e$$

for appropriately defined β_2', and β_3', which converges for arbitrary fixed values of β_1, β_2', and β_3', as p' converges to p, to $y = \beta_1 + \beta_2' \cdot x^p + \beta_3' \cdot x^p \cdot \log(x) + e$.

2.14 Impact of the Intercept

Regression models commonly include an intercept. For example, an intercept is included in the standard polynomial models considered in Sect. 2.9 and in the recommended fractional polynomials considered in Sects. 2.12 and 2.13. Zero intercept models are usually not considered. However, adaptively generated models can have zero intercepts. If desired, such models can be constrained instead to include an intercept. For the model of deathrate as a function of NOindex, the associated constrained model includes the two transforms NOindex$^{0.9}$ and NOindex$^{-0.6}$ with an intercept and LCV score 0.0042849. This score is larger than the score of 0.0042303 for the associated zero intercept model, but the PD is insubstantial at 1.27 %. In this case, considering only models with intercepts provides an improvement, but the zero-intercept model is a parsimonious, competitive alternative. The adaptive modeling process allows for zero-intercept models by default because that can generate at least competitive LCV scores (or the intercept would not be removed), sometimes better scores (see Sect. 3.12), and even substantially better (see Sect. 13.3) with fewer terms and so more parsimoniously.

2.15   Impact of Bounding the Nitric Oxide Pollution Index

The monotonic relationship of Fig. 2.3 suggests that mean deathrate is constant once NOindex gets sufficiently large. Adaptive modeling can be used to assess whether this is a reasonable conclusion and, if so, estimate the cutoff value for NOindex at which its impact becomes constant. The plot for the monotonic model restricted to NOindex ≤ 40 is provided in Fig. 2.5 and suggests that this cutoff occurs somewhere between 5 and 15. Models bounding the impact of NOindex can be generated with predictors

$$NObnded = min(NOindex, bnd)$$

for different settings of bnd. These functions are simple cases of general splines (Ahlberg et al. 1967). NObnded has one knot (or join point) at the value bnd and is linear in NOindex below bnd and constant after that. Adaptively generated models in NObnded are possibly nonlinear in NOindex for values below bnd and constant after that.

Table 2.7 contains models and LCV scores for integer values of bnd ranging from 5 to 15. All models consist of a single transform of NObnded without an

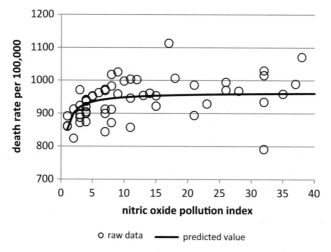

Fig. 2.5 The death rate per 100,000 as a monotonic function of low values for the nitric oxide pollution index

Table 2.7 Alternate bounds for the death rate per 100,000 as a function of the bounded nitric oxide pollution index

Bound	Transform	5-fold LCV score	Percent decrease (%)
5	NObnded$^{0.07}$	0.0041085	2.10
6	NObnded$^{0.06}$	0.0041374	1.42
7	NObnded$^{0.05}$	0.0041437	1.27
8	NObnded$^{0.05}$	0.0041690	0.66
9	NObnded$^{0.05}$	0.0041884	0.20
10	NObnded$^{0.047}$	0.0041948	0.05
11	NObnded$^{0.041}$	0.0041940	0.07
12	NObnded$^{0.04}$	0.0041968	0.00
13	NObnded$^{0.04}$	0.0041931	0.09
14	NObnded$^{0.039}$	0.0041879	0.21
15	NObnded$^{0.037}$	0.0041833	0.32

LCV: likelihood cross-validation
NObnded: bounded nitric oxide pollution index

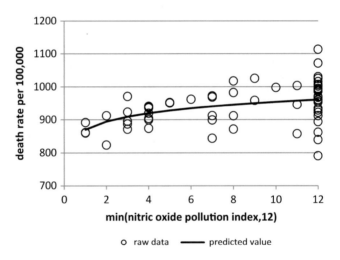

o raw data   —— predicted value

Fig. 2.6 The death rate per 100,000 as a function of the bounded nitric oxide pollution index

intercept. The best score of 0.0041968 is generated by a bound of 12, but all the other bounds generate competitive models. This score is smaller than the LCV score of 0.0042303 (see Table 2.2) generated by the non-monotonic model in NOindex but with insubstantial PD of 0.79 %, indicating that the impact of nitric oxide pollution on the death rate per 100,000 is reasonably considered to be constant for NOindex values of 12 and larger.

The predicted values and raw data for the model with NOindex bounded at bnd = 12 are plotted in Fig. 2.6. The estimated mean death rate per 100,000 increases nonlinearly, from 870.3 per 100,000 for the lowest nitric oxide pollution index of 1 to 961.2 per 100,000 for a nitric oxide pollution index of 12. It then remains at this level for larger values of the nitric oxide pollution index. Variability in the data at the NObnded value of 12 appears larger than for lower values suggesting a possible need for non-constant variances models, but that issue is not addressed here (see Sect. 2.19 for how to address that issue).

2.16   Death Rate as a Function of Other Predictors

So far, only NOindex and its bounded version NObnded has been used to predict deathrate, but other primary predictors are available including SO2index and rain. The adaptive model in SO2index is based on the single transform $SO2index^{0.012}$ without an intercept and LCV score 0.0040239. Figure 2.7 displays predicted values for deathrate as a function of SO2index and the raw data used to compute those estimates. The relationship of Fig. 2.7 is similar to the relationship of Fig. 2.5 for NOindex, suggesting consideration of bounding the effect of SO2index, but that issue is not addressed here. The expanded model generated for this analysis, prior to contraction, is based on the single transform $SO2index^{0.9}$ with an intercept suggesting that deathrate might be close to linear in SO2index, as it is since the linear polynomial model in SO2index has LCV score 0.0041100, larger than for the adaptively generated model. Consequently, although the predicted values of Fig. 2.7 appear curved for low values of SO2index, they are in fact reasonably close to linear in SO2index. An inspection of Fig. 2.7 suggests the possibility that mean deathrate might be constant in and not change with SO2index. This can be assessed by comparing the adaptive model in SO2index for deathrate to the constant model. This latter model has LCV score 0.0038136 and substantial PD compared to

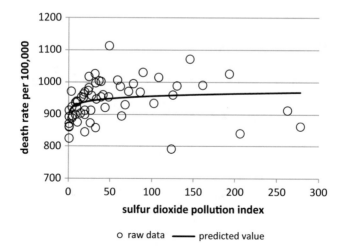

Fig. 2.7   The death rate per 100,000 as a function of the sulfur dioxide pollution index

the adaptive model in SO2index of 5.23 %. Consequently, mean deathrate changes distinctly with SO2index.

The LCV scores for the adaptive and linear models in SO2index are smaller than the score for the adaptive model in NObnded (with bnd = 12), and so NObnded is a more effective singleton predictor of deathrate than SO2index. However, it is possible that SO2index explains aspects of deathrate other than those explained by NObnded. This can be investigated by considering adaptive multiple regression models in NObnded and SO2index in combination. The adaptively generated model contains no transforms of SO2index and is the model based on the transform NObnded$^{0.041}$ without an intercept, nearly the same as the model generated by NObnded alone. This result suggests that, since no transforms of SO2index are in the generated model, NObnded explains essentially all of the effect of SO2index on deathrate. In other words, the dependence of the death rate per 100,000 within the 60 metropolitan statistical areas on the sulfur dioxide pollution index is effectively all accounted for by its dependence on the nitric oxide pollution index bounded to at most 12.

There is a third predictor rain that has not been considered yet. The adaptive model in rain alone includes the single transform rain$^{0.1}$ without an intercept. The LCV score is 0.0044527. Figure 2.8 displays predicted values for deathrate as a function of rain and the raw data used to compute those estimates. Mean deathrate increases at a somewhat faster rate for relatively low values of rain than after that. At first glance, the relationship of Fig. 2.8 does not appear highly curved, suggesting that it might be close to linear. However, the linear polynomial model in rain has LCV score 0.0042690 and substantial PD of 4.13 %, indicating that deathrate is distinctly nonlinear in rain. A closer look indicates that a linear curve over the range 10–20 in. close to the fitted curve of Fig. 2.8 would continue on to a much higher level by 60 in. than the fitted curve.

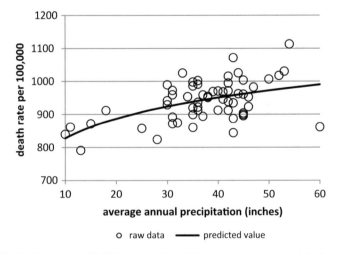

Fig. 2.8 The death rate per 100,000 as a function of the average annual precipitation

The LCV score for the adaptive model in rain is larger than the scores for the adaptive models in NObnded and SO2index, indicating that rain is the most effective singleton predictor for deathrate among these three. As before, joint effects for the predictors can be investigated by considering multiple predictors. Given the earlier result that NObnded explains essentially all of the effect of SO2index, only joint effects for rain and NObnded are considered. The adaptively generated model contains the two predictors $rain^{0.15}$ and $NObnded^{0.3}$ without an intercept, and with LCV score 0.0056386. In comparison, the PD for the adaptive model in rain with the best LCV score of the singleton predictor models is very substantial at 21.03 %, indicating that the two predictor model provides a distinct improvement over the singleton predictor models. Thus, rain and NObnded in combination explain aspects of deathrate distinct from each one separately. Moreover, the model linear in both rain and NObnded has LCV score 0.0053103 with substantial PD of 5.82 %, and so the dependence of deathrate on both rain and NObnded is distinctly nonlinear.

Figure 2.9 displays predicted values for deathrate as a function of rain at selected values of NObnded. For fixed values of NObnded, mean deathrate increases with rain as in the model of Fig. 2.8 for rain unadjusted for NObnded. Mean deathrate is at higher levels for larger values of NObnded with the increases more pronounced for increases in lower NObnded values. Figure 2.10 displays predicted values for deathrate as a function of NObnded at selected values of rain. For fixed values of rain, mean deathrate increases with NObnded as in the model of Fig. 2.6 for NObnded unadjusted for rain. Mean deathrate is at higher levels for larger values of rain with the increases more pronounced for increases in lower rain values.

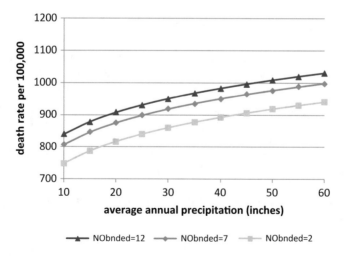

Fig. 2.9 The death rate per 100,000 as a function of the average annual precipitation (rain) at selected values for the nitric oxide pollution index bounded at 12 (NObnded)

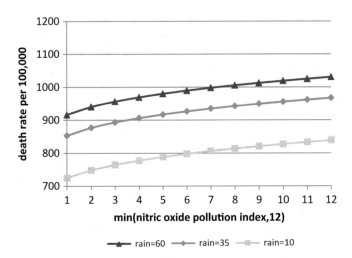

Fig. 2.10 The death rate per 100,000 as a function of the nitric oxide pollution index bounded at 12 (NObnded) at selected values for the average annual precipitation (rain)

Further analyses of the deathrate data are possible including analyses considering interactions between predictors. These are not considered here for brevity, but are addressed in the practice exercises of Chap. 3.

2.17 The Multiple Regression Model

The formulation of Sect. 2.3 only addresses bivariate regression models based on a single predictor, but it extends readily to handle multiple regression models as considered in Sects. 2.6, 2.8–2.10, 2.13, 2.14, and 2.16. Using the notation of Sect. 2.3, for $s \in S$, let $\mathbf{x}_s$ be a $r \times 1$ column vector of r predictor values x_{sj} (including unit predictor values if an intercept is included in the model) with indexes $j \in J = \{j : 1 \leq j \leq r\}$ and $\boldsymbol{\beta}$ the associated $r \times 1$ column vector of coefficients. Setting $y_s = \mathbf{x}_s^T \cdot \boldsymbol{\beta} + e_s$ and $e_s(S) = y_s - \mathbf{x}_s^T \cdot \boldsymbol{\beta}(S)$ for $s \in S$ where $\boldsymbol{\beta}(S)$ is the maximum likelihood estimate of the parameter vector $\boldsymbol{\beta}$, the rest of the formulation of Sect. 2.3 then applies to this more general context. The CV formulations of Sect. 2.5 apply as well. Standardized residuals are computed for these models simply as $\text{stde}_s(S) = e_s(S)/\sigma(S)$ for $s \in S$, that is, by standardizing the residuals by the estimated standard deviation. Studentized residuals can be used instead if desired.

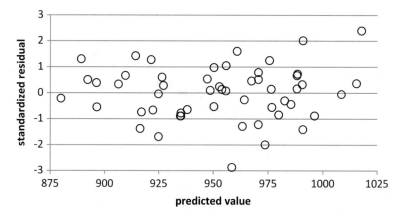

Fig. 2.11 Standardized residual plot for adaptive model of the death rate per 100,000 as a function of the nitric oxide pollution index bounded at 12 (NObnded) and the annual average precipitation (rain)

2.18 Residual Analysis

An adaptive regression model, like any other regression model, is based on assumptions that need to be checked through a residual analysis. Standardized residuals for the adaptive model in NObnded and rain are displayed in Fig. 2.11. These are within ± 3 although there is one standardized residual (with associated observed value 844.0 and predicted value 958.5) that is somewhat lower than the others, but the standardized residual equals -2.87, and so is not distinctly outlying. Also, there may be less variability in the standardized residuals for lower predicted values than for higher ones, suggesting the possibility that the constant variances assumption might not hold, but this issue is not addressed here (it is addressed in Sect. 2.19.2). The normal (probability) plot generated by the standardized residuals is displayed in Fig. 2.12 and is reasonably close to linear except somewhat for the smallest residual. Normality is further supported by a nonsignificant ($P = 0.888$) Shapiro-Wilk test for normality of the standardized residuals.

2.19 Modeling Variances as well as Means

A formulation (which may be skipped) of regression models for variances along with means of univariate continuous outcomes is provided in Sect. 2.19.1. Section 2.19.2 provides an example analysis of means and variances for the death rate data while Sect. 2.19.3 provides an example analysis of means and variances for the simulated data described in Sect. 2.12.

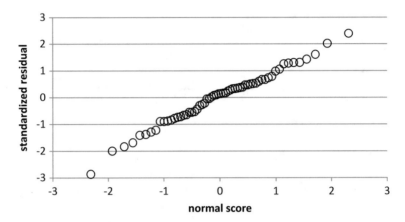

Fig. 2.12 Normal plot generated by the standardized residuals for the adaptive model of the death rate per 100,000 as a function of the nitric oxide pollution index bounded at 12 (NObnded) and the annual average precipitation (rain)

2.19.1   Formulation

Regression models commonly assume that variances are the same for all subjects, but this assumption needs to be assessed. One way to do that is through adaptive modeling of the means and variances in combination. This section provides a formulation (which can be skipped) of regression models for both the means and logs of the variances.

The multiple regression model of Sect. 2.17 can be extended to assess this issue as follows. Using the notation of Sects. 2.3 and 2.17, let the likelihood term L_s for the sth subject satisfy

$$\ell_s = \log(L_s) = -\frac{1}{2} \cdot \frac{e_s^2}{\sigma_s^2} - \frac{1}{2} \cdot \log(\sigma_s^2) - \frac{1}{2} \cdot \log(2 \cdot \pi)$$

and model the log of the variance σ_s^2 as a function of selected predictor variables and associated coefficients. Specifically, let $\log(\sigma_s^2) = \mathbf{v}_s^T \cdot \boldsymbol{\gamma}$ where, for $s \in S$, $\mathbf{v}_s$ is a $q \times 1$ column vector of q predictor values v_{sj} (including unit predictor values if an intercept is to be included) with indexes $j \in Q = \{j : 1 \leq j \leq q\}$ and $\boldsymbol{\gamma}$ is the associated $q \times 1$ column vector of coefficients. The $(r + q) \times 1$ parameter vector $\boldsymbol{\theta} = (\boldsymbol{\beta}^T, \boldsymbol{\gamma}^T)^T$ is estimated through maximum likelihood estimation. Alternative models can be compared with LCV scores. The adaptive modeling process can be extended to search through models for the means and variances in combination (see Chap. 20).

2.19.2   Analysis of Death Rate Means and Variances

As indicated in Sect. 2.18, the residual analysis suggested the possibility of non-constant variances for deathrate as a function of NObnded and rain. This can be addressed by applying the extended adaptive modeling process to the means and variances of deathrate, both as functions of NObnded and rain. The generated model has means depending on the transforms $rain^{0.14}$ and $NObnded^{0.4}$ without an intercept, variances depending on the transform $NObnded^{-0.01}$ without an intercept, and LCV score 0.056157. The model generated for the means assuming constant variances described in Sect. 2.16 has larger LCV score 0.0056386. This indicates that variances for deathrate are reasonably treated as constant in NObnded and rain when means are modeled in terms of those same two variables.

When the LCV score for the non-constant variances model is larger than the score for the constant variances model, a LCV ratio test can be used to assess whether this is a substantial improvement. If the PD for the constant variances model is smaller than the cutoff for a substantial PD, then the variances are reasonably considered to be constant. On the other hand, if the PD is larger than the cutoff, then the variances are distinctly non-constant.

2.19.3   Analysis of Means and Variances for the Simulated Data

For the simulated data of Sect. 2.12, the adaptive model for means and variances has means based the single transform: $xsim^{-6.9}$ with an intercept and variances depending on the one transform: $xsim^{0.02}$ without an intercept. The transform for the means is the same one as was generated for the constant variances model. The LCV score is 0.047783, only slightly larger than the score 0.047782 for the adaptive constant variances model and with insubstantial PD 0.002 %. Consequently, adaptive modeling results in the conclusion that the simulated data are reasonably considered to have constant variances, as they were simulated. This result provides support for the effectiveness of the adaptive modeling process for means and variances in combination.

2.20   Overview of Analyses of Death Rates

1. For the death rate data (Sect. 2.2), analyses use $k = 5$ folds (Sect. 2.8) as chosen with the approach recommended at the end of Sect. 2.8.
2. Standard polynomials are ineffective for addressing nonlinearity in the death rate data (Sect. 2.9).

3. PLCs are effective for modeling the death rate data, but in some cases are more highly influenced by outliers in the data (Sect. 2.10.2).
4. The selected model for the death rate as a function of the nitric oxide pollution index is counterintuitively non-monotonic (Fig. 2.1). However, the adaptive monotonic model is a competitive alternative (Sect. 2.11). As would be expected, the effect on the death rate of the nitric oxide pollution index can reasonably be considered to increase with increasing values of that index. Moreover, that effect can reasonably be treated as being a constant for values of 12 or larger (Sect. 2.15).
5. The adaptive monotonic model for the death rate as a function of the nitric oxide pollution index generates a better LCV score than the recommended degree 1 fractional polynomial models, but not a substantially better score, indicating that consideration of only that limited set of powers can sometimes be effective (Sect. 2.12).
6. The adaptive modeling process does not consider zero powers to avoid deciding whether that corresponds to the constant model (when the model has a zero intercept) or to the natural log transform (when the model has a nonzero intercept). Further consideration of the natural log transform of the nitric oxide pollution index does not substantially improve on the model not considering that transform (Sect. 2.13.1), suggesting that it is reasonable not to consider the natural log transform in general.
7. Regression models commonly include intercepts, but the adaptive modeling process considers models with zero intercepts. The model for the death rate as a function of the nitric oxide pollution index constrained to include an intercept does not substantially improve on the model allowing for a zero intercept (Sect. 2.14), indicating that zero intercept models can be parsimonious, competitive alternatives.
8. The dependence of the death rate on the nitric oxide pollution index is distinctly nonlinear (Sect. 2.9) as is its dependence on the average annual precipitation (Sect. 2.16). On the other hand, its dependence on the sulfur dioxide pollution index is reasonably close to linear (Sect. 2.16).
9. The nitric oxide pollution index explains essentially all of the effect of the sulfur dioxide pollution index on the death rate (Sect. 2.16). On the other hand, the nitric oxide pollution index and the average annual precipitation explain different aspects of the death rate (Sect. 2.16). Results for this model are displayed in Figs. 2.9 and 2.10.
10. The adaptive model in the nitric oxide pollution index and the average annual precipitation generate standardized residuals that are reasonably close to being normally distributed and without distinct outliers (Sect. 2.18). Moreover, they are also reasonably close to having constant variances (Sect. 2.19.2).

2.21   Overview of Analyses of the Simulated Outcome

1. For the simulated data (Sect. 2.12), analyses use k = 10 folds (Sect 2.12) as chosen with the approach recommended at the end of Sect. 2.8.
2. The adaptive process is effective in analyzing this bivariate simulated data set (Sect. 2.12). However, the recommended set of powers is ineffective because the true power is outside of that set (Sect. 2.12). Thus, consideration of only the recommended powers is not always sufficient. In cases where the best power from the recommended set is the lowest (highest) of those powers, it would be better to continue searching through lower (higher) powers.
3. Consideration of the degree 2 recommended set of fractional polynomials distinctly improves on the degree 1 recommended set, but adaptive modeling still generates a substantially better model (Sect. 2.13.1).
4. The simulated data are reasonably considered to have constant variances (Sect. 2.19.3) as they have been simulated.

2.22   Chapter Summary

This chapter has presented a series of analyses of the death rate data, addressing how the death rate per 100,000 depends on the nitric oxide pollution index, the sulfur dioxide pollution index, and the average annual precipitation in inches for 60 metropolitan statistical areas. These analyses demonstrate adaptive regression modeling of univariate continuous outcomes using fractional polynomials, including how to set the number of folds for computing likelihood cross-validation (LCV) scores, how to compare alternative models using LCV ratio tests, and how to model variances as well as means.

The analyses demonstrate how to assess whether relationships are distinctly nonlinear versus not using LCV ratio tests. For example, death rates per 100,000 are distinctly nonlinear in the nitric oxide pollution index. In this case, the slope for the nitric oxide pollution index in the commonly used linear polynomial model is nonsignificant, and so the dependence of the death rates on the nitric oxide pollution index can only be identified through nonlinear relationships. Moreover, this dependence cannot be identified with standard quadratic or cubic polynomial models as well. Identification of that dependence requires consideration of fractional polynomial models. On the other hand, the dependence of death rates on the sulfur dioxide pollution index is reasonably treated as linear, but this conclusion requires a comparison of the linear polynomial and adaptive models in the sulfur dioxide pollution index. Similar assessments can be made to decide if the relationship of an outcome y in terms of a predictor x is distinctly non-constant in x as opposed to not depending on x at all by comparing the adaptive model for y in x to the constant model for y.

Adaptive models and their LCV scores can be used to compare the effects of predictor variables on an outcome variable. For example, the dependence of death rates per 100,000 on the average annual precipitation is stronger than their dependence on the nitric dioxide pollution index. Adaptive models can be also used to assess the dependence of outcome variables on multiple predictors. For example, the nitric oxide pollution index explains essentially all of the effect of the sulfur dioxide pollution index on death rates since the adaptive model in these two predictors depends on only the nitric oxide pollution index. On the other hand, each of the average annual precipitation and the nitric oxide pollution index explains aspects of death rates the other does not since the adaptive model in these two predictors generates a distinctly better LCV score than both of the associated singleton predictor models.

Adaptive models can be used to assess whether relationships are reasonably monotonic or not. For example, the adaptive model in the nitric oxide pollution index counterintuitively suggests that its effect on death rates decreases for large values. However, the adaptive monotonic model based on a single transform of the nitric oxide pollution index provides a competitive alternative leading to the intuitive conclusion that the mean death rate increases with the nitric oxide pollution index. Adaptive modeling further supports the conclusion that this effect is reasonably treated as constant for large nitric oxide pollution index values.

The analyses also demonstrate that adaptive modeling can generate a better degree 1 fractional polynomial model than those based on the pre-specified set of powers recommended by Royston and Altman (1994), but the recommended degree 1 set in that case provides a competitive alternative. However, a simulated data set is also analyzed in the chapter demonstrating that adaptive modeling can distinctly outperform the recommended set of degree 1 transforms. Consideration of the degree 2 transforms recommended by Royston and Altman (1994) provides a distinct improvement for the simulated data over recommended degree 1 transforms, but the adaptive model is still a distinctly better choice. Adaptively generated models for the simulated data, both with constant variances and allowing for non-constant variances, are reasonably close to the true underlying model for these data, providing support for the effectiveness of the adaptive modeling process.

Variances as well as means can be adaptively modeled. These models can be used to assess the usual constant variances assumption by comparing associated adaptive constant and non-constant variances models. For example, the analyses demonstrate that variances for death rates per 100,000 are reasonably considered to be constant in the average annual precipitation and the nitric oxide pollution index when their means are modeled in terms of these two predictors.

The chapter has also provided a formulation for multiple regression models of univariate continuous outcomes and for k-fold LCV scores. Other alternatives for conducting cross-validation are defined as well. Penalized likelihood criteria (PLCs), including the Akaike information criterion (AIC), Bayesian information criterion (BIC), and Takeuchi information criterion (TIC), are defined and their use in model selection compared to using LCV. For the example analyses, the models generated with these three PLCs and with LCV are competitive alternatives. However, the models selected with BIC and TIC scores are more highly influenced by outliers than models selected with LCV and AIC scores.

See Chap. 3 for details on conducting analyses in SAS like those presented in this chapter. See Chaps. 6 and 7 for analyses involving power transformation of outcomes as well as predictors. See Chaps. 4 and 5 for the extension of adaptive modeling to multivariate continuous outcomes. See Chaps. 8 and 9 for the extension of adaptive modeling to univariate discrete outcomes with two or more values and Chaps. 12 and 13 for the extension of adaptive modeling to univariate count/rate outcomes. See Chaps. 16 and 17 for a comparison of adaptive regression modeling to generalized additive modeling for addressing nonlinearity and Chaps. 18 and 19 for a comparison to multivariate adaptive regression splines (MARS) modeling.

References

Ahlberg, J. H., Nilson, E. N., & Walsh, J. L. (1967). *The theory of splines and their applications*. New York: Academic.

Allen, D. M. (1974). The relationship between variable selection and data augmentation and a method of prediction. *Technometrics, 16*, 125–127.

Burman, P. (1989). A comparative study of ordinary cross-validation, ν-fold cross-validation and the repeated learning-testing methods. *Biometrika, 76*, 503–514.

Claeskens, G., & Hjort, N. L. (2009). *Model selection and model averaging*. Cambridge: Cambridge University Press.

Geisser, S., & Eddy, W. F. (1979). A predictive approach to model selection. *Journal of the American Statistical Association, 74*, 153–160.

Gunst, R. F., & Mason, R. L. (1980). *Regression analysis and its applications: A data-oriented approach*. New York: Dekker.

Hastie, T., Tibshirani, R., & Friedman, J. (2009). *The elements of statistical learning* (2nd ed.). New York: Springer.

Knafl, G. J., Dixon, J. K., O'Malley, J. P., Grey, M., Deatrick, J. A., Gallo, A., et al. (2012). Scale development based on likelihood cross-validation. *Statistical Methods in Medical Research, 21*, 599–619.

Knafl, G. J., & Grey, M. (2007). Factor analysis model evaluation through likelihood cross-validation. *Statistical Methods in Medical Research, 16*, 77–102.

McDonald, G. C., & Ayers, J. A. (1978). Some applications of the "Chernoff Faces": A technique for graphically representing multivariate data. In P. C. C. Wang (Ed.), *Graphical representation of multivariate data* (pp. 183–197). New York: Academic.

McDonald, G. C., & Schwing, R. C. (1973). Instabilities of regression estimates relating air pollution to mortality. *Technometrics, 15*, 463–482.

Royston, P., & Altman, D. G. (1994). Regression using fractional polynomials of continuous covariates: Parsimonious parametric modeling. *Applied Statistics, 43*, 429–467.

Sclove, S. L. (1987). Application of model-selection criteria to some problems in multivariate analysis. *Psychometrika, 52*, 333–343.

Stone, M. (1977). An asymptotic equivalence of choice of model by cross-validation and Akaike's criterion. *Journal of the Royal Statistical Society, Series B, 39*, 44–47.

Takeuchi, K. (1976). Distribution of informational statistics and a criterion of model fitting. *Suri-Kagaku (Mathematical Sciences), 153*, 12–18. In Japanese.

Chapter 3
Adaptive Regression Modeling of Univariate Continuous Outcomes in SAS

3.1 Chapter Overview

This chapter describes how to use the genreg macro for adaptive regression modeling, with models for the means linear in their intercept and slope parameters, and its generated output in the special case of univariate continuous outcomes. See Supplementary Materials for a more complete description of the macro. See Freund and Littell (2000) and Littell et al. (2002) for details on standard approaches for regression modeling in SAS. See Carpenter (2004) for details on the SAS macro language.

Code and output are provided for analyzing data on death rates per 100,000 as reported in Chap. 2. Section 3.2 covers loading in the data, Sect. 3.3 modeling death rates in terms of the nitric oxide pollution index, Sect. 3.4 setting the number k of folds for computing k-fold likelihood cross-validation (LCV) scores, Sect. 3.5 standard polynomial modeling, Sect. 3.6 model selection using penalized likelihood criteria (PLCs) rather than LCV, Sect. 3.7 restricting to monotonic models based on a single transform of a primary predictor, Sect. 3.8 comparison of adaptive modeling to recommended fractional polynomial modeling, Sect. 3.9 incorporating log transforms of primary predictors, Sect. 3.10 zero-intercept models, Sect. 3.11 bounding primary predictors, Sect. 3.12 adjusting for multiple primary predictors, Sect. 3.13 residual analyses, and Sect. 3.14 adaptive modeling of variances as well as means. Practice exercises are also provided for conducting analyses similar to those presented in Chaps. 2 and 3.

© Springer International Publishing Switzerland 2016
G.J. Knafl, K. Ding, *Adaptive Regression for Modeling Nonlinear Relationships*,
Statistics for Biology and Health, DOI 10.1007/978-3-319-33946-7_3

3.2   Loading in the Death Rate Data

A data set on death rates for 60 metropolitan statistical areas in the US is analyzed in Chap. 2 (see Sect. 2.2). Assume that this data set has been loaded into the default (work or user) library (for example, by importing it from a spreadsheet file) under the name deathrate. An output title line, selected system options, and labels for the variables can be assigned with the following code.

```
title "Death Rate Data";
options linesize=76 pagesize=53 pageno=1 nodate;
data deathrate;
 set deathrate;
 label id="Metropolitan Statistical Area ID"
       deathrate="Death Rate (deaths/100,000)"
       NOindex="Nitric Oxide Pollution Index"
       SO2index="Sulfur Dioxide Pollution Index"
       rain="Average Annual Precipitation (inches)";
run;
```

3.3   Adaptive Models Based on NOindex

Assuming the genreg macro has been loaded into SAS (see Supplementary Materials), an adaptive model for deathrate as a function of a single trans-form of NOindex can be requested as follows.

```
%genreg(modtype=norml,datain=deathrate,yvar=deathrate,
        expand=y,expxvars=NOindex,multtrns=n);
```

As for all macros, genreg is invoked by prefixing its name with a percent symbol (%) followed by a list of parameter settings in parentheses and separated by commas. Any parameters not given a setting in the invocation have their default settings as specified in the genreg interface code (see Supplementary Materials). The parameter setting "modtype=norml" requests a regression model based on the normal distribution as considered in this chapter. This is the default modtype setting and so it is not needed. The other supported settings are logis for logistic regression (see Chaps. 8–11) and poiss for Poisson regression (see Chaps. 12–15). The datain parameter specifies the input data set. It can be the name of a default library data set as in this case or a two-level SAS data set name when it is in some other library. The yvar parameter specifies the outcome variable, in this case the variable named deathrate. The base model by default is the constant, intercept-only model, but this can be changed if needed. The parameter setting "expand=y" ("y" is short for "yes") requests that the base model be expanded. The model for the means is expanded by adding in transforms of variables listed in the setting for the expxvars parameter. In this case, only NOindex is considered for expansion and only a single transform of NOindex due to "multtrns=n" ("n" is short for "no" and means here that multiple transforms of expxvars variables should not be considered in the expansion). The model for the variances can be expanded as well (see Sect. 3.14).

The adaptive modeling process requested by the above genreg call is controlled by LCV scores that are used to compare models. By default, these LCV scores are based on 10 folds, but the number of folds can be adjusted using the foldcnt macro parameter. For the above call, the selected model for the means is based on the transform NOindex$^{-0.8}$ with an intercept. The expansion process considers powers with arbitrary numbers of decimal digits. In this case, since the selected power is not an integer, there is a benefit (as defined in Chap. 20) to using fractional powers. The 10-fold LCV score for this model is 0.0041051. These analysis results are reported in the genreg output as described in Sect. 3.12.

Consideration of multiple transforms of NOindex can be requested by changing the setting of multtrns to "y". This is the default setting for the multtrns parameter so it can also be requested by just removing "multtrns=n". In this example, the expanded model allowing for multiple transforms of NOindex has three transforms added in the following order: NOindex$^{-0.8}$, NOindex$^{1.1}$, and NOindex^{-6}, together with an intercept. The LCV score is 0.0042534.

It is likely that some transforms of the above expanded model are extraneous. Expanded models can often be improved further by contracting them, removing extraneous transforms, and adjusting the powers of the remaining transforms. This is requested by adding the setting "contract=y". Each term of the model including the intercept is considered for removal. For the analysis of deathrate as a function of NOindex, the expanded and then contracted model has the two transforms NOindex$^{-0.04}$ and NOindex$^{-0.39}$ without an intercept and 10-fold LCV score 0.0042256.

In this case, the expanded model is changed by the contraction. Since the remaining transforms have their powers adjusted, there is no need for further transformation. However, when the contraction leaves the expanded model unchanged, there may be a benefit to adjusting the transforms in the uncontracted expanded model. For this reason, the adaptive process includes a conditional transformation step after a contraction that leaves the expanded model unchanged. This is controlled by the condtrns macro parameter with default setting "condtrns=y". The conditional transformation can be turned off with the setting "condtrns=n". This is not needed in the above code since the condtrns setting only has an effect when a contraction is requested. Turning off the conditional transformation when a contraction has been requested is not recommended since it can sometimes distinctly improve an uncontracted expanded model (see Sect. 10.4.1 for an example).

An output data set named dataout is created in the default library containing a copy of the datain data set along with several generated variables. The dataout macro parameter can be used to change the name of this data set. One of the generated dataout variables is named yhat and is loaded with predicted values (that is, estimated mean values) for subjects, computed with estimated parameters of the final model selected by genreg. The macro parameter yhatvar can be used to change the name of this variable. The dataout data set can be used to generate an internal SAS plot of yhat versus NOindex to visualize the relationship between deathrate and NOindex. Alternately, it can be exported to a graphics tool (like Excel if working in Windows) and used to generate that plot. A third option is to compute estimated means directly over a range of predictor values in a spreadsheet using estimated coefficients and powers reported in the genreg output, and then use those estimates to generate the plot. Figure 2.1 displays predicted values generated by the adaptive model for deathrate as a function of NOindex (using an expansion followed by a contraction) together with the raw data.

3.4 Setting the Number of Cross-Validation Folds

The Table 2.2 models for different numbers of folds can be generated with the genreg foldcnt macro parameter, for example, by varying the setting of the kfold macro variable in the following code.

```
%let kfold=5;
%genreg(modtype=norml,datain=deathrate,yvar=deathrate,
        expand=y,expxvars=NOindex,contract=y,
        foldcnt=&kfold);
```

The macro reference &kfold is translated to the current setting of this macro variable, 5 in this case as set with the %let statement, prior to executing the subsequent code containing that reference. Since $k = 5$ generates the largest LCV score over multiples of 5-folds up to $k = 15$ (see Sect. 2.8), the kfold macro variable is assumed to be set to 5 in what follows. The Table 2.2 LCV scores for $k = 5$ folds can be generated by varying the setting of the xpwrs macro variable in the following code.

```
%let xpwrs=-0.04 -0.39;
%genreg(modtype=norml,datain=deathrate,yvar=deathrate,
        xintrcpt=n,xvars=NOindex NOindex,
        xpowers=&xpwrs,foldcnt=&kfold);
```

The xpowers macro parameter is used along with the xvars macro parameter by genreg to specify fractional polynomial base models. The "xintrpct=n" option is used to request a zero intercept (the default setting "xintrcpt=y" requests the inclusion of an intercept in the base model). The above code generates the model for deathrate in terms of NOindex$^{-0.04}$ and NOindex$^{-0.39}$ without an intercept as adaptively generated with k=10 along with its 5-fold LCV score. The 5-fold score for the k=15 solution can be obtained by changing to "%let xpwrs=−0.04 − 0.40". A LOO LCV can be requested by setting "loo=y" along with an empty or missing foldcnt setting (i.e., "foldcnt=" or "foldcnt=.") as follows.

```
%genreg(modtype=norml,datain=deathrate,yvar=deathrate,
        expand=y,expxvars=NOindex,contract=y,
        foldcnt=,loo=y);
```

3.5 Standard Polynomial Models in NOindex

Standard polynomial models as in Table 2.3 are generated with the xvars and xpowers macro parameters. For example, the fully-specified cubic polynomial model in NOindex is generated as follows.

```
%genreg(modtype=norml,datain=deathrate,yvar=deathrate,
        xintrcpt=y,xvars=NOindex NOindex NOindex,
        xpowers=1 2 3,foldcnt=&kfold);
```

3.6 Selecting Models in NOindex Using Penalized Likelihood Criteria

An adaptive model for deathrate versus NOindex using adjusted AIC (AIC'; see Sect. 2.10) scores (as defined in Sect. 2.10.1) is generated as follows.

```
%genreg(modtype=norml,datain=deathrate,yvar=deathrate,
        expand=y,expxvars=NOindex,contract=y,
        scretype=AIC);
```

The scretype macro parameter is used to specify the type of scores to be used by genreg to evaluate and compare models. The default setting is "scretype=LCV" so that models are evaluated and compared with LCV scores (or generalized LCV scores when appropriate). Changing to "scretype=AIC" requests that AIC' scores be used instead to control the adaptive modeling process. The same heuristics are used to generate models, but the scores for those models change and so different

models can be selected. BIC$'$ (TIC$'$) scores are requested by changing to
"scretype=BIC" ("scretype=TIC"). The setting of the foldcnt macro parameter is
ignored when scores are based on an adjusted PLC.

3.7 Monotonic Model in NOindex

An adaptive monotonic relationship for deathrate in terms of NOindex can
be generated as follows.

```
%genreg(modtype=norml,datain=deathrate,yvar=deathrate,
        expand=y,expxvars=NOindex,multtrns=n,
        contract=y,foldcnt=&kfold);
```

As before, "multtrns=n" restricts the expansion to at most one transform
of NOindex, which adds in the single transform NOindex$^{-0.8}$. The contraction
leaves the model unadjusted and the 5-fold LCV score for the final model is
0.0041005. Even though the default setting "condtrns=y" is requested, further
transformation can have no effect in cases like this with only one transform in the
uncontracted expanded model, and so the conditional transformation step is not
executed.

3.8 Recommended Fractional Polynomials in NOindex

The following code can be used to assess the impact of restricting to the
recommended degree 1 set of powers (see Sect. 2.12) for modeling the relationship
of deathrate with NOindex. The power transforms t1–t3 and t5–t8 are computed
using the SAS exponentiation operator "**". The macro variable trnsform can be
changed from t1 to t8 to generate LCV scores for each recommended degree
1 fractional polynomial.

```
data extended;
  set deathrate;
  t1=NOindex**(-2); t2=NOindex**(-1); t3=NOindex**(-0.5);
  t4=log(NOindex); t5=NOindex**(0.5); t6=NOindex**(1);
  t7=NOindex**(2); t8=NOindex**(3);
run;
%let trnsform=t1;
%genreg(modtype=norml,datain=extended,yvar=deathrate,
        xvars=&trnsform,foldcnt=&kfold);
```

Several support macros have been developed for iteratively invoking the genreg macro (see Supplementary Materials). One of these is the RA1compare macro, which invokes genreg to generate the adaptive degree 1 monotonic fractional polynomial model for a single predictor and compare its LCV score to LCV scores for the constant model and the Royston and Altman (1994) recommended set of degree 1 fractional power transforms in that predictor. It can be used to generate the complete results of Table 2.5 as follows.

```
%RA1compare(modtype=norml,datain=deathrate,yvar=deathrate,
            xvar=NOindex,foldcnt=&kfold,scorefmt=9.7);
```

The modtype, datain, yvar, and foldcnt macro parameters have the same meaning as for the genreg macro. The xvar macro parameter is like the xvars macro parameter of genreg, but it can only specify a single predictor variable for the means. The scorefmt macro parameter requests that LCV scores generated by RA1compare be formatted with the SAS w.d format (where w is the width and d is the number of decimal digits) with value 9.7, that is, with scores printed out in 9 character positions and rounded to 7 decimal digits. Generated results are displayed in Table 3.1. The only differences from Table 2.5 are that powers are ordered by LCV scores and the percent decrease (PD) for the 0.5 power is rounded differently. The constant model is the one with power specified as "--".

Table 3.1 Results generated by the RA1compare macro comparing the recommended degree 1 fractional polynomial models for the mean death rate per 100,000 in the nitric oxide pollution index (NOindex) and the constant model (--) to the associated adaptive monotonic model (adapt) using likelihood cross-validation (LCV) scores

Power for Transform of NOindex	LCV Score	Percent Decrease
adapt	0.0041005	0.00%
-1	0.0040929	0.19%
-0.5	0.0040684	0.78%
-2	0.0039949	2.58%
0	0.0038741	5.52%
2	0.0038597	5.87%
--	0.0038136	7.00%
3	0.0037732	7.98%
1	0.0036979	9.82%
0.5	0.0036775	10.3%

3.9 Impact of the Log Transform of NOindex

The impact of the log transform can be assessed by including both a predictor xvar and its log transform log(xvar) in the expxvars list. For the analysis of deathrate as a function of NOindex, the impact of the log transform of NOindex can be addressed as follows.

```
%genreg(modtype=norml,datain=deathrate,yvar=deathrate,
        expand=y,expxvars=NOindex log_NOindex,
        contract=y,foldcnt=& kfold);
```

It is not necessary to compute the log transform in the datain data set before running genreg. Variable names of the form "log_xvar" starting with the prefix "log_" followed by the name xvar of a variable in the datain data set are computed by genreg as "log_xvar=log(xvar)" and also loaded into the dataout data set. This assumes that xvar is positive valued so that log(xvar) is well-defined. See Sect. 4.6 on how genreg computes log transforms for general real valued predictors xvar.

A macro called RA2compare is available for comparing adaptive models to the recommended degree 2 fractional polynomial models (see Sect. 2.13). The adaptive model that is generated is based on power transforms of both the predictors NOindex and log(NOindex) since these two variables are also considered in the recommended degree 2 models. However, it also considers products of powers of these two predictors since such products are included in the recommended degree 2 set (these products generalize standard interactions; see Sect. 4.5.4 for details). The following code generates LCV scores for all 36 recommended degree 2 models for deathrate as a function of NOindex, comparing them to LCV scores for the constant model and the associated adaptive model.

```
%RA2compare(modtype=norml,datain=deathrate,yvar=deathrate,
            xvar=NOindex,foldcnt=&kfold,scorefmt=9.7);
```

The modtype, datain, yvar, xvar, foldcnt, and scorefmt macro parameter have the same meaning as for RA1compare. The best LCV score for the recommended degree 2 fractional polynomial models is 0.0043085 generated with $p = p' = 0$ (as defined in Sect. 2.13) corresponding to the model in log(NOindex) and $(\log(\text{NOindex}))^2$.

3.10 Zero-Intercept Models in NOindex

The genreg macro considers zero-intercept models as part of its adaptive modeling process. The base model has a zero intercept when "xintrcpt=n", but by default "xintrcpt=y" so that then the base model includes an intercept. Consequently, the expanded model in that case also includes an intercept. By default, the contraction considers removal of the intercept as well as the other terms of the model so that a zero-intercept model can be generated. It may be desirable to restrict to models with intercepts and not consider zero-intercept alternatives. This is possible by adjusting the contraction not to consider removing the intercept from the expanded model. For the analysis of deathrate as a function of NOindex, this can be requested as follows.

```
%genreg(modtype=norml,datain=deathrate,yvar=deathrate,
        expand=y,expxvars=NOindex,contract=y,
        nocnxint=y,foldcnt= &kfold);
```

The setting "nocnxint=y" in the above code means do not contract the intercept parameter of the model for the means (corresponding to the "x" in "nocnxint=y") while the default setting "nocnxint=n" means allow the removal of that intercept. The model for the variances is constant by default and so based on an intercept term, but by default this is not changed (see Sect. 3.14 for how to model the variances).

3.11 Models Bounding the Impact of NOindex

Models bounding the impact of NOindex can be generated with the following code.

```
%let bnd=12;
data bounded;
 set deathrate;
 NObnded=min(NOindex,&bnd);
 label NObnded="NOindex Bounded to At Most &bnd";
run;
%genreg(modtype=norml,datain=bounded,yvar= deathrate,
        expand=y,expxvars=NObnded,contract=y,
        foldcnt= &kfold);
```

The setting of the macro variable bnd is varied over selected values to generate the variable NObnded equaling NOindex for values below &bnd and equaling &bnd after that. The call to genreg generates an adaptive model based on transforms of NObnded, which are nonlinear in NOindex for values below &bnd and constant after that. The above label is enclosed in double quote marks ("") rather than single quote marks (") since then the macro processor resolves macro references in the label, in this case, the reference &bnd in the label for the variable NObnded. The best LCV score over &bnd ranging from 5 to 15 occurs when &bnd = 12. This setting is used in subsequent analyses.

3.12   Models in Other Available Predictors

So far, only NOindex and its bounded version NObnded have been used to predict deathrate, but other predictors are available. Alternate adaptive models can be generated by changing the expxvars setting. An adaptive model in SO2index is generated using "expxvars=SO2index". An adaptive model in NObnded and SO2index is generated using "expxvars=NObnded SO2index". The order variables are listed in expxvars has no effect on the results. The order they are entered into the model in the expansion is determined by LCV scores. The estimates displayed in Figs. 2.9 and 2.10 are generated as follows.

```
%genreg(modtype=norml,datain=bounded,yvar=deathrate,
        expand=y,expxvars=rain NObnded,contract=y,
        foldcnt=&kfold);
```

The first two pages of the output generated by this code (not provided here) document a variety of macro parameter settings like the version of the macro, the model type, the name of the datain data set and names of variables generated in the dataout data set. They also document the form of cross-validation requested including the number of folds, range of sizes of the folds, and the cutoff for a substantial PD in the LCV scores for the data. The third page documents the base model. Table 3.2 contains part of the third page. The estimated constant mean is 940.3, the estimated constant variance parameter is 3804.6, and the LCV score is 0.0038136. Note that the LCV score is described in Table 3.2 as an mth root but is defined in Sect. 2.5.3 as an nth root. The genreg macro uses the symbol m to denote the number of total measurements, which is the same for univariate data as the number n of subjects. However, this is not the case in the more general repeated measurement case also supported by genreg (see Chaps. 4, 5, 10, 11, 14, and 15).

The fourth page of the output (not provided here) documents the parameter settings controlling the expansion and the fifth page the expanded model. Table 3.3

Table 3.2 Estimates and likelihood cross-validation score for the base model for the mean death rate per 100,000 in terms of only an intercept (XINTRCPT)

```
                       base expectation component

                    predictor      power    estimate

                    XINTRCPT          1     940.31333
...
MLE of outcome variance:                              3804.5931
...
mth root of the likelihood using deleted predictions:   0.0038136
```

Table 3.3 Expansion steps, estimates, and likelihood cross-validation score for the expanded model for the mean death rate per 100,000 in terms of an intercept (XINTRCPT) and transforms of the average annual precipitation (rain) and the nitric oxide pollution index bounded at 12 (NObnded)

```
                     expanded expectation component

          predictor      power     estimate         score   order

          XINTRCPT            1    1264.9051     0.0038136       0
          rain             -0.2    -1051.786     0.0044433       1
          NObnded           0.3    105.39914     0.0055678       2
...
MLE of outcome variance:                                     1588.5599
...
mth root of the likelihood using deleted predictions:        0.0055678
```

contains part of the fifth page. The transform rain$^{-0.2}$ is added to the constant model first increasing the LCV score from 0.0038136 to 0.0044433. The transform NObnded$^{0.3}$ is added next increasing the LCV score to 0.0055678 and then the expansion stops. The expansion allows the LCV score to decrease as long as the PD is not larger than the amount controlled by the expansion stopping tolerance, but that does not happen here (see Chap. 20 for details). Estimates for this model are 1264.9 for the intercept, -1051.8 for the slope of the rain transform, 105.4 for the slope of the NObnded transform, and 1588.6 for the constant variance parameter. New transforms are added without adjusting or removing transforms already in the model, and so improvements are possible by adjusting the expanded model. This is addressed by contraction.

The sixth page of the output (not provided here) documents the parameter settings controlling the contraction and the seventh page the contracted model. Table 3.4 contains part of the seventh page. The intercept is removed first, increasing the LCV score from 0.0055678 to 0.0056386. This provides an example of a zero intercept model improving on the associated model with an intercept, but the PD for the expanded model of 1.26 % is insubstantial (since it is lower than the cutoff of 3.15 % for a substantial PD for the data reported in Sect. 2.7). The contraction then stops resulting in a final LCV score of 0.0056392. In this case, the contraction produces an increased LCV score. In general, the contraction allows removal of transforms that decrease the LCV score as long as the decrease is not too large as controlled by the contraction stopping tolerance. By default, this tolerance parameter is calculated so that the decision to continue or stop the contraction is based on a LCV ratio test (see Sects. 2.7 and 4.4.2). In this case, the contraction stops because removal of each of the two remaining transforms results in a PD (not reported in the output) greater than the cutoff for the data. It also stops when there is only one transform left in the model, but that does not happen in this case. With each contraction of the model, the powers of remaining transforms are adjusted to improve the LCV score. For the final contracted model, the power for the remaining

Table 3.4 Contraction steps, estimates, and likelihood cross-validation score for the contracted model for the mean death rate per 100,000 in terms of transforms of the average annual precipitation (rain) and the nitric oxide pollution index bounded at 12 (NObnded)

```
                    contracted expectation component

              predictor old power new power     estimate

              rain               -0.2     0.15   440.03464
              NObnded             0.3      0.3    103.12287

              discarded   old power          score order

                                 .    0.0055678     0
              XINTRCPT            1    0.0056386     1
...
MLE of outcome variance:                                   1590.6721
...
mth root of the likelihood using deleted predictions:      0.0056386
```

rain transform is changed to 0.15 with estimated slope 440.0 and the power for NObnded remains at 0.3 with estimated slope 103.1. The estimated constant variance parameter is 1590.7 while the LCV score is 0.0056386.

The adaptive modeling process is not instantaneous and can take considerable amounts of time for complex modeling situations and/or large data sets. The amount of clock time in seconds can be requested by the macro parameter setting "rprttime=y". However, the adaptive model in rain and NObnded requires only about 4.9 s (the amount of time is not always the same for each execution of the same code but is close and can be different for different computers and can be affected by other processes running at the same time). The adaptive modeling process can be monitored as it proceeds if the SAS log window is visible where details on models generated at the various steps of the expansion and contraction are displayed. In SAS version 9.3 or later, issue the output delivery system (ODS) command: "ods listing;" first, otherwise these details do not appear in the log. As an example, Table 3.5 contains reported progress for the expansion steps of the adaptive modeling process for deathrate as a function of NObnded and rain. The contraction steps are also reported in the SAS log window, but are not provided here.

3.13 Residual Analysis

Residual analysis is supported by the genreg macro and can be requested for the final selected adaptive model depicted in Figs. 2.9 and 2.10 as follows.

Table 3.5 Adaptive expansion progress reported in the SAS log window for models for the mean death rate per 100,000 in terms of an intercept (XINTRCPT) and transforms of the average annual precipitation (rain) and the nitric oxide pollution index bounded at 12 (NObnded)

```
                    initial x/v expansion solution

        xvars     xpowers vvars     vpowers       score

        XINTRCPT  1       VINTRCPT  1       0.0038136


                    current x/v expansion solution

        xvars     xpowers vvars     vpowers       score

        XINTRCPT  1       VINTRCPT  1       0.0044433
        rain      -0.2


                    current x/v expansion solution

        xvars     xpowers vvars     vpowers       score

        XINTRCPT  1       VINTRCPT  1       0.0055678
        rain      -0.2
        NObnded   0.3
```

```
%genreg(modtype=norml,datain=bounded,yvar=deathrate,
       xintrcpt =nxvars=rain NObnded,
       xpowers=0.15 0.3,foldcnt=&kfold,ranlysis=y);
```

The setting "ranlysis=y" requests a residual analysis (as opposed to the default setting of "ranlysis=n"). Standardized residuals are generated in the dataout data set in a variable named stdres. This variable name can be changed with the stdrsvar macro parameter. Normal scores for the standardized residuals are also produced in a variable named nscore, which can be changed with the nscrevar macro parameter. Standardized residual and normal (probability) plots are also generated by genreg using PROC PLOT. These plots can be generated as well by exporting the dataout data set to a graphics tool (as for Figs. 2.11 and 2.12). The P-value for the Shapiro-Wilk test of normality of the standardized residuals is also generated. Normal scores, the normal plot, and the test for normality are only generated for "modtype=norml" since they are not relevant for other settings of the modtype macro parameter. The stdrsvar and nscore variables are generated whatever the setting for ranlysis is.

If studentized residuals are desired instead, add the "procmod=y" option to the genreg code. The procmod macro parameter is used to have genreg invoke the associated SAS PROC for the current analysis, PROC REG in this case. A data set named procmod is generated, inputted to PROC REG which adds two variables using the SAS output statement with SAS-generated names predict and studres, containing the predicted values and the studentized residuals, respectively. These latter two variables can be used to generate studentized residual and normal plots similar to Figs. 2.11 and 2.12. The procmod data set is always created. Its name can be changed with the prmodout macro parameter. The predict and studres variables are only added to this data set if "procmod=y", and only for "modtype=norml" with a univariate continuous outcome like deathrate. Currently, the names of these latter two variables cannot be changed through genreg.

Untransformed predictors in the adaptive model are generated in the procmod data set with their names in the datain data set. Transformed predictors in the adaptive model need to be given new names. Transforms used to model the means are included in both the procmod and dataout data sets with names starting with the prefix XTR_ (short for x transform) followed by an index number (that is, 1, 2, . . .). When "procmod=y", the genreg output includes a description of the variables passed to PROC REG as well as the output generated by PROC REG. Table 3.6 displays part of this output for the adaptive model for deathrate as a function of NObnded and rain. There are two predictors for the means named XTR_1 and XTR_2 corresponding to $rain^{0.15}$ and $NObnded^{0.3}$, respectively (with "**" denoting exponentiation as in SAS code). These are the predictor names listed in the PROC REG output. Transforms used to model the variances are also generated in the procmod data set, in this case just a constant predictor named VINTRCPT corresponding to a variance intercept since the variances for this model are

Table 3.6 Results of the "procmod=y" option for the adaptive model of the mean death rate per 100,000 as a function of the annual average precipitation (rain) and the nitric oxide pollution index bounded at 12 (NObnded)

```
          transforms passed in the dataout and procmod data sets:

                  names        transforms

                  XTR_1        rain**(0.15)
                  XTR_2        NObnded**(0.3)
                  VINTRCPT     --
...

                      The REG Procedure
                        Model: MODEL1
                  Dependent Variable: deathrate
...

                      Parameter Estimates

                  Parameter        Standard
      Variable    DF   Estimate        Error     t Value    Pr > |t|

      XTR_1       1    440.03464     15.62254      28.17     <.0001
      XTR_2       1    103.12287     14.47457       7.12     <.0001
```

constant. Note that slopes for XTR_1 and XTR_2 are highly significant at $P < 0.001$ (and with the same estimated values as generated by genreg in Table 3.4). Coefficients for adaptively generated models are usually all significant, and often highly significant as in this case. Consequently, standard t tests for zero coefficients of adaptive regression models are usually inappropriate. LCV ratio tests are in most cases more appropriately used to compare adaptive models to alternative models (see Sect. 1.3 for an example where it is reasonable to conduct t tests for some of an adaptive model's coefficients).

3.14 Modeling Variances as Well as Means

Both variances and means for deathrate can be modeled in terms of NObnded and rain as follows.

```
%genreg(modtype=norml,datain=bounded,yvar= deathrate,
        expand=y,expxvars=rain NObnded,
        expvvars=rain NObnded,contract=y,
        foldcnt=&kfold,rprttime=y);
```

The expvvars macro parameter provides a list of primary predictors to consider for modeling variances. The list in this case is the same as for expxvars, but it can be different. Other macros parameters are supported for modeling the variances including vvars, vpowers, and vintrcpt, which work like xvars, xpowers, and xintrcpt but address the logs of the variances rather than the means.

The expanded model (output not provided) for the above code has means based on the same two transforms as the expanded constant variances model: $\text{rain}^{-0.2}$ and $\text{NObnded}^{0.3}$ with an intercept and variances based on the two transforms: $\text{NObnded}^{1.1}$ and rain^5 also with an intercept. The LCV score is 0.0054405. Table 3.7 contains part of the output for the contraction of this expanded model. The intercept for the variances is removed first increasing the LCV score to 0.0056895. Next the intercept for the means is removed followed by the rain transform for the variances, and then the contraction stops. The final model has means based on the two transforms: $\text{rain}^{0.14}$ and $\text{NObnded}^{0.4}$ without an intercept and with estimated slopes 481.7 and 65.0 as well as variances based on the single transform: $\text{NObnded}^{-0.01}$ also without an intercept and with estimated slope 7.5. The LCV score is 0.0056157 (as also reported in Sect. 2.19.2). Since this is smaller than the score for the constant variances model of Table 3.4, the variances for deathrate are reasonably considered to be constant.

The clock time for this non-constant variances model is about 39.7 s, or about 0.7 min, compared to about 4.9 s for the associated constant variances model as reported in Sect. 3.12, or about 8.1 times as long. While the actual time for this constant variances model is not very long at 0.7 min, in general non-constant variances models can require substantially longer processing times than associated constant variances models. However, non-constant variances models are important to consider. They can provide substantial improvements over associated constant

Table 3.7 Contraction steps, estimates, and likelihood cross-validation score for the contracted model for both the means and variances of death rate per 100,000 in terms of transforms of the average annual precipitation (rain) and the nitric oxide pollution index bounded at 12 (NObnded)

```
             contracted expectation component

      predictor old power new power     estimate

      rain            -0.2      0.14   481.72042
      NObnded          0.3       0.4   64.962741

      discarded    old power         score order

                           .   0.0054405       0
      XINTRCPT             1   0.0057782       2

             contracted log variance component

      predictor old power new power     estimate

      NObnded          1.1     -0.01   7.5231897

      discarded    old power         score order

                           .   0.0054405       0
      VINTRCPT             1   0.0056895       1
      rain                 5   0.0056157       3
...
mth root of the likelihood using deleted predictions:        0.0056157
```

variances models. Constant variances models can be reasonable alternatives in some cases (as for the death rate data), but that conclusion is only possible by generating the non-constant variances model and comparing it to the constant variances model.

3.15   Practice Exercises

For Practice Exercises 3.1–3.4, first create a data set called extended containing all the variables of the deathrate data set as well as NObnded (computed as in Sect. 3.11 with "%let bnd=12") and the three possible interactions NO_SO2, NO_rain, and SO2_rain created as follows.

```
NO_SO2=NObnded*SO2index;
NO_rain=NObnded*rain;
SO2_rain=SO2index*rain;
```

Consideration of interaction terms addresses the issue called moderation (see Sect. 4.5.3). Note that an adaptive model containing interaction terms does not necessarily provide a distinct improvement over the associated additive model without interactions. This is only the case if the LCV score for the additive model generates a substantial PD in LCV scores compared to the interaction-based model.

3.1 In the analysis of deathrate in terms of NObnded and SO2index reported in Sect. 2.16, the generated model depends only on NObnded. However, this is an additive model and does not account for possible interaction between NObnded and SO2index. Repeat the analysis also considering the interaction NO_SO2 and assess the results. Use k = 5 folds as justified in Sect. 2.8.

3.2 In the analysis of deathrate in terms of NObnded and rain reported in Sect. 2.16, the generated model depends on both NObnded and rain. However, this is an additive model and does not account for possible interaction between NObnded and rain. Repeat the analysis also considering the interaction NO_rain and assess the results. Use k = 5 folds as justified in Sect. 2.8.

3.3 In the analyses of deathrate reported in Sect. 2.16, the additive model in NObnded and SO2index does not depend on SO2index, and so SO2index has not been considered yet in analyses involving NObnded and rain. However, it is possible that SO2index has an effect when rain is also considered in the analysis. First address this issue by generating the adaptive additive model in the three predictors NObnded, SO2index, and rain and assess the results. Then address this issue further by generating the adaptive model in these three predictors along with the three possible interactions between them and assess the results. Use k = 5 folds as justified in Sect. 2.8.

3.4 In Sect. 2.11, it is noted that there are two outlying observations with NOindex values of 171 and 319 compared to NOindex values of 1–66 for the other observations. Conduct a sensitivity analysis assessing whether these two observations have a highly influential effect on modeling the full data. First create a data set called reduced containing all the extended data except the observations with the two highest NOindex values. Use the adaptive analysis of death rates for these reduced data in terms of NOindex as a benchmark analysis for setting the number k of folds. Using the reduced data and this value for k, generate the model in NOindex selected adaptively for the full data, the monotonic model in NOindex generated adaptively for the full data, and the model in NObnded selected adaptively for the full data. Compare these models to the adaptive model in NOindex generated adaptively for the reduced data. Are the two outlying observations highly influential in the sense that some of the models generated for the full data are substantially inferior to the adaptively generated model for the reduced data? Note that the cutoff for a substantial PD for these data with 58 observations is 3.26 %.

For Practice Exercises 3.5–3.8, use the body fat data set available on the Internet (see Supplementary Materials). The outcome variable for this data set is called bodyfat and contains body fat values in gm/cm^3 for 252 men. The file contains several predictors. Practice Exercises 3.4–3.6 use only three of these predictors, called weight, height, and BMI containing weights in pounds, heights in inches, and body mass index values in kg/cm^2, respectively.

3.5. Use the adaptive analysis of bodyfat in weight with constant variances as a benchmark for determining an appropriate number of folds for computing LCV scores. Use this number of folds in all subsequent analyses of the body fat data. Assess whether the generated adaptive model is distinctly nonlinear in weight or not. Generate an adaptive model for bodyfat as a function of height with constant variances and assess if there is a substantial nonlinear relationship in height. Generate an adaptive model in terms of BMI with constant variances and assess if there is a substantial nonlinear relationship in BMI. Which of these three singleton-predictor models is the best for predicting bodyfat?

3.6. Generate the adaptive model in the three predictors: weight, height, and BMI with constant variances. Use the number of folds determined as part of Practice Exercise 3.5. Compare this model to the best singleton predictor model of Practice Exercise 3.4. Does consideration of weight, height, and BMI together distinctly improve on results for each separately?

3.7. Generate the adaptive model for both means and variances in the three pre-dictors: weight, height, and BMI. Use the number of folds determined as part of Practice Exercise 3.5. Compare this model to the constant variances model with the best LCV score generated for Practice Exercises 3.5 and 3.6. Does account-ing for non-constant variances provide a substantial improvement or not?

3.8. Conduct a residual analysis for the model identified in Practice Exercise 3.7 as preferable. Are there any outliers with standardized residuals outside the range of ±3? If so, conduct a sensitivity analysis as in Practice Exercise 3.5 to determine if these outliers are highly influential on the conclusions for the full data. If the adaptive reduced-data model provides a distinct improvement over the full-data model, conduct a residual analysis for it and iterate this process until no outliers are identified. Finally, for the full data, plot BMI on the y-axis versus height on the x-axis. Are there any anomalous observations in this plot that are not identified as outliers in the residual analysis?

References

Carpenter, A. (2004). *Carpenter's complete guide to the SAS macro language* (2nd ed.). Cary, NC: SAS Institute.

Freund, R., & Littell, R. (2000). *SAS system for regression* (3rd ed.). Cary, NC: SAS Institute.

Littell, R. C., Stroup, W. W., & Freund, R. J. (2002). *SAS for linear models* (4th ed.). Cary, NC: SAS Institute.

Royston, P., & Altman, D. G. (1994). Regression using fractional polynomials of continuous covariates: Parsimonious parametric modeling. *Applied Statistics, 43*, 429–467.

Chapter 4
Adaptive Regression Modeling of Multivariate Continuous Outcomes

4.1 Chapter Overview

This chapter formulates and demonstrates adaptive regression modeling of means and variances for repeatedly measured continuous outcomes treated as multivariate normal. A description of how to generate these models in SAS is provided in Chap. 5. Standard models for this context are addressed in several texts (e.g., Brown and Prescott 1999; Fitzmaurice et al. 2011; Verbeke and Molenberghs 2000).

Section 4.2 describes the dental measurement data to be used in analyses. Section 4.3 formulates marginal modeling of means for multivariate continuous outcomes using maximum likelihood (ML) to estimate parameters. Section 4.4 extends likelihood cross-validation (LCV) to marginal modeling (see Sect. 2.5.3 for the univariate case) including LCV ratio tests in Sect. 4.4.2. Section 4.5 provides example analyses of the dental measurement data using marginal ML-based modeling with order 1 autoregressive (AR1) correlations including adaptive moderation analyses in Sect. 4.5.3 and analyses based on geometric combinations, generalizing standard interactions, in Sect. 4.5.4. Section 4.6 provides a formulation for general power transforms of possibly negative or zero valued predictors. Section 4.7 formulates transition modeling for multivariate continuous outcomes in terms of prior outcome measurements while Sect. 4.8 provides example analyses of the dental measurement data using these models. Section 4.9 generalizes transition modeling to general conditional modeling for multivariate continuous outcomes in terms of the other outcome measurements, not just the prior measurements, while Sect. 4.10 provides example analyses of the dental measurement data using these models. Section 4.11 formulates parameter estimation using generalized estimating equations (GEE) for marginal models of means of multivariate continuous outcomes and provides example GEE analyses of the dental measurement data including a comparison of LCV and the quasi-likelihood information criterion (QIC) specially developed for GEE-based model selection. Section 4.12 provides a description of

© Springer International Publishing Switzerland 2016
G.J. Knafl, K. Ding, *Adaptive Regression for Modeling Nonlinear Relationships*,
Statistics for Biology and Health, DOI 10.1007/978-3-319-33946-7_4

the exercise data and example analyses using marginal and transition modeling. The dental measurement data have no missing outcomes but the exercise data do. Section 4.13 formulates the extension to LCV scoring to account for missing outcome measurements. Section 4.14 reanalyzes the exercise data using this alternative form of LCV. Section 4.15 extends marginal modeling of means to marginal modeling of both means and variances and also provides example analyses of the dental measurement and exercise data using these models. The extensions to modeling of means and variances for transition and general conditional models are straightforward and similar to the extension of Sect. 2.19.1 for the univariate case. Sections 4.16 and 4.17 provide overviews of the results of the analyses of the dental measurement and exercise data, respectively. The dental measurement and exercise data are longitudinal, but analyses of clustered data can be conducted similarly. Formulations can be skipped to focus on analyses.

4.2   The Dental Measurement Data

A data set on dental measurements for 27 children, including 16 boys and 11 girls, over four ages is available on the Internet (see Supplementary Materials). These data were analyzed by Potthoff and Roy (1964) in their classic growth curve modeling paper. They are reanalyzed here to demonstrate how to conduct regression analyses that account for nonlinearity in predictor variables for means of correlated continuous outcome measurements (in this case, longitudinal). The variable dentmeas is the outcome for these analyses and contains values for each child's dental measurements, the distance in mm from the center of the pituitary to the pterygomaxillary fissure. The possible predictor variables are age (with values 8, 10, 12, and 14 years), male (the indicator for the child being a boy), and their interaction agemale = age·male. There are 108 outcome measurements with four measurements available for each child, and so none missing. The cutoff for a substantial percent decrease (PD) in the LCV scores for these data with 108 measurements is 1.76 % (see Sect. 4.4.2). Prior to analyzing these data in Sect. 4.5, models are formulated in Sect. 4.3 for data like these along with LCV scoring for such models in Sect. 4.4.

4.3   The Marginal Multivariate Regression Model and Its Parameter Estimates

This section provides a formulation (which can be skipped) for models of outcome variables for matched sets (for example, subjects or families) measured repeatedly over specific conditions (e.g., time or family member), with outcomes possibly measured over different subsets of conditions for different matched sets (for example, outcomes measured at different times for different subjects). For the dental measurement data, the matched sets correspond to children and the conditions to the ages at which those children are measured. A marginal approach (Fitzmaurice et al. 2011) is considered with the outcome means depending only on predictors of interest and not on random effects or other outcome values and with the covariance structure (or, equivalently, the variances and correlations) for outcomes within the same matched set modeled directly. For example, compound symmetry is the covariance structure with the same variance for all conditions and the same correlation for all pairs of distinct conditions. These are also called covariance pattern models (Brown and Prescott 1999). Outcomes are considered multivariate normally distributed. Only marginal models with constant variances are considered here. See Sect. 4.15 for the generalization to non-constant variances. Parameters are estimated with ML. See Sect. 4.11 for the formulation of GEE parameter estimation for marginal models.

4.3.1   Complete Data

Let $\mathbf{y}_s$ be a column vector of m outcome measurements y_{sc} under alternative conditions with indexes $c \in C = \{c : 1 \leq c \leq m\}$ for n matched sets of measurements with indexes $s \in S = \{s : 1 \leq s \leq n\}$. The indexes s are often considered to represent different subjects, but the matched sets may contain outcome measurements for clusters of subjects like multiple members of the same family and so are more general. For $s \in S$ and $c \in C$, let $\mathbf{x}_{sc}$ be a column vector of r predictor values x_{scj} with indexes $j \in J = \{j : 1 \leq j \leq r\}$ and $\mathbf{X}_s$ the $m \times r$ predictor matrix with rows $\mathbf{x}_{sc}^T$. Note that sc denotes a pair of indexes s and c and does not involve multiplication.

4.3.2   Incomplete Data

While data sets like the dental measurement data can be complete with outcome measurements available for all possible conditions for all matched sets, multivariate outcome data often consist of different sets of outcome measurements within the matched sets, for example, due to missing data as for the exercise data of Sect. 4.12 or due to studying different sized clusters of subjects. Consequently, the formulation considers this more general case.

Let $\mathbf{y}_{s,C'}$ denote the vector $\mathbf{y}_s$ with its entries y_{sc} restricted to the indexes $c \in C'$, an arbitrary, possibly empty subset of C. Also, let $\mathbf{X}_{s,C'}$ denote the matrix $\mathbf{X}_s$ with its rows restricted to the indexes $c \in C'$.

To account for different subsets of outcome measurements for matched sets, let C(s) denote the subset of C consisting of the $m(s) \leq m$ conditions for which y_{sc} and $\mathbf{x}_{sc}$ are actually measured for each matched set $s \in S$. Let $O_{s,C(s)} = (\mathbf{y}_{s,C(s)}, \mathbf{X}_{s,C(s)})$ denote the observed data for each $s \in S$. Also, let $SC = \{sc: c \in C(s), s \in S\}$ be the set of indexes sc for the observed measurements and $m(SC) = \sum_{s \in S} m(s) \leq n \cdot m$ the total number of observed measurements.

4.3.3 Marginal Maximum Likelihood Modeling of Dependence

For $s \in S$, assume that conditioned on the values for the predictor matrices $\mathbf{X}_{s,C(s)}$, the outcome vectors $\mathbf{y}_{s,C(s)}$ are independent and multivariate normally distributed with mean vectors $\boldsymbol{\mu}_{s,C(s)}$ having entries μ_{sc} for $c \in C(s)$ and covariance matrices $\boldsymbol{\Sigma}_{s,C(s)}$ having entries $\Sigma_{scc'}$ for $c, c' \in C(s)$. Model the means as $\boldsymbol{\mu}_{s,C(s)} = \mathbf{X}_{s,C(s)} \cdot \boldsymbol{\beta}$ for a $r \times 1$ vector $\boldsymbol{\beta}$ of fixed effects coefficients and the covariance matrices as $\boldsymbol{\Sigma}_{s,C(s)} = \sigma^2 \cdot \mathbf{R}_{s,C(s)}(\boldsymbol{\rho})$ for a constant variance parameter σ^2 and a vector $\boldsymbol{\rho}$ of parameters determining the correlation matrices $\mathbf{R}_{s,C(s)}(\boldsymbol{\rho})$ for $\mathbf{y}_{s,C(s)}$. Let $\boldsymbol{\theta} = (\boldsymbol{\beta}^T, \sigma^2, \boldsymbol{\rho}^T)^T$ denote the vector of all the model parameters.

For each $s \in S$, the likelihood term $L(O_{s,C(s)}; \boldsymbol{\theta})$ satisfies

$$\ell(O_{s,C(s)}; \boldsymbol{\theta}) = \log\left(L\left(O_{s,C(s)}; \boldsymbol{\theta}\right)\right) = -\frac{1}{2} \cdot \mathbf{e}_{s,C(s)}^T \cdot \boldsymbol{\Sigma}_{s,C(s)}^{-1} \cdot \mathbf{e}_{s,C(s)}$$
$$- \frac{1}{2} \cdot \log(|\boldsymbol{\Sigma}_{s,C(s)}|) - \frac{1}{2} \cdot m(s) \cdot \log(2 \cdot \pi),$$

where $\mathbf{e}_{s,C(s)} = \mathbf{y}_{s,C(s)} - \boldsymbol{\mu}_{s,C(s)}$ is the error vector, $|\boldsymbol{\Sigma}_{s,C(s)}|$ the determinant of the covariance matrix $\boldsymbol{\Sigma}_{s,C(s)}$, and π the usual constant. The likelihood $L(SC; \boldsymbol{\theta})$ is the product of the likelihood terms $L(O_{s,C(s)}; \boldsymbol{\theta})$ over $s \in S$. The maximum likelihood estimate $\boldsymbol{\theta}(SC)$ of $\boldsymbol{\theta}$ is obtained by maximizing the log-likelihood $\ell(SC; \boldsymbol{\theta}) = \log(L(SC; \boldsymbol{\theta}))$ over all possible parameter vectors $\boldsymbol{\theta}$. This is achieved by solving the estimating equations $\partial \ell(SC; \boldsymbol{\theta})/\partial \boldsymbol{\theta} = \mathbf{0}$ obtained by differentiating $\ell(SC; \boldsymbol{\theta})$ with respect to $\boldsymbol{\theta}$. For simplicity of notation, parameter estimates $\boldsymbol{\theta}(SC)$ are denoted as functions of the index set SC for the observed data used in their computation without hat (^) symbols.

For $s \in S$, error vectors $\mathbf{e}_{s,C(s)}$ can be scaled (using the terminology of PROC MIXED, SAS Institute 2004) as follows. Let $\mathbf{U}_{s,C(s)}$ be the upper triangular matrix satisfying $\boldsymbol{\Sigma}_{s,C(s)} = \mathbf{U}_{s,C(s)}^T \cdot \mathbf{U}_{s,C(s)}$. In other words, $\mathbf{U}_{s,C(s)}$ is the square root of the covariance matrix $\boldsymbol{\Sigma}_{s,C(s)}$ determined by its Cholesky decomposition. The associated scaled errors are $\mathbf{sclde}_{s,C(s)} = \left(\mathbf{U}_{s,C(s)}^T\right)^{-1} \cdot \mathbf{e}_{s,C(s)}$. The covariance matrix for $\mathbf{sclde}_{s,C(s)}$ is

$$(\mathbf{U}_{s,C(s)}{}^T)^{-1} \cdot \mathbf{\Sigma}_{s,C(s)} \cdot ((\mathbf{U}_{s,C(s)}{}^T)^{-1})^T = (\mathbf{U}_{s,C(s)}{}^T)^{-1} \cdot (\mathbf{U}_{s,C(s)}{}^T \cdot \mathbf{U}_{s,C(s)})$$
$$\cdot \, \mathbf{U}_{s,C(s)}{}^{-1} = \mathbf{I}_{m(s)},$$

where $\mathbf{I}_{m(s)}$ is the $m(s) \times m(s)$ identity matrix. Hence scaled residual vectors can be computed as

$$\mathbf{sclde}_{s,C(s)}(SC) = (\mathbf{U}_{s,C(s)}{}^T(SC))^{-1} \cdot \mathbf{e}_{s,C(s)}(SC)$$

from the unscaled residual vectors

$$\mathbf{e}_{s,C(s)}(SC) = \mathbf{y}_{s,C(s)} - \boldsymbol{\mu}_{s,C(s)}(SC) = \mathbf{y}_{s,C(s)} - \mathbf{X}_{s,C(s)} \cdot \boldsymbol{\beta}(SC)$$

and the estimate $\mathbf{U}_{s,C(s)}(SC)$ of $\mathbf{U}_{s,C(s)}$ computed from the estimate $\mathbf{\Sigma}_{s,C(s)}(SC) = \sigma^2(SC) \cdot \mathbf{R}_{s,C(s)}(\boldsymbol{\rho}(SC))$. Scaled residuals can be used similarly to standardized residuals for univariate continuous outcomes.

4.4 LCV for Marginal Models

This section provides an extension of the LCV formulation of Sect. 2.5.3 to marginal multivariate normal models (which can be skipped). LCV ratio tests as described in Sect. 2.7 are also extended and formally defined including how to compute the cutoff for a substantial PD in the LCV scores.

4.4.1 LCV Formulation

As in Sect. 2.5.2, randomly partition the index set SC into k disjoint folds F(h) for $h \in H = \{h : 1 \le h \le k\}$ with all C(s) measurements for a matched set s assigned to the same fold F(h(s)) where $h(s) = \text{int}(k \cdot u_s) + 1$ for independent, uniform random values u_s in (0, 1). LCV scores are defined as

$$LCV = \prod_{h \in H} \prod_{s \in F(h)} L\big(O_{s,C(s)}; \boldsymbol{\theta}(SC \backslash F(h))\big)^{\frac{1}{m(SC)}}.$$

The LCV score is normalized by the total number m(SC) of observed measurements over all matched sets $s \in S$ rather than by the total number n of matched sets. For the univariate outcome case of Chap. 2, $m(SC) = n$, but this does not hold for the more general multivariate case considered here.

4.4.2   *LCV Ratio Tests*

Stone (1977) provided an argument supporting χ^2-based LCV ratio tests in analogy to likelihood ratio tests under leave-one-out (LOO) fold assignment. A similar argument holds for k-fold LCV. This result depends on the fact that the computation of LCV scores is consistent with how associated likelihoods $L(\cdot; \theta)$ are calculated so that $LCV^{m(SC)}$ equals $L(SC; \theta)$ when computed with parameter estimates $\theta(SC)$ for the whole set of data with indexes in SC rather than with deleted estimates $\theta(SC\backslash F(h))$. As long as the sizes of the complements $SC\backslash F(h)$ of the index sets $F(h)$ increase to infinity with the number $m(SC)$ of measurements, the deleted estimates $\theta(SC\backslash F(h))$ will converge to the same limit as the undeleted estimates $\theta(SC)$ (assuming random fold assignment independent of the observed data). Consequently, $LCV^{m(SC)}$ is asymptotically the same as the likelihood.

    Thus, k-fold LCV ratio tests can be used to assess whether or not a change in the LCV score is substantial. Specifically, if model M_1 is nested within model M_2, with DF the difference in the number of parameters and with LCV scores $LCV(M_1)$ and $LCV(M_2)$, respectively, then the difference

$$\delta = 2 \cdot \log\left(LCV(M_2)^{m(SC)}\right) - 2 \cdot \log\left(LCV(M_1)^{m(SC)}\right)$$

is asymptotically χ^2 distributed with DF degrees of freedom. The associated PD in the LCV scores is

$$PD(\delta, m(SC)) = \frac{LCV(M_2) - LCV(M_1)}{LCV(M_2)} \cdot 100\% = \left(1 - e^{-\delta/(2 \cdot m(SC))}\right) \cdot 100\%$$

and is significant when δ exceeds the cutoff determined by the 95th percentile $\delta(95 \%, DF)$ of the χ^2 distribution with DF degrees of freedom. The percent increase (PI) can also be used, satisfying

$$PI(\delta, m(SC)) = \frac{LCV(M_2) - LCV(M_1)}{LCV(M_1)} \cdot 100\% = \left(e^{\delta/(2 \cdot m(SC))} - 1\right) \cdot 100\%.$$

    For a penalized likelihood criterion $PLC = -2 \cdot \log(L(SC; \theta(SC))) + PF$, where PF is the penalty factor, its adjusted score $PLC' = \exp(-1/2 \cdot PLC/m(SC))$ is used in the adaptive modeling process. For associated adjusted PLC ratio tests, δ as defined above for the LCV case becomes

$$\delta = 2 \cdot \log(PLC'(M_2)^{m(SC)}) - 2 \cdot \log(PLC'(M_1)^{m(SC)})$$
$$= -PLC(M_2) + PLC(M_1) = \chi^2(M_1, M_2) - PF(M_2) + PF(M_1),$$

where $\chi^2(M_1, M_2)$ is the usual likelihood ratio statistic with approximate χ^2 distribution with DF degrees of freedom. Consequently, δ exceeds the cutoff determined by the 95th percentile $\delta(95 \%, DF)$ when $\chi^2(M_1, M_2)$ exceeds the cutoff

$\delta(95\%, \mathrm{DF}) + \mathrm{PF}(M_2) - \mathrm{PF}(M_1)$. Since $\mathrm{PF}(M_2) - \mathrm{PF}(M_1) > 0$ (i.e., the penalty is smaller for the nested model), PLC' ratio tests use larger cutoffs for significance than standard likelihood ratio tests and so are more conservative. A leave-one-out (LOO) LCV is asymptotically equivalent (eq. 2.30, Claeskens and Hjort 2009) to using the special PLC called the Takeuchi information criterion (TIC; eq. 2.20, Claeskens and Hjort 2009), which is also asymptotically equivalent to using AIC when the model is correctly specified. Consequently, a LOO LCV ratio test is also more conservative than the associated likelihood ratio test. These results explain prior observations that k-fold LCV ratio tests are similar in effect to multiple comparisons procedures in sometimes not considering the effect of a term in a model significant even though its coefficient is significantly nonzero using standard tests for zero coefficients (for examples see Riegel and Knafl 2014; Knafl and Riegel 2014).

Alternative models, however, are often not nested, but there is still a need to compare their LCV scores. For example, a model with an untransformed predictor can have a smaller LCV score than the model with the predictor replaced by its log transform. How substantive a change this is can be assessed by the PD (or PI) in the LCV scores. When the PD is substantive, the nonlinear, log transform model with the higher score distinctly outperforms the linear model with the lower score. Otherwise, the linear model is preferable as a simpler, competitive alternative. A measure of what constitutes a substantive PD is needed to make such assessments. A PD is treated as substantial when it is larger than the value at the cutoff given by the 95th percentile $\delta(95\%, 1) = 3.84146$ of the χ^2 distribution with $\mathrm{DF} = 1$ (but see Sect. 9.8 for an exception when the cutoff is based on $\mathrm{DF} = 2$). Thus, a substantive PD exceeds what would be a significant amount for nested models differing by the smallest possible nonzero integer number of parameters. This is called substantial (or distinct) rather than significant since it might not involve nested models. For the dental measurement data with $m(\mathrm{SC}) = 108$, the cutoff for a substantial PD is 1.76 % (computed as PD(3.84146, 108) with the formula given above for PD($\delta, m(\mathrm{SC})$)).

4.5   Marginal Order 1 Autoregressive Modeling of the Dental Measurement Data

4.5.1   Order 1 Autoregressive Correlations

Since the dental measurement data are longitudinal, order 1 autoregressive (AR1) correlations weakening the further apart outcome measurements are in time are natural to start with to model their dependence. Specifically, for indexes c satisfying $1 \le c \le 4$, the four ages (8, 10, 12, and 14) for each child are given by $t(c) = 6 + 2 \cdot c$. Then, the correlations, depending on the single autocorrelation parameter ρ, have values $\rho^{|t(c)-t(c')|}$ where $|t - t'|$ denotes the absolute value of $t - t'$ and hence the distance between t and t'. Since all $t(c)$ are integers in this case,

$\rho^{|t(c)-t(c')|}$ is well-defined for $-1 < \rho < 1$. In other cases where the observed times t(c) are not all integers, $\rho^{|t(c)-t(c')|}$ can be guaranteed to be well-defined by restricting to $0 \leq \rho < 1$. Such a restriction can be removed (see p. 2728, SAS Institute 2004), but that more general case is not considered here. Note that this is a spatial autoregression with distance apart measured by the actual ages t(c) rather than their indexes c as often used in autoregression. For equally spaced data like the dental measurements, these two approaches are equivalent, but not for unequally spaced data.

4.5.2   Setting the Number of Cross-Validation Folds

Modeling the mean dental measurements as a function of the child's age under AR1 correlations is used as the benchmark analysis for setting the number k of folds for LCV scores (see Sect. 2.8). With $k = 5$ folds, the adaptively generated model includes the transform $age^{0.3}$ without an intercept and LCV score 0.10552. With $k = 10$ folds, the same model is generated with smaller LCV score 0.10534. This result suggests using $k = 5$ for subsequent analyses, but this choice may not always be best in such cases. However, with $k = 15$ folds, the same model is generated again with even smaller LCV score 0.10434. Since $k = 5$ generates the largest LCV score over these three cases, it seems reasonable to use $k = 5$ for subsequent analyses of these data, and so $k = 5$ is used in what follows. The number of measurements in the 5 folds ranges from 12 to 32 with average 21.6 for 3–8 matched sets (children in this case) with average 5.4.

The linear polynomial model (i.e., the model based on untransformed age) for the mean dental measurements has 5-fold LCV score 0.10539 and insubstantial PD compared to the adaptively selected model of 0.12 % (that is, less than the cutoff of 1.76 % for the data). Thus, the mean dental measurements are reasonably close to linear in the child's age.

4.5.3   Moderation of the Effect of Age by Gender

It is possible that mean dental measurements change differently for boys than for girls as they age. This can be addressed by adaptively modeling those means in terms of the three predictors: age, male, and their interaction agemale. The generated model includes the two transforms $agemale^{2.2}$ and $age^{0.18}$ without an intercept and LCV score 0.11465. The PD for the model in age by itself is substantial at 7.96 %, suggesting that mean dental measurements do change with age differently for boys than for girls.

The fact that a power transform of the interaction agemale is included in the model suggests that the pattern for the means for boys as they age is different from the associated pattern for girls. In other words, this supports the conclusion that gender of the child moderates the effect of age on the mean dental measurements (Baron and Kenny 1986). However, it is possible that the model with only a covariate effect to gender, that is, with the pattern over ages the same for boys and girls but shifted up or down by a constant amount, provides a competitive alternative. If this is the case, the interaction effect is not substantial and moderation (also called modification) has not really occurred. This is addressed by the adaptive model with the mean dental measurements changing only with age and male but not with agemale. The associated model has two terms: $age^{0.31}$ and male without an intercept, and has LCV score 0.11065 with substantial PD of 3.49 % compared to the model accounting for an interaction effect. Consequently, gender distinctly moderates the effect of age on the mean dental measurements.

Moderation in the continuous outcome context involves three variables: the continuous outcome variable y, the predictor variable x, and the moderator variable z. It is commonly addressed using the linear moderation model with the expected outcome Ey satisfying

$$Ey = \beta_1 + \beta_2 \cdot x + \beta_3 \cdot z + \beta_4 \cdot x \cdot z.$$

A significant slope β_4 for the interaction term x·z in this model indicates that moderation holds. Alternately, for the special case with y univariate, moderation can be assessed by comparing R^2 for the moderation model to R^2 for the linear covariate model with

$$Ey = \beta_1 + \beta_2 \cdot x + \beta_3 \cdot z.$$

A partial F-test (see, for example, Sect. 9.4, Kleinbaum et al. 1998) can then be used to test for a significant change in R^2. The assessment of nonlinear moderation cannot be addressed by a test for a zero interaction coefficient. It can be assessed instead with a LCV ratio test, as in the above example, comparing the adaptively generated moderation model to the adaptively generated covariate model, and so is analogous to testing in the univariate linear moderation context for a significant change in R^2.

When linear moderation analyses are based on continuous x and/or z, these variables are sometimes first centered, usually by subtracting their observed means, and the centered variables are used in the linear moderation model in place of associated uncentered variables (e.g., Aiken and West 1991). Centering of the variables of the linear moderation model generates an equivalent model and has no effect on the coefficient β_4 of the interaction term x·z for that model. Centering does have an effect on the other coefficients of the linear moderation model, and so its use can impact the interpretation of the estimates for that model. Nonlinear moderation models can also be based on centered variables, but those are not equivalent in general to models based on uncentered variables. For the dental measurement data, the adaptively generated model based on male, the variable centage = age − 11 with age centered at its mean value of 11, and their interaction cagemale = centage·male is based on the transforms: centage$^{-0.07}$, cagemale$^{-0.25}$, and centage$^{1.6}$ without an intercept. The LCV score is 0.11554. While the adaptive uncentered model has smaller LCV score 0.11465, the PD is insubstantial at 0.77 % and it is simpler based on two compared to three transforms both without an intercept. The adaptively generated additive model in male and centage is based on the two transforms centage$^{0.7}$ and male with LCV score 0.11218 with substantial PD 2.91 % compared to the model based also on cagemale. Consequently, moderation is also established using centered age values. It is possible that improvements can be obtained by centering at other values than the mean. LCV can be used to choose the best centering value and to compare those results to uncentered results (see Practice Exercise 5.3).

For the dental measurement data, the test for zero slope β_4 for the interaction term age·male of the linear moderation model is nonsignificant $(P = 0.116)$. Moreover, the LCV score for the linear covariate model is 0.11056 with insubstantial PD of 0.77 % compared to the LCV score of 0.11142 for the linear moderation model. Thus, the addition of the linear interaction term does not substantially improve on the linear covariate model. Consequently, a linear moderation analysis leads to the conclusion that gender does not moderate the effect of age on the mean dental measurements. Furthermore, the linear moderation model generates a substantial PD of 2.82 % compared to the adaptive moderation model indicating that the moderated effects of age on mean dental measurement by gender are distinctly nonlinear. In this case, moderation can only be identified through an adaptive nonlinear analysis.

4.5.4 Geometric Combinations

Using an interaction x·x′, like agemale, as one of the primary predictors for an adaptive analysis does not address the most general nonlinear interaction model. Associated power transforms then have the form $(x \cdot x')^p$, and so each term of the interaction is always raised to the same power. More general interactions with each term of the interaction raised to its own power, for example, $x^p \cdot x'^{p'}$, can be considered as part of the adaptive modeling process in possibly transformed form $(x^p \cdot x'^{p'})^{p''}$. These are called geometric combinations (GCs) since their logs are linear combinations, for example, $\log(x^p \cdot x'^{p'}) = p \cdot \log(x) + p' \cdot \log(x')$. There is no difference for interactions like agemale between a general predictor and an indicator variable since indicator variables are unaffected by power transforms, but there is a difference for general interactions.

Prior analyses have used the directly specified interactions agemale or cagemale. Alternately, adaptive models can be generated by only specifying non-interaction primary predictors (for example, age and male but not agemale) and requesting that

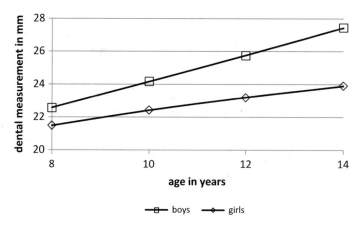

Fig. 4.1 Estimated mean dental measurements based on adaptive marginal AR1 modeling

GCs between those predictors be generated as part of the adaptive modeling process. For primary predictors age and male, the associated adaptive GC-based model is based on age$^{0.19}$ and the automatically generated transformed GC

$$\left(\text{male} \cdot \text{age}^{-14}\right)^{-0.15} = \text{male} \cdot \text{age}^{2.1}$$

without an intercept. The LCV score is 0.11467, a little larger than the LCV score for the model based on agemale. This result supports the validity of the heuristics for generating GCs (see Chap. 20). For this GC-based AR1 marginal model, the estimated autocorrelation is 0.78 so that correlations decrease from 0.61 at 2 years apart to 0.23 at 6 years apart. The estimated constant standard deviation is 2.2. Estimated means are displayed in Fig. 4.1. They appear only mildly nonlinear, and so a competitive linear model might exist. This can be assessed by generating an adaptive model constrained to consider only the untransformed, linear terms in age, male, and the simple GC age·male. The generated model is based on age, age·male, and an intercept with LCV score 0.11246. The PD compared to the associated adaptive nonlinear GC-based model is substantial at 1.93 %, indicating that the moderation relationships of Fig. 4.1 are distinctly nonlinear (but perhaps more so for girls than boys).

4.6 General Power Transforms

Power transforms for positive valued primary predictors, like age, are well-defined for all real valued powers p, but primary predictors can have zero values, as for indicator variables like male and interactions like agemale based on those indicators, or even negative values, as for centered variables like centage or log transforms of variables with some values between 0 and 1. Section 4.6.1 provides a formulation (which can be skipped) for defining power transforms of general primary predictors with possible negative or zero values and for incorporating those power transforms and GCs computed from them in fractional polynomial models. Specifically, transformed zero values are left as zero, transformed positive values are computed as usual, and transformed negative values are set equal to the transform of their absolute values weighted by a cosine function to switch signs between positive and negative values. Log transforms of real valued predictors are defined similarly. Section 4.6.2 addresses the approach recommended by Royston and Sauerbrei (2008) for handling negative predictors.

4.6.1   Formulation

So that power transforms are well defined in all cases, they are defined as $f(u, p)$ with value u^p when $u > 0$, 0 when $u = 0$, and $\cos(\pi \cdot p) \cdot |u|^p$ when $u < 0$ where u is a primary predictor variable and $|u|$ denotes its absolute value. Note that when $u < 0$, the multiple $\cos(\pi \cdot p)$ equals 1 for even integer powers p, -1 for odd integer powers p, and oscillates between ± 1 otherwise. The validity of this approach for transforming negative values is supported by centered analyses reported in Sect. 4.5.3 providing competitive results to uncentered analyses. A primary predictor may be a log transform of another primary predictor u' corresponding to the power $p = 0$. So that this log is well-defined, it is defined as $\log(u')$ when $u' > 0$, 0 when $u' = 0$, and $\cos(\pi \cdot 0) \cdot \log(|u'|) = \log(|u'|)$ when $u' < 0$. Note that, for a primary predictor u with some 0 values and otherwise positive valued, the transform $f(u, p)$ with a small value of p like 0.0001 approximates the indicator $I(u > 0)$ for u being positive when $I(u > 0)$ is not already in the model and approximates the log transform for positive values of u when $I(u > 0)$ is already in the model (the argument is similar to those of Sect. 2.13.2).

Let u_i for $1 \leq i \leq I$ be one of I primary predictors. Let u_{sci} be the observed values for u_i for $c \in C(s)$ and $s \in S$ and $\mathbf{u}_{sc}$ the $I \times 1$ vectors with entries u_{sci}. The primary predictors generate fractional polynomial models with associated $r \times 1$ predictor vectors $\mathbf{x}_{sc} = \mathbf{F}(\mathbf{u}_{sc})$ with entries $x_{scj} = F_j(\mathbf{u}_{sc})$ for $j \in J = \{j : 1 \leq j \leq r\}$ where F_j are r real valued functions of $I \times 1$ vectors $\mathbf{u}$. The choices for F_j include simple power transforms $f(u, p)$ of one of the primary predictors u as well as GCs $f(u, p) \cdot f(u', p') \cdots$, that is, products of simple power transforms of multiple distinct primary predictors using possibly different powers. Once a GC $f(u, p) \cdot f(u', p') \cdots$ is generated by the adaptive modeling process, it is transformed as $f(f(u, p) \cdot f(u', p') \cdots, q)$, adjusting all of its powers p, $p', \cdots$ by a common power q rather than adjusting each of those powers separately (thereby, reducing the complexity of the heuristics of the adaptive modeling process).

4.6.2   The Royston and Sauerbrei Approach

Royston and Sauerbrei (2008; Sect. 4.7) suggest adjusting a nonpositive valued primary predictor u to the positive valued primary predictor $u' = u - \min(u) + \eta$ where $\min(u)$ is the minimum observed value for u and η is a positive constant. If a positive valued primary predictor u is adjusted to the centered variable $cent(u, u_c) = u - u_c$ for some centering constant u_c within the range of observed values for u, it becomes nonpositive valued, and so would be adjusted under the Royston and Sauerbrei approach to

$$cent(u, u_c)' = u - u_c - (\min(u) - u_c) + \eta = u - \min(u) + \eta,$$

and so there would then be no effect to the centering constant u_c.

One suggested choice for η is the minimum distance between successive ordered observed values for u. Using this choice, $\eta = 2$ for the centered primary predictor age $- 11$, so that

$$adjcage = (age - 11)' = age - 8 + 2 = age - 6.$$

The adaptive model for dentmeas in terms of adjcage, male, and GCs is based on the two transforms: $(male \cdot adjcage^{1.5})^{0.6}$ and $adjcage^{0.07}$. The LCV score is 0.11378 with insubstantial PD 0.78 % compared to the associated adaptive model in the uncentered primary predictor age. Consequently, a competitive model is generated, but there is no need for considering this adjustment since age is positive valued to start with. Another alternative for centering is to center a fractional polynomial transform $x = u^p$ of a positive valued primary predictor u rather than u itself, subtracting from x the average of its observed values (Royston and Sauerbrei 2008; Sect. 4.11.1).

4.7   Transition Modeling of Dependence

This section provides a formulation (which can be skipped) of a conditional approach of transition (or autoregressive or Markov) type for modeling the dependence within outcomes of the same matched set (e.g., within dental measurements at different ages for each child). For transition models of continuous outcomes, conditioned on the values of available predictors and on values of prior outcome measurements, current outcome measurements are considered to be univariate normal with means a function of the available predictors and of the prior outcomes measurements. The conditions for repeated outcome measurements need to be ordered (e.g., time or age) to use such transition modeling. The formulation incorporates prior outcome measurements into the model for the means by considering averages of fixed numbers (e.g., 1, 2, $\cdots$) of them as well as indicator variables for when there are no prior outcome measurements to average (e.g., at the youngest age of 8 years for the dental measurements). LCV scores for transition models can be compared to LCV scores for marginal models to assess which are more appropriate for the data.

4.7.1 Formulation Using Averages of Prior Outcome Measurements

For $s \in S$ and $c \in C(s)$, define $\mathrm{PRE}(s,c) = \{c' : c' \in C(s), c' < c\}$ as the possibly empty set of indexes in $C(s)$ prior to the index c. The likelihood $L(O_{s,C(s)}; \boldsymbol{\theta})$ can be written as the product of conditional likelihoods

$$L(O_{s,C(s)}; \boldsymbol{\theta}) = \prod_{c \in C(s)} L(O_{sc} | y_{s,\mathrm{PRE}(s,c)}; \boldsymbol{\theta}),$$

where $O_{sc} = (y_{sc}, \mathbf{x}_{sc})$ denotes the observed data corresponding to the cth measurement for the matched set s. For the smallest index $c^\circ(s) = \min(C(s))$ in $C(s)$ and so also in $\mathrm{PRE}(s,c)$ when $c > c^\circ(s)$, $\mathrm{PRE}(s,c^\circ(s)) = \varnothing$, and so $L(O_{sc^\circ(s)} | y_{s,\mathrm{PRE}(s,c^\circ(s))}; \boldsymbol{\theta})$ in the above product is set to the unconditional likelihood $L(O_{sc^\circ(s)}; \boldsymbol{\theta})$.

For complete data like the dental measurement data, the conditional distribution $L(O_{sc} | y_{s,\mathrm{PRE}(s,c)}; \boldsymbol{\theta})$ under AR1 correlations for $c > c^\circ(s) = 1$ is univariate normal and depends only on the prior outcome measurement with index $\mathrm{prior}(s,c) = c - 1$. This suggests consideration of transition models (Diggle et al. 2002) with current outcome measurements depending on values of prior outcome measurements, but in this case just the prior outcome measurement. Define the dependence predictor variable $\mathrm{PRE}(y,1)$ as having values $\mathrm{PRE}(y,1)_{sc^\circ(s)} = 0$ and $\mathrm{PRE}(y,1)_{sc} = y_{s\mathrm{prior}(s,c)}$ for $c \in C(s)$, $c > c^\circ(s)$ where $\mathrm{prior}(s,c) = \max(\mathrm{PRE}(s,c))$ is the largest index in $\mathrm{PRE}(s,c)$. Extend the predictor vectors $\mathbf{x}_{sc}$ to include values for transforms of $\mathrm{PRE}(y,1)$ along with transforms for standard predictors as used with marginal models as well as GCs in both kinds of primary predictors. For $sc \in SC$, let $y^{\#}_{sc} = y_{sc} | y_{s,\mathrm{PRE}(s,c)}$ denote an outcome measurement conditioned on the associated prior measurements where $y^{\#}_{sc^\circ(s)} = y_{sc^\circ(s)}$ is the unconditional initial measurement for s. Model the associated observations $O^{\#}_{sc} = (y^{\#}_{sc}, \mathbf{x}_{sc})$ as independent and normally distributed with constant variances as in Chap. 2. Cases $sc^\circ(s)$ can require special treatment. To cover the need for an adjustment in these cases, adaptive models can also be based on the special transform of $\mathrm{PRE}(y,1)$ given by the indicator variable $\mathrm{PRE}(y,1,\varnothing)$ for cases when the prior measurement has not been measured, that is, when $\mathrm{PRE}(s,c) = \varnothing$ or, equivalently, when $c = c^\circ(s)$.

In analogy to higher order autoregressive models, adaptive transition models can also be based on primary predictors computed from subsets of the prior outcome measurements, not just from the prior measurement. Let m(PRE(s,c)) be the number of conditions in PRE(s,c). For $1 \le i \le$ m(PRE(s,c)), let PRIOR(s,c,i) be the subset of PRE(s,c) containing just the ith largest index in PRE(s,c). For example, for $c > c°(s)$, PRIOR(s,c,1) = {prior(s,c)}. For i > m(PRE(s,c)), define PRIOR(s,c,i) = $\varnothing$. For $i \le j$, let

$$PRE(s,c,i,j) = \bigcup_{i \le i' \le j} PRIOR(s,c,i').$$

In other words, PRE(s,c,i,j) is the subset of PRE(s,c) consisting of its ith to jth largest indexes. Define the dependence predictors PRE(y,i,j) to have values PRE(y,i,j)$_{sc}$ equal to the average of $y_{sc'}$ over the indexes c' in PRE(s,c,i,j) and equal to 0 when PRE(s,c,i,j) = $\varnothing$. Also define the indicator variables PRE(y,i,j,$\varnothing$) for cases when PRE(s,c,i,j) = $\varnothing$. The variables PRE(y,i,j,$\varnothing$) are not all distinct. For example, when there are no missing outcome measurements as for the dental measurement data, PRE(y,1,j,$\varnothing$) = PRE(y,1,1,$\varnothing$) for all j. PRE(y,1) = PRE(y,1,1) is the special case with $i = j = 1$.

For time-varying primary predictors u not based on the outcome variable y, associated dependence predictors PRE(u,i,j) are also possible with values PRE(u,i,j)$_{sc}$ equal to the average of prior values for u, as are the indicator variables PRE(u,i,j,$\varnothing$) for cases with missing PRE(u,i,j) values. It can also be reasonable to include the current value of u in averages. These are denoted by PRE(u,0,j) and PRE(u,0,j,$\varnothing$) with $i = 0$. For dependence predictors based on the outcome variable y, i should be a positive integer so that the value of the current outcome measurement is not used to predict that outcome measurement.

For sc $\in$ SC, $y^{\#}_{sc}$ are independent and normally distributed with means $\mu^{\#}_{sc} = \mathbf{x}_{sc}^{T} \cdot \boldsymbol{\beta}$ with $\mathbf{x}_{sc}$ possibly depending on dependence predictors for a $r \times 1$ vector $\boldsymbol{\beta}$ of coefficients and variances $\Sigma^{\#}_{sc} = \sigma^2$ assumed for now to be constant. Let $\boldsymbol{\theta} = (\boldsymbol{\beta}^{T}, \sigma^2)^{T}$ denote the vector of all the model parameters. The likelihood L(SC; $\boldsymbol{\theta}$) is the product of the conditional likelihoods L(O$_{sc}$|$\mathbf{y}_{s,PRE(sc)}$; $\boldsymbol{\theta}$) = L(O$^{\#}_{sc}$; $\boldsymbol{\theta}$) over sc $\in$ SC. The maximum likelihood estimate $\boldsymbol{\theta}$(SC) of $\boldsymbol{\theta}$ is obtained by solving the estimating equations $\partial \ell(SC; \boldsymbol{\theta})/\partial \boldsymbol{\theta} = \mathbf{0}$ where $\ell(SC; \boldsymbol{\theta}) = \log(L(SC; \boldsymbol{\theta}))$.

Transition models as formulated in this section are based on univariate normal likelihoods for the conditional measurements $y^{\#}_{sc}$. Consequently, adaptive models can be generated for their means $\mu^{\#}_{sc}$ using the adaptive regression modeling methods of Chap. 2 extended to handle the dependence predictors PRE(y,i,j) and PRE(y,i,j,$\varnothing$) (and other dependence predictors PRE(u,i,j) and PRE(u,i,j,$\varnothing$) as well). Moreover, those conditional likelihoods multiply up to true marginal likelihoods for the outcome vectors $\mathbf{y}_{s,C(s)}$ so that LCV scores generated for transition models are comparable to LCV scores for multivariate normal marginal models.

4.7.2 Transition Model Induced by the Marginal AR1 Model with Constant Means

This section (which can be skipped) demonstrates that the marginal AR1 model with constant means and variances induces a transition model with non-constant variances, and so in general non-constant variances models may be needed in order to make a full comparison of marginal and transition models.

For complete data like the dental measurement data, consider the simple case of a marginal AR1 model with constant means $\mu_{sc} = \mu$ for $sc \in SC$. Assume further that outcome measurements are equally spaced so that the correlation $\rho_{scc-1} = \rho'$ between consecutive measurements for $c > 1$ is constant (for example, for the dental measurement data with outcomes 2 years apart, $\rho' = \rho^2$). For $c > 1$, the outcome measurements satisfy

$$y_{sc} = \mu + \rho' \cdot (y_{sc-1} - \mu) + e_{sc} = (1 - \rho') \cdot \mu + \rho' \cdot y_{sc-1} + e_{sc},$$

where the errors e_{sc} are independent of y_{sc-1} and of each other and have zero means and constant variances σ_e^2. Since y_{sc} have constant variances σ^2, $\sigma_e^2 = (1 - \rho'^2) \cdot \sigma^2$. Thus, the constant means marginal AR1 model induces the conditional model

$$y^{\#}_{sc} = \beta_1 + \beta_2 \cdot PRE(y,1)_{sc} + e^{\#}_{sc},$$

where $\beta_1 = (1 - \rho') \cdot \mu$ and $\beta_2 = \rho'$ and the errors $e^{\#}_{sc}$ are independent and normally distributed. However, $y^{\#}_{s1}$ requires special treatment since $y^{\#}_{s1} = y_{s1}$ and so has mean μ. This can be accounted for with the model

$$y^{\#}_{sc} = \beta_1 + \beta_2 \cdot PRE(y,1)_{sc} + \beta_3 \cdot PRE(y,1,\varnothing)_{sc} + e^{\#}_{sc},$$

where $\beta_3 = \mu - (1 - \rho') \cdot \mu = \rho' \cdot \mu$. Furthermore, $y^{\#}_{s1}$ has variance σ^2 and not $\rho'^2 \cdot \sigma^2 + \sigma_e^2$ as for $c > 1$, and so the associated constant variances model is still not equivalent. Thus, in general, non-constant variances transition models may be needed to be competitive with AR1 marginal models (see Sects. 4.15.3–4.15.4).

4.7.3 Using Weighted Averages of Prior Outcome Measurements

The transition models of Sect. 4.7.1 use simple averages of prior outcome measurements, and so do not account for the distance between prior and current outcome measurements. Prior outcome measurements closer to the current outcome measurement may be more important for predicting current outcome measurements than farther ones. This can be addressed with weighted averages of prior outcome measurements. Denote such weighted averages as WPRE(y,i,j). The weights used in analyses equal $\exp(-d(c',c))$, where c indexes the current outcome measurement, c' a prior outcome measurement, and $d(c',c) = |c' - c|$ the distance between them. Note that WPRE(y,i,j,$\varnothing$) = PRE(y,i,j,$\varnothing$).

4.8 Transition Modeling of the Dental Measurement Data

4.8.1 Using the Prior Dental Measurement

An adaptive transition model for the mean dental measurements can be generated by considering the standard primary predictors age and male, the dependence predictors PRE(y,1) (set equal to the previous value for y when one exists and 0 otherwise) and PRE(y,1,$\varnothing$) (the indicator for the case when no previous value for y exists) where y = dentmeas, and automatically generated GCs between these four primary predictors. The associated adaptive model is based on the three predictors: $(\text{male} \cdot \text{PRE}(y,1)^{-7})^{0.7}$, $(\text{PRE}(y,1)^{3.4} \cdot \text{age})^{2}$, and $(\text{PRE}(y,1)^{3} \cdot \text{age}^{0.1})^{-2}$ with an intercept. The LCV score is 0.12813 and the PD for the GC-based AR1 marginal model of Sect. 4.5.4 is a substantial 10.50 %. Consequently, for the dental measurement data, an adaptive transition model with dependence based on the prior outcome measurement distinctly outperforms the associated adaptive AR1 marginal model.

4.8.2 Comparison to the Marginal Model with Exchangeable Correlations

Marginal models can also be based on exchangeable correlations (EC) as used in standard repeated measures modeling. Under EC, all pairs of distinct outcome measurements have the same correlation ρ. For the dental measurement data with 4 measurements per child, there are $4 \cdot 3/2 = 6$ pairs of distinct measurements for each child, all assumed to have the same correlation ρ. Using EC, the adaptive model in age, male, and automatically generated GCs is based on two transforms, $\text{age}^{0.21}$ and $(\text{age}^2 \cdot \text{male})^{0.903}$ without an intercept, correlation estimate 0.62, and improved LCV score 0.12975. This model for the means is similar to the GC-based model generated with AR1 correlations and the plot of estimated mean values (not displayed) is very similar to the plot for the AR1 model of Fig. 4.1, but the LCV score for that model has the very substantial PD of 11.62 %. In this case, exchangeable correlations provide a very substantial improvement over order 1 autoregressive correlations even though the data are longitudinal. The linear moderation model using EC correlations has LCV score 0.12539 with substantial PD of 6.82 % compared to the nonlinear moderation model. Hence, the conclusion of substantial nonlinear moderation of the effect of age by gender still holds for the EC case. However, the interaction term in the linear moderation model is now significant ($P = 0.013$) and the linear covariate model has LCV score 0.12175 with substantial PD of 2.90 % compared to the linear moderation model, supporting the conclusion of linear moderation in contrast to results for the AR1 case. For these data, the conclusion of linear moderation changes with the correlation structure, indicating the need in general to identify an appropriate correlation structure before conducting tests for zero fixed effects. Since the LCV score for the linear AR1-based moderation model has substantial PD of 11.14 % compared to the linear EC-based moderation model, the EC-based model is more appropriate for the data, and so there is substantial linear moderation of the effect of age by gender of the child.

4.8.3   Using Multiple Prior Dental Measurements

The EC-based marginal model also has a larger LCV score than the transition model based on PRE(y,1), but with insubstantial PD of 1.25 %. While this is a competitive score, more general transition models can be generated with dependence based on multiple prior outcome measurements, rather than on just the prior outcome measurement, and with the potential for outperforming the EC-based marginal model. The model based on the prior two dental measurements is determined by the primary predictors age, male, PRE(y,1,2) (set equal to the average of the up to two previous values for y when at least one previous value exists and 0 otherwise), and PRE(y,1,2,$\varnothing$) (the indicator for the case when there are no values to average for PRE(y,1,2) and so the same as PRE(y,1,$\varnothing$) since there are no missing dental measurements), and GCs based on these primary predictors. The associated adaptive model includes the four transforms: $(\text{age}^{1.5} \cdot \text{PRE}(y,1,2)^5)^{0.99}$, $(\text{male} \cdot \text{age}^2)^{1.2}$, $(\text{PRE}(y,1,2)^{-3} \cdot \text{age}^2)^7$, and $(\text{male} \cdot \text{PRE}(y,1,2)^{-1} \cdot \text{age}^{-1})^{-1.9}$ with an intercept and improved LCV score 0.13363. The adaptive marginal EC model generates a substantial PD of 2.90 %. Consequently, this more general transition model provides a distinct improvement over both types of marginal models and over the simpler transition model. It uses simple averages of prior outcome measurements, and so might be improved by consideration of weighted prior measurements WPRE(y,1,2) with weights decreasing with the distance from the current measurement (as defined in Sect. 4.7.3). However, the adaptive weighted transition model for these data has smaller LCV score 0.12414, and so simple averages are more effective in this case.

Improvements may also be possible by using PRE(y,1,3), based on the maximal number three of prior outcome measurements. The adaptive model based on age, male, PRE(y,1,3), PRE(y,3,$\varnothing$), and GCs is based on the four transforms:

$(PRE(y,1,3)^{5.6} \cdot age^{1.7})^{0.9}$, $(male \cdot age^2)^{1.2}$, $(male \cdot PRE(y,1,3)^{1.8} \cdot age^{1.4})^{1.3}$, and $(PRE(y,1,3)^{-2} \cdot age)^5$ with an intercept. It has smaller LCV score 0.13324, but with insubstantial PD of 0.29 %. However, it is not less complex. Models can also be generated considering all three of PRE(y,1), PRE(y,1,2), and PRE(y,1,3) together, but these more general transition models are not considered here.

Under the adaptive transition model based on PRE(y,1,2), the estimated standard deviation is 1.8 mm. Estimated means are displayed in Fig. 4.2 for girls and boys at ages 10, 12, and 14 years old as a function of the average PRE(y,1,2) of the prior two outcome measurements. Mean outcome measurements for boys increase nonlinearly with the average of the prior two outcome measurements, are shifted up as they age, and are mainly larger than for girls at the same age. The patterns for girls are similar but with less difference across ages except that they start out counterintuitively at lower values for larger ages. Individual-child predicted dental measurements at ages 10–14 years are displayed in Fig. 4.3 for each of the 11 girls and in Fig. 4.4 for each of the 16 boys. With the exception of one girl, children's predicted values tend to increase with age following different patterns for different

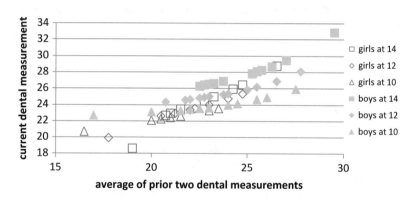

Fig. 4.2 Estimated mean dental measurements based on transition modeling

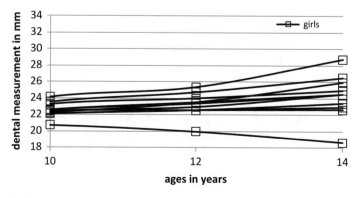

Fig. 4.3 Girls' individual predicted dental measurements based on transition modeling

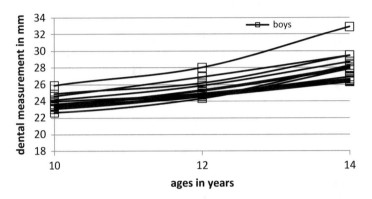

Fig. 4.4 Boy's individual predicted dental measurements based on transition modeling

children and with more of an increase for boys than for all but the girl with the largest predicted values. The one girl with the exceptional decreasing pattern in Fig. 4.3 has predicted values lower than for all the other girls and decreasing with age, resulting in the counterintuitive decrease with age in the lowest predicted values for girls of Fig. 4.2.

4.8.4 *Transition Model Selection with Penalized Likelihood Criteria*

Adaptive transition modeling can be conducted using penalized likelihood criteria (PLCs; Sect. 2.10). In the multivariate outcome context, the sample size used in computing the penalty for Bayesian information criterion (BIC) scores can be taken to be the number of measurements, as used in SPSS® (IBM, Armonk, NY), or the number of matched sets, as used by SAS PROC MIXED. Table 4.1 provides a comparison of results for the adaptive transition models in the primary predictors age, male, PRE(y,1,2), PRE(y,1,2,∅), and GCs generated through LCV and alternative PLCs, including BIC scores computed with the number of measurements, BIC scores computed with the number of matched sets, Akaike information criterion (AIC) scores with penalty based only on the number of parameters, and Takeuchi information criterion (TIC) scores with a more complex penalty factor. Adaptive models generated using all four of these PLCs generate LCV scores with substantial PDs compared to the LCV-based model. This indicates that adaptive modeling based on these PLCs can generate distinctly inferior models compared to LCV-based models, and so adaptive modeling based on PLCs should usually be avoided, at least for transition modeling of continuous outcomes, with possible exception highly time-consuming analyses.

Table 4.1 Comparison of penalized likelihood criteria to likelihood cross-validation for generating the adaptive transition model for dental measurements as a function of age, the indicator male for being a male child, and the average of the prior two dental measurements

Model selection criterion	Model transforms[a]	5-fold LCV score	Percent decrease (%)
AIC	$1, \left(\mathrm{PRE}(y,1,2)^6 \cdot \mathrm{age}^{1.2}\right)^{0.84}, \left(\mathrm{male} \cdot \mathrm{age}^{0.6}\right)^2,$ $\left(\mathrm{male} \cdot \mathrm{PRE}(y,1,2)^4\right)^{0.6}$	0.12934	3.21
BIC—number of matched sets	$1, \left(\mathrm{PRE}(y,1,2)^6 \cdot \mathrm{age}^{1.2}\right)^{0.84}, \left(\mathrm{male} \cdot \mathrm{age}^{0.6}\right)^2,$ $\left(\mathrm{male} \cdot \mathrm{PRE}(y,1,2)^4\right)^{0.6}$	0.12934	3.21
BIC—number of measurements	$1, \left(\mathrm{PRE}(y,1,2)^6 \cdot \mathrm{age}^{1.2}\right)^{0.91}, \left(\mathrm{male} \cdot \mathrm{age}^{0.6}\right)^{1.6}$	0.12295	7.99
TIC	$1, (\mathrm{age}^{-4} \cdot \mathrm{male})^{0.87}, \mathrm{PRE}(y,1,2)^{5.8919},$ $\left(\mathrm{male} \cdot \mathrm{PRE}(y,1,2)^{-2.9} \cdot \mathrm{age}^2\right)^{1.9196},$ $\left(\mathrm{age}^{-4.1} \cdot \mathrm{PRE}(y,1,2)^{-3.3}\right)^{0.7001}$	0.02410	81.97
5-fold LCV	$1, \left(\mathrm{age}^{1.5} \cdot \mathrm{PRE}(y,1,2)^5\right)^{0.99}, \left(\mathrm{male} \cdot \mathrm{age}^2\right)^{1.2},$ $\left(\mathrm{PRE}(y,1,2)^{-3} \cdot \mathrm{age}^2\right)^7,$ $(\mathrm{male} \cdot \mathrm{PRE}(y,1,2)^{-1} \cdot \mathrm{age}^{-1})^{1.1}$	0.13363	0.00

AIC: Akaike information criterion, BIC: Bayesian information criterion, LCV: likelihood cross-validation, PRE (y,1,2): average of prior two dental measurements, TIC: Takeuchi information criterion
[a]The predictor 1 corresponds to including an intercept in the model

4.9 General Conditional Modeling of Dependence

This section generalizes the special conditional modeling case of transition modeling formulated in Sect. 4.7 to general conditional modeling. Conditioned on the values of available predictors and on the values of the other outcome measurements, current outcome measurements are considered to be univariate normal with means a function of the available predictors and of the other outcome measurements. The conditions for repeated outcome measurements do not need to be ordered to use general conditional modeling. However, it is more appropriately used when conditions are not ordered (e.g., members of a family or patients of the same health care provider) while transition modeling is more appropriate when the conditions are naturally ordered as for the dental measurements. The formulation incorporates prior, post, or both prior and post outcome measurements into the model for the means by considering simple or weighted averages of fixed numbers (e.g., 1, 2, $\cdots$) of them as well as indicator variables for when there are no such other outcome measurements to average. CV scores for general conditional models are based on pseudolikelihoods (and so denoted as PLCV scores) rather than on true likelihoods, and so these cannot be directly compared to LCV scores for marginal models unless the model is a transition model (since the PLCV score is then actually a LCV score). However, marginal models induce general conditional models whose PLCV scores can be compared to those of other general conditional models, and a formulation for such induced models is also provided in this section. The formulations of Sects. 4.9.1 and 4.9.2 can be skipped to focus on analyses.

4.9.1 Formulation

Let $O^{\#}_{sc} = (y^{\#}_{sc}, \mathbf{x}_{sc})$ be the observed data for measurement $sc \in SC$ where $\mathbf{x}_{sc}$ is determined as before by standard primary predictors, conditional primary predictors based on subsets of the other outcome measurements not just the prior ones, and GCs. Define $POST(s,c) = \{c' : c' \in C(s), c' > c\}$ as the possibly empty set of indexes in $C(s)$ subsequent to the index c. For the largest index $c^*(s) = \max(C(s))$ in $C(s)$, and so also in $POST(s,c)$ when $c < c^*(s)$, $POST(s, c^*(s)) = \varnothing$. Let $m(POST(s,c))$ be the number of conditions in $POST(s,c)$. For $1 \le i \le m(POST(s,c))$, let $NEXT(s,c,i)$ be the subset of $POST(s,c)$ containing just the ith smallest index in $POST(s,c)$. For $i > m(POST(s,c))$, define $POST(s,c,i) = \varnothing$. For $i \le j$, let

$$POST(s, c, i, j) = \bigcup_{i \le i' \le j} NEXT(s, c, i').$$

Define the primary conditional predictors $POST(y,i,j)$ to have values $POST(y,i,j)_{sc}$ equal to the average of $y_{sc'}$ over the indexes c' in $POST(s,c,i,j)$ and equal to 0 when $POST(s,c,i,j) = \varnothing$. Also define the indicator variables $POST(y,i,j,\varnothing)$ for cases when $POST(s,c,i,j) = \varnothing$. Primary predictors can also include the conditional predictors $OTHER(y,i,j)$ with values $OTHER(y, i, j)_{sc}$ equal to the average of $y_{sc'}$ over the indexes c' in the set

$$OTHER(s,c,i,j) = PRE(s,c,i,j) \cup POST(s,c,i,j)$$

and as 0 when $OTHER(s,c,i,j) = \varnothing$ as well as on the indicator variables $OTHER(y,i,j,\varnothing)$ for cases when $OTHER(s,c,i,j) = \varnothing$. For complete data with $m > 1$, like the dental measurement data, $OTHER(s,c,i,j)$ are never empty when $i < m$ and so then $OTHER(y,s,c,i,j,\varnothing)$ have all 0 values and are not needed. Weighted averages can be used in place of simple averages (using the weights of Sect. 4.7.3) generating the dependence predictors $WPOST(y,i,j)$, $WPOST(y,i,j,\varnothing)$, $WOTHER(y,i,j)$, and $WOTHER(y,i,j,\varnothing)$.

For time-varying primary predictors u not based on outcome variable y, associated primary predictors POST(u,i,j) are also possible with values POST(u,i,j)$_{sc}$ equal to the average of subsequent values for u as are the indicator variables POST(u,i,j,∅) for cases with missing POST(u,i,j) values. Also possible are associated primary predictors OTHER(u,i,j) with values OTHER(u,i,j)$_{sc}$ equal to the average of other values for u and the indicator variables OTHER(u,i,j, ∅) for cases with missing OTHER(u,i,j) values. It can also be reasonable to include the current value of u giving POST(u,0,j), POST(u,0,j,∅), OTHER(u,0,j), and OTHER(u,0,j,∅) with i = 0. For conditional predictors based on the outcome variable y, i should be a positive integer so that the value of the current outcome measurement is not used to predict that outcome measurement.

Exact likelihoods for general conditional models are often difficult to compute, and so pseudolikelihoods are used instead. The pseudolikelihood PL(SC;θ) is the product over sc ∈ SC of the conditional likelihoods

$$L\left(O_{sc} \middle| \mathbf{y}_{s,C(s)\backslash\{c\}}; \boldsymbol{\theta}\right) = L\left(O^{\#}{}_{sc}; \boldsymbol{\theta}\right)$$

for the conditional measurements $y^{\#}{}_{sc} = y_{sc}|\mathbf{y}_{s,C(s)\backslash\{c\}}$, treated as independent and normally distributed with means $\mu^{\#}{}_{sc} = \mathbf{x}_{sc}{}^{T} \cdot \boldsymbol{\beta}$ for a r × 1 vector $\boldsymbol{\beta}$ of coefficients and variances $\Sigma^{\#}{}_{sc} = \sigma^2$ assumed for now to be constant. Let $\boldsymbol{\theta} = (\boldsymbol{\beta}^{T}, \sigma^2)^{T}$ denote the vector of all the model parameters. The maximum pseudolikelihood estimate θ(SC) is obtained by solving the estimating equations $\partial\ell(SC;\boldsymbol{\theta})/\partial\boldsymbol{\theta} = \mathbf{0}$ where $\ell(SC;\boldsymbol{\theta}) = \log(PL(SC;\boldsymbol{\theta}))$.

As for LCV scores in Sect. 4.4.1, define k-fold pseudolikelihood CV (PLCV) scores by randomly partitioning the index set S into k disjoint folds F(h) for h ∈ H = {h : 1 ≤ h ≤ k} with all C(s) measurements for a matched set s assigned to the same fold F(h(s)) where h(s) = int(k · u$_s$) + 1 for independent, uniform random values u$_s$ in (0, 1). Then set

$$PLCV = \prod_{h\in H} \prod_{s\in F(h)} \prod_{c\in C(s)} L(O_{sc}; \boldsymbol{\theta}(S\backslash F(h)))^{1/m(SC)}.$$

These scores can be used in PLCV ratio tests with the cutoff for a substantial PD computed as in Sect. 4.4.2. The LCV score for a transition model equals its PLCV score, and so transition models can be compared to general conditional models using PLCV ratio tests.

4.9.2   Conditional Models Induced by Marginal Models

Suppose a model was estimated using likelihood terms L(O$_{s,C(s)}$; θ) based on the multivariate normal likelihood of Sect. 4.3.3 with mean vectors $\boldsymbol{\mu}_{s,C(s)}$ and covariance matrices $\Sigma_{s,C(s)}$ for s ∈ S determined by the vector of parameters θ. LCV scores for this model can be compared to PLCV scores for normally distributed transition models since pseudolikelihoods for transition models are actual likelihoods, but not to more general conditional models. However, marginal multivariate normal models induce general conditional models whose PLCV scores can be compared to those for other normally distributed conditional models.

Let $\Sigma_{s,c',c''}$ denote the submatrix of $\Sigma_{s,C(s)}$ with row entries $c' \in C'$ and column entries $c'' \in C''$. The conditional density for $y^{\#}_{sc} = y_{sc}|y_{s,C(s)\backslash\{c\}}$ equals the ratio of the density $L(O_{s,C(s)}; \boldsymbol{\theta})$ for $\mathbf{y}_{s,C(s)}$ divided by the density $L(O_{s,C(s)\backslash\{c\}}; \boldsymbol{\theta})$ for $\mathbf{y}_{s,C(s)\backslash\{c\}}$. It is well-known (e.g., eq. 6, p. 88, Morrison 1967) that the log of this ratio equals the univariate normal log-likelihood

$$\log\left(L\left(O^{\#}_{sc}; \boldsymbol{\theta}\right)\right) = -\frac{1}{2} \cdot e^{\#}_{sc}{}^2 / \Sigma^{\#}_{sc} - \frac{1}{2} \cdot \log(\Sigma^{\#}_{sc}) - \frac{1}{2} \cdot \log(2 \cdot \pi),$$

where

$$e^{\#}_{sc} = y_{sc} - \mu_{sc} - \Sigma_{s,\{c\},C(s)\backslash\{c\}} \cdot \Sigma_{s,C(s)\backslash\{c\},C(s)\backslash\{c\}}^{-1} \cdot (\mathbf{y}_{s,C(s)\backslash\{c\}} - \mu_{s,C(s)\backslash\{c\}}) \quad \text{and}$$
$$\Sigma^{\#}_{sc} = \Sigma_{s,\{c\},\{c\}} - \Sigma_{s,\{c\},C(s)\backslash\{c\}} \cdot \Sigma_{s,C(s)\backslash\{c\},C(s)\backslash\{c\}}^{-1} \cdot \Sigma_{s,C(s)\backslash\{c\},\{c\}}.$$

The associated conditional model then has variances $\Sigma^{\#}_{sc}$ and means $\mu^{\#}_{sc}$ chosen so that $e^{\#}_{sc} = y_{sc} - \mu^{\#}_{sc}$, that is, satisfying

$$\mu^{\#}_{sc} = \mu_{sc} + \Sigma_{s,\{c\},C(s)\backslash\{c\}} \cdot \Sigma_{s,C(s)\backslash\{c\},C(s)\backslash\{c\}}^{-1} \cdot (\mathbf{y}_{s,C(s)\backslash\{c\}} - \mu_{s,C(s)\backslash\{c\}}).$$

PLCV scores computed using $y^{\#}_{sc} = y_{sc}$, $\mu^{\#}_{sc}$, and $\Sigma^{\#}_{sc}$ can be compared to PLCV scores for other general conditional models to assess how well general conditional models induced by marginal models perform compared to other general conditional models.

4.10   General Conditional Modeling of the Dental Measurement Data

The adaptively generated conditional model based on age, male, OTHER(y,1,2) (set equal to the average of the up to two prior and post values for y), and GCs (the indicator OTHER(y,1,2,∅) for no other values to average in OTHER(y,1,2) is always 0 in this case and so not used) is based on the two transforms: $(\text{OTHER}(y,1,3)^{-0.5} \cdot \text{age}^{-0.19})^{-1.52}$ and $(\text{age}^{10} \cdot \text{male} \cdot \text{OTHER}(y,1,3)^{-4})^{2.15}$ without an intercept and with PLCV score 0.15347. The PD for the transition model based on PRE(y,1,2) with PLCV = LCV score 0.13363 (see Sect. 4.8.3) is very substantial at 12.93 %. Consequently, present dental measurements can be much better predicted from combined future and past values than with only past values. As for transition models, the weighted model based on WOTHER(y,1,3) generates a smaller LCV score (0.14347). The marginal EC model induces a general conditional model with PLCV = 0.14782 and substantial PD of 3.68 %, and so the induced general conditional model in this case is distinctly inferior to the model based directly on PLCV.

The above analyses are included to demonstrate general conditional models. The results indicate that such models with individual outcome measurements a function of other outcome measurements can generate distinctly better PLCV scores than transition models for the same data. However, general conditional models seem inappropriate for use with longitudinal data like the dental measurement data. For longitudinal data, transition models with individual outcome measurements a function of only prior outcome measurements are more intuitive, providing useful information on how the present depends on the past. Consequently, the transition model depicted in Figs. 4.2–4.4 seems to provide the more appropriate description of the mean dental measurements, and so results of the adaptive general conditional model for these data have not been plotted. On the other hand, general conditional models can be appropriately used to model clustered data without an inherent ordering to the measurements within the matched sets (e.g., measurements for members of the same family, nurses on the same unit, and mice born in the same litter).

4.11   Adaptive GEE-Based Modeling of Multivariate Continuous Outcomes

So far marginal models for multivariate continuous outcomes have been estimated using maximum likelihood (ML). Alternately, estimation can be conducted using generalized estimating equations (GEE) that circumvent the computation of the likelihood (Liang and Zeger 1986). This is more important for general multivariate outcomes, for which the computation of likelihoods can be overly complex (see Chaps. 10 and 14 for multivariate discrete and count/rate outcomes, respectively). In the multivariate normal context, likelihoods are readily computed, and so GEE parameter estimation would often not be considered. However, LCV scores can also be readily computed in this case and used to control the adaptive GEE-based modeling process. Thus, comparison of the impact of ML and GEE parameter estimation on the adaptive modeling process is possible in the multivariate normal context, and so is addressed in this section. Section 4.11.1 provides a formulation (which can be skipped) for GEE-based modeling of multivariate continuous outcomes. Section 4.11.2 provides example adaptive GEE analyses of the dental measurements. General GEE-based modeling of possibly non-continuous outcomes requires alternative model selection approaches. For this reason, Pan (2001) proposed the quasi-likelihood information (QIC) criterion for evaluating GEE-based models with smaller scores indicating better models. The effectiveness of model selection for the dental measurement data based on QIC compared to LCV is assessed in Sect. 4.11.3.

4.11.1 Formulation

Using the notation of Sects. 4.3.1, 4.3.2 and 4.3.3, the generalized estimating equations, that is, generalized from the estimating equations for the independent case to incorporate covariance without considering the likelihood, correspond to

$$\mathbf{H}(SC; \boldsymbol{\beta}) = \sum_{s \in S} \mathbf{D}_{s,C(s)}{}^{T} \cdot \boldsymbol{\Sigma}_{s,C(s)}(\boldsymbol{\beta})^{-1} \cdot \mathbf{e}_{s,C(s)}$$

with $\mathbf{D}_{s,C(s)} = \partial \boldsymbol{\mu}_{s,C(s)} / \partial \boldsymbol{\beta}$ and $\boldsymbol{\Sigma}_{s,C(s)}(\boldsymbol{\beta}) = \phi(\boldsymbol{\beta}) \cdot \mathbf{R}_{s,C(s)}(\boldsymbol{\rho}(\boldsymbol{\beta}))$ where $\phi(\boldsymbol{\beta})$ is a constant dispersion parameter, in this case the same as the constant variance parameter $\sigma^2(\boldsymbol{\beta})$. The GEE estimate $\boldsymbol{\beta}_{GEE}(SC)$ of $\boldsymbol{\beta}$ is obtained by solving $\mathbf{H}(SC; \boldsymbol{\beta}) = \mathbf{0}$.

In GEE modeling, the constant dispersion parameter $\phi(\boldsymbol{\beta})$ and the working correlation matrices $\mathbf{R}_{s,C(s)}(\boldsymbol{\rho}(\boldsymbol{\beta}))$ are estimated using the errors $e_{sc}(\boldsymbol{\beta})$ with estimates determined by the structure R for the matrices $\mathbf{R}_{s,C(s)}(\boldsymbol{\rho}(\boldsymbol{\beta}))$. For example, under exchangeable correlations (R = EC), all the off-diagonal entries of $\mathbf{R}_{s,C(s)}(\boldsymbol{\rho}(\boldsymbol{\beta}))$ are the same with common value $\rho(\boldsymbol{\beta})$ (and so the vector $\boldsymbol{\rho}(\boldsymbol{\beta})$ consists of the single entry $\rho(\boldsymbol{\beta})$). Given a value $\boldsymbol{\beta}$ for the expectation parameter vector, $\rho(\boldsymbol{\beta})$ is estimated as

$$\rho_{GEE}(\boldsymbol{\beta}) = \frac{1}{m(CC) - r} \sum_{c'c \in CC} \text{stde}_{sc'}(\boldsymbol{\beta}) \cdot \text{stde}_{sc}(\boldsymbol{\beta}),$$

where $CC = \{c'c \ : \ c' < c, \ c',c \in C(S), \ s \in S\}$, $m(CC)$ is the number of pairs $c'c$ of indexes in CC, and the errors $\text{stde}_{sc'}(\boldsymbol{\beta})$ and $\text{stde}_{sc}(\boldsymbol{\beta})$ are computed by standardizing the errors $e_{sc'}(\boldsymbol{\beta})$ and $e_{sc}(\boldsymbol{\beta})$, respectively, by the square root of the estimate $\phi_{GEE}(\boldsymbol{\beta})$ of $\phi(\boldsymbol{\beta})$ given by

$$\phi_{GEE}(\boldsymbol{\beta}) = \frac{1}{m(SC) - r} \sum_{sc \in SC} e_{sc}(\boldsymbol{\beta})^2.$$

These are bias-corrected estimates since the denominators are adjusted for bias by subtracting the number r of expectation parameters. Unadjusted estimates are also possible by not subtracting r in the denominators. Similar estimates of the correlation matrices can be obtained under other structures R like autoregressive (R = AR) and unstructured (R = UN) correlations (for details, see SAS Institute 2004). The estimating equations are solved to obtain the estimate $\boldsymbol{\beta}_{GEE}(SC)$ using a Gauss-Newton-like iterative algorithm. The Hessian matrix used in this algorithm is given by $\mathbf{H}'(SC; \boldsymbol{\beta}) = \sum_{s \in S} \mathbf{D}_{s,C(s)}{}^{T} \cdot \boldsymbol{\Sigma}_{s,C(s)}(\boldsymbol{\beta})^{-1} \cdot \mathbf{D}_{s,C(s)}$. Using the notation of SAS Institute (2004, p. 1676), the model-based estimator, assuming the working correlation matrix is the true correlation matrix, of the covariance matrix of the estimate $\boldsymbol{\beta}_{GEE}(SC)$ of $\boldsymbol{\beta}$ is $\boldsymbol{\Sigma}_M(\boldsymbol{\beta}_{GEE}(SC)) = \mathbf{I}_0{}^{-1}$ where $\mathbf{I}_0 = \mathbf{H}'(SC; \boldsymbol{\beta}_{GEE}(SC))$.

The robust empirical estimator of that covariance matrix is $\Sigma_E(\boldsymbol{\beta}_{GEE}(SC)) = I_0^{-1} \cdot I_1 \cdot I_0^{-1}$ where $I_1 = \sum_{s \in S} \mathbf{H}(SC; \boldsymbol{\beta}_{GEE}(SC)) \cdot \mathbf{H}(SC; \boldsymbol{\beta}_{GEE}(SC))^T$. P-values reported for GEE models are based on the empirical estimator.

The QIC score equals -2 times the log of the quasi-likelihood $QL(\boldsymbol{\beta}_{GEE}(SC), \phi_{GEE}(SC))$ (that is, the likelihood adjusted to account for dispersion) computed under the independent correlation structure $R = IND$ with estimates $\boldsymbol{\beta}_{GEE}(SC)$ and $\phi_{GEE}(SC)$ determined using the actual working correlation structure R penalized by two times the trace of the product of the inverse of the model-based estimator $\Sigma_M(\boldsymbol{\beta}_{GEE}(SC); IND)^{-1} = I_0(IND)$ under the independent working correlation structure $R = IND$ and the robust empirical estimator $\Sigma_E(\boldsymbol{\beta}_{GEE}(SC); R) = I_0^{-1}(R) \cdot I_1(R) \cdot I_0(R)^{-1}$ under the actual working correlation matrix R. Formally,

$$QIC(SC; R) = -2 \cdot \log(QL(\boldsymbol{\beta}_{GEE}(SC), \phi_{GEE}(\boldsymbol{\beta}(SC)))) + 2 \cdot tr\left(I_0(IND) \cdot I_0^{-1}(R) \cdot I_1(R) \cdot I_0(R)^{-1}\right)$$

with smaller scores indicating better models, where $tr(\mathbf{A})$ denotes the trace of a square matrix $\mathbf{A}$ equal to the sum of its diagonal entries. The QIC score can be converted to the larger is better score

$$QIC' = \exp\left(-\frac{1}{2} \cdot QIC/m(SC)\right).$$

4.11.2 Adaptive GEE-Based Modeling of the Dental Measurement Data

Although general GEE-based modeling does not require computation of likelihoods, likelihoods and LCV scores based on those likelihoods are readily computed for GEE-based models in the multivariate normal context. Consequently, adaptive GEE-based modeling of multivariate continuous outcomes can be conducted with estimates based on GEE and model comparisons on LCV. GEE generates marginal models with correlations and variances (the same as dispersions for this case) estimated as functions of estimates of the means. In contrast, the marginal models formulated in Sect. 4.3 use maximum likelihood (ML) estimation of all the parameters determining means, variances, and correlations. For these ML-based marginal models, the EC correlation structure generates the adaptive model in age, male, and GCs with LCV score of 0.12975 (as described in Sect. 4.8.2, which is also better than the LCV score for the ML-based model with AR1 correlation structure). Using this same EC correlation structure, the adaptive GEE-based model in age, male, and GCs with constant variances has the two transforms $age^{0.2}$ and $(age^7 \cdot male)^{0.4} = age^{2.8} \cdot male$ without an intercept, correlation estimate 0.61, and a plot of estimated mean values (not displayed) that is very similar to Fig. 4.1 (as is the plot for the ML-based model using EC). The LCV score is 0.13124, and so the ML-based marginal model is a competitive alternative with insubstantial PD of 1.14 %. Since both models are based on two transforms, the GEE approach for estimating the marginal model provides somewhat better results compared to the ML approach. However, the PD of 1.79 % compared to the transition model based on age, male, PRE(y,1,2), PRE(y,1,2,∅), and GCs of Sect. 4.8.3 with LCV score 0.13363 is substantial. Consequently, while adaptive marginal GEE-based modeling for these data provides a competitive alternative to adaptive ML-based modeling, it generates a distinctly inferior model compared to adaptive transition modeling.

Adaptive GEE-based modeling supports the use of unstructured (UN) correlation matrices with correlations between different outcome measurements all treated as distinct parameters. There are $4 \cdot 3/2 = 6$ different correlations for the dental measurement data. The adaptive GEE-based model for the dental measurements using UN correlations is the constant model with LCV score 0.02201 and very substantial PD 83.23 % compared to the GEE-based adaptive model using EC correlations. In this case, using six distinct correlation parameters appears to overfit the data to the extent that it is not possible to identify a non-constant model for the means. This result suggests that UN correlation structures may often be ineffective, at least for GEE-based marginal modeling and most likely also for ML-based marginal modeling, and are reasonably not considered in adaptive modeling of multivariate outcomes.

4.11.3   Assessment of the Quasi-Likelihood Information Criterion

Table 4.2 reports QIC' scores (converting the QIC score from smaller is better to larger is better) and LCV scores for alternative correlation structures for the linear moderation model based on age, male, and the interaction age·male and with correlations estimated by GEE. There is very little difference between the QIC' scores for the 4 correlation structures (all PDs are less than the cutoff of 1.76 % for the data). The best QIC' score is achieved for both the independent case with zero correlation and the exchangeable case with estimated correlation 0.61 (value not reported in Table 4.2), suggesting counterintuitively that this latter correlation estimate, while quite large, is not of substance. In contrast, LCV scores indicate that the EC correlation structure is the best choice and substantially better than the other three correlation structures (with all PDs greater than the cutoff of 1.76 %). The same QIC' scores are generated for the independent and EC correlation structures because GEE estimates of the mean parameters of the model are the same for these two cases. However, these estimates are not the same for the complements of the folds considered in the LCV computations so that the LCV

Table 4.2 Comparison of QIC and LCV for assessing the correlation structure for the dental measurement data using the linear moderation model for the means[a]

Correlation structure	QIC		5-fold LCV	
	Adjusted score[b]	Percent decrease from best (%)	Score	Percent decrease from best (%)
Independent	0.58229	0.00	0.09782	22.53
Autoregressive	0.58162	0.12	0.11405	9.68
Exchangeable	0.58229	0.00	0.12627	0.00
Unstructured	0.57729	0.86	0.00256	97.97

LCV: likelihood cross-validation, QIC: quasi-likelihood criterion
[a]With means based on the three predictors age, male, and their interaction age·male
[b]$QIC' = \exp(-\frac{1}{2} \cdot QIC/m(S))$ where $m(S) = 108$, the number of measurements

scores indicate that the independent case is very inferior to the EC case with PD 22.53 %. In this case, QIC scores provide little discrimination between alternative correlation structures in contrast to LCV scores. This may hold more generally since QIC scores are based in part on the independent correlation structure even when that is not the assumed correlation structure.

Table 4.3 reports QIC' and LCV scores for alternative submodels of the linear moderation model for the means based on subsets of the three predictors: age, male, and their interaction age·male, with EC correlations as suggested by Table 4.2 results. Under the full linear moderation model, the effects of age $(P < 0.001)$ and age·male $(P = 0.009)$ are significant while the effect of male $(P = 0.454)$ is nonsignificant. The submodel of this linear moderation model with the best QIC' score is the constant model with all three predictors removed from the model. On the other hand, the best LCV score is achieved for the model based on age and age·male with male removed, and the constant model is distinctly inferior to this submodel with PD in the LCV scores of 31.59 %. For the submodel based on age and age·male, both effects are highly significant at $P < 0.001$. The QIC' analysis counterintuitively suggests that the model based on these two highly significant terms can be improved by removing both of them, which results in a substantial improvement due to a PD in the QIC' scores of 2.32 % for the model based on age and age male. In contrast, the LCV analysis supports the intuitive conclusion that the full model can be improved by removing its one nonsignificant term giving a submodel whose two highly significant terms are best kept in the model.

As implemented in SAS by PROC GENMOD, the QIC score for a given model is computed using the dispersion estimate for that model. Pan (2001, p. 122) recommended instead that the dispersion estimate for the largest possible model for the means be used in computing QIC scores for all models for the means under consideration. The QIC' scores of Table 4.3 are computed using the built-in SAS approach, which may explain why they generate counterintuitive conclusions. However, QIC scores as recommended by Pan are not generated directly by SAS and require extra complex computations so that this is not a practical option for most applied researchers. Moreover, while there is a largest possible model for the

Table 4.3 Comparison of QIC and LCV for assessing means for the dental measurement data using submodels of the linear moderation model using the exchangeable correlation structure

			QIC		5-fold LCV	
Predictors for the means			Adjusted score[a]	Percent decrease from best (%)	Score	Percent decrease from best (%)
Age	Male	Age·male	0.58229	2.44	0.12627	0.70
Age	Male	–	0.58143	2.58	0.12241	3.74
Age	–	Age·male	0.58301	2.32	0.12716	0.00
–	Male	Age·male	0.58316	2.29	0.11515	9.44
Age	–	–	0.59324	0.60	0.11893	6.47
–	Male	–	0.59042	1.08	0.08953	29.59
–	–	Age·male	0.58229	2.44	0.12627	0.70
–	–	–	0.59685	0.00	0.08699	31.59

LCV: likelihood cross-validation, QIC: quasi-likelihood criterion
[a]QIC′ = exp(−½·QIC/m(S)) where m(S) = 108, the number of measurements

analyses of Table 4.3, this is not always the case, for example, when the models under consideration include any number of any real valued powers of one or more continuous predictors as in adaptive modeling.

4.12   Analysis of the Exercise Data

A data set on strength measurements for 37 subjects undergoing one of two weightlifting programs is available on the Internet (see Supplementary Materials). For 11 subjects, the number of repetitions increased over time while, for the remaining 26 subjects, the weight increased over time. Strength measurements are available at baseline and every 2 days after that up to 12 days for a total of seven measurement times. The variable strength is the outcome for these analyses. The possible predictor variables are time (with equally spaced values 0, 2, $\cdots$, 12 days), incrwgts (the indicator for having the weights increase), and their interaction time·incrwgts. There are a total of 239 outcome measurements with an average of 6.5 measurements per subject. Of the 37 subjects, 23 (62.2 %) had no missing outcome measurements while eight (21.6 %) had one missing and six (16.2 %) had two missing. The cutoff for a substantial PD in the LCV scores for these data with 239 measurements is 0.80 %.

The benchmark analysis used to set the number of folds is adaptive modeling of mean strength as a function of time under a ML-based marginal AR1 model. For $k = 5$ folds, the adaptively generated model includes an intercept and the transform time$^{0.5}$ with LCV score 0.18678. For $k = 10$ folds, the same model is generated with LCV score 0.18627. Since this is a lower score, $k = 5$ might be an appropriate choice to use in subsequent analyses. However, for $k = 15$ folds, the same model is generated but with larger LCV score 0.18688 while, for $k = 20$ folds, the same model is generated once again with decreased LCV score 0.18649. Since the same model is generated for all these choices of k, using k = 5 may be a reasonable choice. However, since k = 15 is a local maximum with a larger LCV score than for k = 5, this seems like a better choice for these data and, consequently, k = 15 is used in all subsequent analyses. The number of measurements in the 15 folds ranges from 6 to 33 for 1–5 matched sets (subjects in this case).

Using 15 folds, the marginal model under the EC correlation structure is similar and based on an intercept and the transform time$^{0.4}$. However, the LCV score for the EC model is 0.15807 with very substantial PD of 15.42 %, and so AR1 provides a much better depiction of the dependence over time and is used in subsequent analyses of the exercise data. The linear polynomial model has LCV score 0.18373 with substantial PD of 1.69 %, and so mean strength changes distinctly nonlinearly with time. The adaptive transition model based on time, PRE(y,1), PRE(y,1,∅), and GCs has LCV score 0.14789 with very substantial PD of 20.86 %. In this case, the marginal AR1 model very distinctly outperforms the associated transition model, and so other transition models for the exercise data are not considered here (but see Sects. 4.15.3, 4.15.4 for the impact of constant variances on this result). The adaptive marginal AR1 moderation model based on incrwgts, time, and GCs does not depend on incrwgts and is the same model as generated for time alone, thereby indicating that mean strength does not change distinctly differently for subjects on the two weightlifting programs.

The adaptive GEE-based model based on incrwgts, time, and GCs using the AR1 correlation structure generates a better LCV score of 0.18430 than the associated GEE-based model using the EC correlation structure (with LCV score 0.15640). In contrast to the adaptive AR1 ML-based model, the adaptive AR1 GEE-based model does depend on incrwgts. However, the PD 1.38 % is substantial compared to the associated ML-based model, indicating that in this case ML estimation provides a distinct improvement over GEE estimation and that the more appropriate conclusion is that mean strength does not depend on incrwgts.

Under the final selected model for mean strength, the estimated constant standard deviation is 4.4. Estimated correlations decrease from 0.95 at 2 years apart to 0.74 at 12 years apart. Estimated means are plotted in Fig. 4.5; they are distinctly nonlinear up to 4 weeks but appear quite linear after that.

Conclusions about the exercise data have been based so far on LCV scores computed with all of a subject's measurements assigned to the same fold. This seems reasonable for complete data like the dental measurement data. For incomplete data like the exercise data, it seems more appropriate to base LCV scores on folds that reflect the possibility for missing outcome measurements. This is achieved using measurement-wise deletion as formulated in the next section.

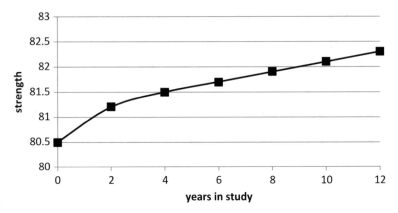

Fig. 4.5 Estimated mean strength based on adaptive marginal AR1 modeling

4.13   LCV with Measurement-Wise Deletion

So far, LCV scores have been computed using matched-set-wise deletion with all measurements for a matched set assigned to the same fold. This seems reasonable when all matched sets have no missing measurements. On the other hand, when some matched sets have missing measurements, LCV scores seem more appropriately computed in a way that accounts for such missingness. This can be achieved through measurement-wise deletion with the measurements of each matched set randomly spread out over the folds. Moreover, the effect of missingness on conclusions can be assessed by comparing results based on LCV scores computed using matched-set-wise deletion to results based on LCV scores computed using measurement-wise deletion. This section provides a formulation (which can be skipped) for LCV scores extending them to the measurement-wise deletion context.

For a subset SC' of SC, let $C(s, SC') = \{c : sc \in SC'\}$, the set of condition indexes c with sc in SC', for each $s \in S$. The associated observed data $O_{s, C(s, SC')}$ have likelihood $L(O_{s, C(s, SC')}; \theta)$ which is defined equal to 1 when $C(s, SC') = \varnothing$. Randomly partition the index set SC into k disjoint folds $F(h)$ for $h \in H = \{h : 1 \le h \le k\}$ with measurement indexes sc assigned to the fold $F(h(sc))$ where $h(sc) = \text{int}(k \cdot u_{sc}) + 1$ for independent, uniform random values u_{sc} in $(0, 1)$. For $h \in H$, let $U(h) = \cup_{h' \le h} F(h')$ denote the union of the fold index sets $F(h')$ for $h' \le h$ and $U(0)$ the empty set. Define revised LCV terms using conditional likelihoods as

$$LCV_{sh} = L\big(O_{s, C(s, F(h))} \big| O_{s, C(s, U(h-1))}; \theta(SC \backslash F(h))\big)$$
$$= L\big(O_{s, C(s, U(h))}; \theta(SC \backslash F(h))\big) / L\big(O_{s, C(s, U(h-1))}; \theta(SC \backslash F(h))\big).$$

In other words, the contribution to the LCV score for measurements of the matched set s within the hth fold F(h) is the conditional likelihood for those data given the measurements for that matched set in prior folds evaluated at parameter estimates based on data in the complement SC\F(h) of the hth fold. The associated LCV score is

$$\text{LCV} = \prod_{s \in S} \prod_{h \in H} \text{LCV}_{sh}{}^{1/m(SC)}.$$

With this definition, $\text{LCVM}^{(SC)}$ equals $L(SC; \boldsymbol{\theta})$ when computed with parameter estimates $\boldsymbol{\theta}(SC)$ rather than with the deleted estimates $\boldsymbol{\theta}(SC\backslash F(h))$ as needed to use measurement-wise deletion LCV ratio tests (see Sect. 4.4.2). Note that when fold assignment is matched-set-wise with all the measurements for matched set s in the same fold $F(h(s))$ for all $s \in S$, $\text{LCV}_{sh(s)} = L(O_{s,C(s)}; \boldsymbol{\theta}(SC\backslash F(h)))$ while $\text{LCV}_{sh} = 1$ for $h \neq h(s)$ so that the above definition of the LCV score for that case agrees with the definition given in Sect. 4.4.1.

The above formulation addresses the extension of LCV scores for marginal models to the measurement-wise deletion context using conditional likelihoods. The extension of PLCV scores to that context does not require a special formulation since they are based on conditional likelihoods to start with. However, measurement-wise deletion for conditional models requires that conditional predictors of PRE, POST, and OTHER types need to be recomputed for the complements of all of the folds to obtain appropriate deleted parameter estimates. This is not required for matched-set-wise deletion. An intermediate alternative requiring less computation is to use a partial measurement-wise deletion approach, computing deleted parameter estimates from conditional predictors based on the complete data rather than on the data in the complements of folds.

4.14   Revised Analysis of the Exercise Data

Analyses reported in this section use LCV scores with measurement-wise deletion to assess the effect of missingness on adaptive marginal modeling of the exercise data. The first local maximum in the LCV score for the adaptive ML-based AR1 model in time occurs for 10 folds, and so 10-fold LCV is used in subsequent analyses. The number of measurements in the 10 folds ranges from 15 to 34 for 12 to 23 matched sets (subjects in this case). The generated model has LCV score 0.18842 and includes an intercept and the transform $time^{0.5}$ as do the models for 5 and 15 folds. The same adaptive model was generated using the EC correlation structure, but the LCV score is 0.16059 with very substantial PD of 14.77 %. The linear polynomial model with AR1 correlation structure has LCV score 0.18556 with substantial PD 1.52 % so that mean strength is distinctly nonlinear in time. The adaptive transition model based on time, PRE(y,1), PRE(y,1,∅), and GCs has LCV score 0.15147 with substantial PD 18.95 %. The adaptive AR1-based marginal model in time, incrwgts, and GCs depends only on time and is the same model as generated for time by itself. The adaptive GEE-based model based on incrwgts, time, and GCs using the AR1 correlation structure generates a better LCV score of 0.17205 than the associated GEE-based model using the EC correlation structure (with LCV score 0.16047). The means of this model depend on incrwgts through the single predictor incrwgts· time$^{1.9}$ together with an intercept, suggesting the possibility of a dependence on incrwgts not identified through ML estimation. However, the PD compared to the ML-based model is substantial at 7.94 %, indicating as before that ML estimation provides a distinct improvement over GEE estimation and that the more appropriate conclusion is that mean strength does not depend on incrwgts. Thus, the same conclusions are reached using measurement-wise deletion LCV as with matched-set-wise deletion LCV, indicating that missingness has not affected conclusions based on LCV.

However, missingness may have an effect on mean strength, which can be assessed by investigating the impact of missingness predictor variables. For example, this can be addressed using the adaptive ML-based AR1 model in time, incrwgts, and the variable nmiss set to the number of missing outcome measurements for subjects along with GCs of these three variables. The associated adaptive model is the same model as generated without consideration of missingness, suggesting that missingness has not affected the prior conclusion on how mean strength depended on time and incrwgts. This analysis treats the number of missing measurements as a continuous predictor. It can also be treated as a categorical predictor by considering the two indicators nmiss1 and nmiss2 for having 1 and 2 missing measurements in place of the variable nmiss. The adaptively generated model is again the model generated without consideration of missingness, further supporting the conclusion of no impact to missingness on mean strength.

4.15   Modeling Variances as Well as Means

Variances are commonly assumed to be constant. As an alternative, PROC MIXED allows in some cases for heterogeneous variances with variance estimates changing with the repeated measurement conditions (e.g., ages of a child). The genreg macro supports more general variance modeling as described for univariate continuous outcomes in Sect. 2.19. This extends to multivariate continuous outcomes, and the extension is formulated in Sect. 4.15.1 (which can be skipped) and demonstrated in Sects. 4.15.2, 4.15.3 and 4.15.4.

4.15.1   Formulation

For marginal ML-based models, the covariance matrices $\Sigma_{s,C(s)}$ are assumed to satisfy

$$\Sigma_{s,C(s)} = B_{s,C(s)} \cdot R_{s,C(s)}(\rho) \cdot B_{s,C(s)},$$

where $B_{s,C(s)}$ are the diagonal matrices with diagonal entries σ_{sc} denoting the standard deviations of the outcome measurements y_{sc} for $c \in C(s)$ and $s \in S$. The logs of the variances σ_{sc}^2 are then modeled as functions of selected predictor variables and associated coefficients. Specifically, let $\log(\sigma_{sc}^2) = v_{sc}^T \cdot \gamma$ where, for $s \in S$ and $c \in C(s)$, v_{sc} is a $q \times 1$ column vector of q predictor values v_{scj} (including unit predictor values if an intercept is to be included) with indexes $j \in Q = \{j : 1 \leq j \leq q\}$ and γ is the associated $q \times 1$ column vector of coefficients. The parameter vector $\theta = (\beta^T, \gamma^T, \rho^T)^T$ is estimated through ML estimation. Define $V_{s,C(s)}$ to be the $m(s) \times q$ matrix with rows v_{sc}^T for $c \in C(s)$ and $s \in S$ and let

$$O_{s,C(s)} = \left(y_{s,C(s)}, X_{s,C(s)}, V_{s,C(s)} \right)$$

denote the observed data for each $s \in S$. With this notation, the formulations of Sects. 4.3 and 4.4 extend to combined adaptive marginal ML-based modeling of means and variances for multivariate continuous outcomes. A similar extension for modeling of dispersions along with means can be formulated for GEE-based models with the GEE equations for estimating mean parameters augmented with ML equations for estimating variances. Since transition modeling (Sect. 4.7) and general conditional modeling (Sect. 4.9) use pseudolikelihoods, equal to products of pseudolikelihood terms for the conditional measurements $y_{sc}^\#$, the associated extensions are generated analogously to the extension for univariate outcomes given in Sect. 2.19.1.

4.15.2 Analysis of Dental Measurement Means and Variances

An adaptive marginal ML-based model can be generated for the dental measurements with both means and variances functions of age, male, and associated GCs under exchangeable correlations (EC). Order 1 autoregressive correlations (AR1) are not considered since AR1-based constant variances models are not competitive with EC-based constant variances models (Sect. 4.8.2). The generated EC model has means depending on the transforms $age^{0.23}$ and $age^2 \cdot male$ without an intercept, variances depending on the indicator male with an intercept, and LCV score 0.13570. In contrast, the marginal EC model generated for the means assuming constant variances described in Sect. 4.8.2 has LCV score 0.12975 and substantial PD of 4.38 %, indicating that the variances for dental measurements are distinctly non-constant in male, under EC correlations. Means for the constant variances model are based on a similar set of transforms: $age^{0.21}$ and $(age^2 \cdot male)^{0.903}$ without an intercept, suggesting that estimated means have not changed much after accounting for non-constant variances. This can be assessed by starting from the model for the means generated with constant variances and generating the adaptive model for the variances holding the model for the means fixed. The generated model for the variances is based on the transforms: male and $age^{0.1}$ without an intercept. The LCV score is 0.13528 with insubstantial PD of 0.31 %, indicating that the model for the means has not changed substantially by considering non-constant variances.

An adaptive transition model can be generated with both means and variances depending on the primary predictors age, male, PRE(y,1,2), and PRE(y, 1, 2, ∅) as well as GCs based on these primary predictors. Models based on weighted averages are not considered since they did not improve on simple averages for constant variances analyses (Sect. 4.8). The generated model for means includes $(age^{1.5} \cdot PRE(y,1,2)^5)^{0.95}$, $(male \cdot age^2)^{1.1}$, $(male \cdot PRE(y,1,2)^{1.7} \cdot age^{1.6})^{1.1}$, and $(PRE(y,1,2)^{-3} \cdot age^2)^{4.3}$ with an intercept. The generated model for the variances includes $(age^{2.5} \cdot PRE(y,1,2))^{0.9}$ and $(male \cdot age^4 \cdot PRE(y,1,2))^{0.9}$ also with an intercept. The LCV score is 0.14264. In contrast, the transition model generated for the means assuming constant variances (see Sect. 4.8) has LCV score 0.13363 and substantial PD of 6.32 %, indicating that the variances for dental measurements are distinctly non-constant in age, male, and the average of the previous two dental measurements. Moreover, the adaptive marginal ML-based model with non-constant variances and EC correlations generates a substantial PD in LCV scores of 4.87 %, indicating that transition modeling outperforms marginal ML-based modeling of means and variances of the dental measurements as it did for modeling of means with constant variances. The adaptive transition model for the variances holding the model for the means fixed at the adaptive constant variances model is based on the transforms: $PRE(y,1,2)^{0.6}$ and $(male \cdot age^3 \cdot PRE(y,1,2)^2)^{2.04}$ with an intercept. The LCV score is 0.14215 with insubstantial PD 0.34 %, indicating that the transition model for the means has not changed substantially by considering non-constant variances.

An adaptive GEE-based model can be generated for the dental measurements with both means and variances functions of age, male, and associated GCs under marginal GEE-based models with EC correlations. The associated GEE-based model has means depending on the transforms $age^{0.22}$ and $(age^7 \cdot male)^{0.5}$ without an intercept, variances depending on the transform $(male \cdot age)^{-1}$ with an intercept, and LCV score 0.13670. In contrast, the marginal GEE-based model generated for the means assuming constant variances and EC correlations described in Sect. 4.11.2 has LCV score 0.13124 and substantial PD of 3.99 %, indicating as for ML-based models that the variances for dental measurements are distinctly non-constant in age and male. The adaptive ML-based model for both means and variances has a smaller LCV score than the associated GEE-based model, but the PD for the ML-based model is insubstantial at 0.73%. However, the non-constant variances GEE-based model generates a substantial PD of 4.16 % compared to the associated non-constant variances transition model, indicating that transition modeling outperforms marginal GEE-based modeling for these data as long as variances are modeled along with means as it did for marginal ML-based modeling.

4.15.3 Transition Modeling of Strength Measurement Means with Adjusted Variances

As demonstrated in Sect. 4.7.2, marginal models with constant variances and AR1 correlations have associated transition models with a different variance for the first measurement of a matched set than for subsequent measurements. Thus, transition models may require variances adjusted for this difference to be competitive with marginal AR1 models. For the case of transition modeling of the means in terms of time, PRE(y,1), and PRE(y,1,$\varnothing$), and GCs with LCV scores based on measurement-wise deletion as considered in Sect. 4.14, this issue can be addressed by starting the adaptive modeling process with the log variance model based on an intercept and the indicator PRE(y,1,$\varnothing$) and allowing contraction of these terms as well as those of the expanded model for the means. The generated model for the means is based on the three transforms: $(\text{PRE}(y,1)^{6.1} \cdot \text{time}^{-0.03})^{0.921}$, $\text{PRE}(y,1)^{-43}$, and $\text{PRE}(y,1)^{-9}$ with an intercept and variances depending on PRE(y,1,$\varnothing$) without an intercept. It has LCV score 0.18479, in contrast to 0.15147 for the constant variances transition model as reported in Sect. 4.14. Thus, it can be very important to adjust the log variance model to generate the best alternative transition model for the means. However, this model generates a substantial PD of 2.03 % compared to the associated marginal AR1 model with constant variances and larger LCV score 0.18842.

4.15.4 Analysis of Strength Measurement Means and Variances

This section conducts a more complete assessment of means and variances for the exercise data than the assessment of Sect. 4.15.3. Measurement-wise deletion is used to compute reported LCV scores as in Sect. 4.14. The adaptive marginal ML-based model for strength measurements with both means and variances functions of time, incrwgts, and GCs and with AR1 correlations (since they outperformed EC correlations in earlier analyses) is the same as the adaptive constant variances model described in Sect. 4.14 with LCV score 0.18842, suggesting that the strength measurements are reasonably treated as having constant variances. The associated adaptive GEE-based model has means depending on time and incrwgts, but with constant variances, reduced LCV score 0.17205, and substantial PD of 8.69 %, and so this marginal GEE-based model is distinctly outperformed by the associated marginal ML-based model.

The adaptive transition model for means and variances in time, incrwgts, PRE(y,1), PRE(y,1,∅), and GCs has means based on the two transforms: PRE(y,1)$^{6.13}$ and time$^{0.4}$ · PRE(y,1)$^{-6}$ with an intercept and variances based on the three transforms: time$^{-0.09}$, time^{-7}, (incrwgts · PRE(y,1)$^{6.2}$)$^{1.01}$ with an intercept. It has an improved LCV score of 0.19089, which is a substantial improvement over the constant variances marginal ML-based model with the largest LCV score so far and PD 1.29 %. Furthermore, the adaptive transition model for means and variances in time, PRE(y,1), PRE(y,1,∅), and GCs, that is, without considering incrwgts, has LCV score 0.18905 with substantial PD 0.96 %. Thus, transition models for the exercise data outperform marginal models as long as both means and variances are modeled. Moreover, they are needed to identify effects of incrwgts on the variances not identifiable with marginal models. The means for this best model do not depend on incrwgts but the variances do. The estimated slope for the one transform for the variances involving incrwgts is negative, indicating that the strength variances are smaller for subjects with the weight increasing over time at post-baseline times (when PRE(y,1) > 0) than for subjects with the number of repetitions increasing over time, with more of a decrease with increasing prior strength measurements (since the power 6.2 · 1.01 for PRE(y,1) is positive).

While these analyses address missingness as it affects LCV scores for models of means and variances, it is possible that the means and/or variances might change with the amount of missing strength measurements. This can be addressed using marginal ML-based modeling with AR1 correlations and means and variances based on time, incrwgts, nmiss (the number of missing strength measurements), and GCs. GEE-based marginal modeling is not considered since it is outperformed by ML-based modeling in analyses not considering nmiss. The generated model for the means is based on the two transforms: time$^{0.5}$ and (incrwgts · time^{8} · nmiss$^{-1.7}$)$^{1.93}$ with an intercept while the model for the variances is based on the two transform: (nmiss$^{1.5}$ · time)$^{0.8}$ and (incrwgts · nmiss · time$^{1.1}$)$^{0.9}$ with an intercept. The LCV score is 0.19545, which is a substantial improvement over the associated adaptive ML-based model not considering nmiss with PD 3.60 %, suggesting that missingness has an effect on the means and variances. Moreover, the transition model generated without considering nmiss has substantial PD of 2.33 %.

The transition model with means and variances based on time, incrwgts, nmiss, PRE(y,1), PRE(y,1,∅), and GCs has means based on the three transforms: (time$^{0.04}$ · PRE(y,1)$^{-6}$)$^{-0.3}$, PRE(y,1)$^{-1.1}$, and (incrwgts · time^{-1} · PRE(y,1)$^{-11}$)$^{-1.1}$ with an intercept and variances based on the four transform: time$^{0.03}$, (nmiss$^{0.6}$ · time$^{1.2}$ · PRE(y,1)^{2})$^{0.8}$, (nmiss^{-7} · incrwgts)$^{0.4}$, and time^{-6} with an intercept. The LCV score is 0.20016, which is a substantial improvement over the associated transition model not considering nmiss with PD 2.84 %, indicating that missingness has a direct effect on the variances but only an indirect effect on the means since they do not change with nmiss but now change with incrwgts. It is also

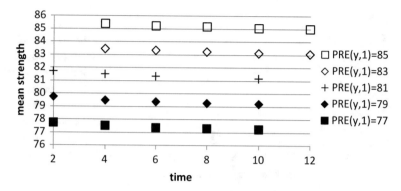

Fig. 4.6 Estimated post-baseline strength means for the increasing number of repetitions group based on adaptive transition modeling of means and variances in terms of time and the prior strength measurement (PRE(y,1))

a substantial improvement over the ML-based marginal model considering nmiss with PD 2.35 %. This model includes an effect to incrwgts on the means and variances. Whether this is substantial can be assessed by comparing results to the model with means and variances depending on time, nmiss, $PRE(y,1), PRE(y,1,\varnothing)$, and GCs, not including incrwgts. The generated model has LCV score 0.19313 with substantial PD of 3.51 %, and so incrwgts has a substantial effect. These results indicate that both the means and variances differ for the two weightlifting program.

Estimated post-baseline strength means for the increasing number of repetitions group based on the adaptive transition model for means and variances are plotted in Fig. 4.6. At each given prior strength measurement value, mean strength decreases somewhat over time, but at higher levels for higher prior strength measurements. For the increased number of weights group, the estimates are in all cases about 0.02 units larger (see Sect. 20.4.10 for an explanation of why this is a constant value). While the effect of the increased number of groups may be substantial in terms of LCV ratio tests, an increase of about 0.02 units may not be a substantively meaningful improvement.

Estimated post-baseline strength standard deviations for the increasing number of repetitions group based on this model are plotted in Fig. 4.7. The variability in post-baseline strength measurements increases as prior strength measurements increase but only for larger prior strength measurements. The variability also increases over time but more so as the number of missing strength measurements increases. For subjects in the increased weight group, the only differences occur when they have missing strength measurements with a decrease in dispersion of 1.07 units when nmiss = 1 and of 0.15 units when nmiss = 2.

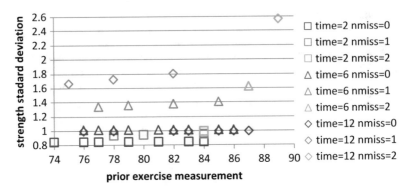

Fig. 4.7 Estimated post-baseline strength standard deviations for the increasing number of repetitions group based on adaptive transition modeling of means and variances in terms of time, the prior strength measurement and the number of missing exercise measurements (nmiss)

4.16   Overview of Analyses of Dental Measurements

1. For the dental measurement data (Sect. 4.2), analyses use $k = 5$ folds (Sect. 4.5.2).
2. Using AR1 correlations and constant variances, the mean dental measurements are reasonably close to linear in the child's age (Sect. 4.5.2).
3. Using AR1 correlations,constant variances, and the interaction agemale, the dependence of the mean dental measurements on the child's age is distinctly nonlinearly moderated by the gender of the child (Sect. 4.5.3). A linear moderation analysis in this case leads to the conclusion that moderation does not occur (Sect. 4.5.3). Hence, moderation in this case can only be identified through an adaptive nonlinear analysis.
4. Linear moderation analyses commonly start by centering variables like the child's age at their observed means. This has no effect on the significance of the interaction effect. However, centering can have an effect for nonlinear models. For the dental measurement data, the model based on centered age also leads to the conclusion that moderation has occurred, but the model based on uncentered age (Sect. 4.5.3) is a parsimonious,competitive alternative.
5. Adaptive modeling supports generation of geometric combinations (GCs), that is, products of power transforms of different primary predictors possibly with different powers, generalizing interactions and their power transforms. The adaptive model in age, gender, and GCs has LCV score a little larger than the one for the model based on age, gender, and the interaction agemale (Sect. 4.5.4), supporting the validity of the heuristics for generating GCs (see Sect. 18.4.6).
6. Adaptive modeling supports power transforms of primary predictors with nonpositive values. Transformed zero values are left as zero, transformed positive values are computed as usual, and transformed negative values are set equal to the transform of their absolute values weighted by a cosine function

to switch signs between positive and negative values. The Royston and Sauerbrei (2008) recommended approach is to add a value to nonpositive valued predictors just large enough to make them positive valued. For centered age, this generates a competitive model to using uncentered age, but it negates the effect of centering (Sect. 4.6.2).

7. Assuming constant variances, the adaptive transition model in age, gender, PRE(y,1) (the prior outcome measurement), PRE(y, 1, ∅) (the indicator for there being no prior outcome measurement; in which case PRE(y, 1) is set to 0), and GCs distinctly outperforms the adaptive AR1-based marginal model (Sect. 4.8.1). The adaptive EC-based marginal model generates a larger LCV score than this transition model, but not substantially larger (Sect. 4.8.3). However, it does substantially improve on the AR1-based marginal model (Sect. 4.8.2). The adaptive transition model in age, gender, PRE(y,1,2) (the average of the up to two prior outcome measurements), PRE(y, 1, 2, ∅), and GCs distinctly outperforms the EC-based marginal model (Sect. 4.8.3). It also generates a better LCV score than the model using PRE(y,1,3) (the average of the up to three prior outcome measurements; Sect. 4.5.3). Results for this model are displayed in Figs. 4.2–4.4.

8. Assuming constant variances, adaptive transition modeling based separately on the four PLCs: AIC, BIC using the number of measurements, BIC using the number of matched sets, and TIC generates substantially inferior models to adaptive transition modeling based on LCV scores (Sect. 4.8.4). Adaptive modeling based on PLCs should usually be avoided, at least for transition modeling of continuous outcomes with possible exception highly time-consuming analyses.

9. General condition modeling with current outcome measurements depending on averages of other outcome measurements occurring either before or after the current one distinctly outperforms transition modeling for the dental measurement data (Sect. 4.10). However, general conditional modeling does not seem appropriate for longitudinal data. It is more appropriately used with clustered data.

10. Assuming constant variances and EC correlations, adaptive GEE-based marginal modeling generates a better LCV score than the associated ML-based model, but not substantially better (Sect. 4.11.2). However, the GEE-based model is distinctly inferior to the associated transition model (Sect. 4.11.2). These results suggest that consideration of GEE-based models may not be necessary in general, at least for modeling continuous outcomes.

11. The adaptive GEE-based model using unstructured (UN) correlations is the constant model with distinctly smaller LCV score than the associated EC-based model (Sect. 4.11.2). UN correlations can overfit the data.

12. Using the full factorial model in age, gender, and agemale, the quasi-likelihood information criterion (QIC) score, commonly used in model selection for GEE-based models, leads to the conclusion that the data may reasonably be considered to be independent even though the EC-based correlation estimate has the substantial value 0.61 (this and the following results reported in

Sect. 4.11.3). Moreover, there is little difference in the QIC scores for alternate correlation structures. Using LCV scores instead leads to the conclusion that the EC correlation structure is the distinctly best choice for these data and that the correlation of 0.61 is substantial. Furthermore, using EC correlations, the QIC score is best for the model constant in age, gender, and agemale even though age and agemale are highly significant ($P < 0.001$ and $P = 0.009$, respectively) in the full factorial model while the LCV score selects the submodel with these two terms included and the nonsignificant ($P = 0.454$) term gender removed. The QIC score can generate counterintuitive results.

13. The adaptive ML-based marginal model with AR1 correlations allowing for non-constant variances distinctly outperforms the associated constant variances model (this and the following results reported in Sect. 4.15.2). This also holds for GEE-based marginal modeling and for transition modeling. As for constant variances, the non-constant variances transition model distinctly outperforms both the ML-based and GEE-based marginal models, which are competitive alternatives to each other.

4.17 Overview of Analyses of Strength Measurements

1. For the exercise data (Sect. 4.12), using LCV scores based on matched set-wise deletion (Sect. 4.4.1) and constant variances, $k = 15$ folds are chosen for analyses of those data (this and the following results reported in Sect. 4.12). Using ML parameter estimation, the AR1-based marginal model for strength in terms of time distinctly outperforms the associated EC-based marginal model and the transition model based on PRE(y, 1). Mean strength is distinctly nonlinear in time and is reasonably considered not to depend on the type of exercise program. Using GEE parameter estimation, the AR1-based marginal model for strength in terms of time once again distinctly outperforms the associated EC-based marginal model. However, this GEE-based model is distinctly outperformed by the associated ML-based model.

2. Using LCV scores based on measurement-wise deletion (Sect. 4.13) and constant variances, $k = 10$ folds are chosen for analyses of the exercise data (this and the following results reported in Sect. 4.14). The results using LCV with matched set-wise deletion as reported above still hold using LCV scores based on measurement-wise deletion. When a possible effect to missingness on the means is addressed by also including predictors measuring the number of missing values for each matched set, the generated models do not depend on these missingness predictors. These results suggest that missingness has not affected the conclusions for constant variances models.

3. The constant variances transition model in PRE(y, 1) is very inferior with PD 18.95 % (Sect. 4.14), but even simple AR1 models induce transition models with variances that are non-constant depending on PRE(y, 1, $\varnothing$) (Sect. 4.7.2), which explains the poor performance of transition modeling in this case (this and the

following results reported in Sect. 4.15.3). Using LCV scores based on measurement-wise deletion and variances based on a constant term and the indicator $PRE(y, 1, \varnothing)$, the generated model has dramatically improved LCV score. However, it is still distinctly inferior to the ML-based marginal model, but now the PD is only 2.03 %.

4. Using LCV scores based on measurement-wise deletion, non-constant variances, and AR1 correlations, the adaptive ML-based marginal model distinctly outperforms the adaptive GEE-based marginal model and is the same as the associated constant variances model (this and the following results reported in Sect. 4.15.4). However, the adaptive transition model distinctly outperforms the adaptive ML-based marginal model. Moreover, it also outperforms the associated constant variances transition model. Consequently, transition modeling is needed to identify non-constant variances including an effect on the variances of the type of exercise program. While transition models are distinctly inferior in this case using constant variances, they become distinctly superior with consideration of non-constant variances. When a possible effect to missingness on the means is addressed by also including the number of missing values for each matched set as a predictor, the generated model depends on this missingness predictor and the model distinctly outperforms the transition model not considering that predictor. Moreover, effects to the exercise program on both the means and variances can only be identified with non-constant transition modeling. Results for this model are displayed in Figs. 4.6–4.7.

4.18   Chapter Summary

This chapter has presented analyses of the dental measurement data, addressing how means and variances for the dental measurements change with the age and gender of the child while accounting for dependence of dental measurements for the same child. These analyses use marginal models based on order 1 autoregressive (AR1) correlations and exchangeable correlations (EC), estimated with maximum likelihood (ML) or generalized estimating equations (GEE), as well as transition models and general conditional models. Analyses have also been presented of the exercise data, addressing how mean strength changes with time and type of weightlifting program. The EC-based marginal model outperforms the AR1-based marginal model for the dental measurement data while AR1 outperforms EC for the exercise data, indicating the importance of considering alternative correlation structures for marginal models. Transition models outperform marginal models for the dental measurement data for both the constant and non-constant variances cases. When variances are constant, marginal models outperform transition models for the exercise data, indicating the importance of considering both types of models. With an appropriate adjustment to the log variance model, as suggested by the transition model induced by the marginal AR1-based model with constant means, transition models for the exercise data can be distinctly improved.

Moreover, with consideration of general non-constant variances for the exercise data, transition models can outperform marginal models. Adaptive marginal models with more complex correlation structures (e.g., autoregressive moving average models of arbitrary orders) might provide distinct improvements, but they have not yet been implemented in the genreg macro. Adaptive modeling of means and variances in combination is also considered and generates distinct improvements over constant variances models for both the dental measurement and exercise data, demonstrating the need in general to consider such models. Adaptive marginal ML-based and GEE-based models are competitive alternatives for analyzing the dental measurement data, but adaptive marginal ML-based models distinctly outperform adaptive marginal GEE-based models for the exercise data. It seems reasonable to consider only marginal ML-based models for continuous multivariate outcomes.

General conditional models distinctly outperform transition models for the dental measurement data, indicating that dental measurements at present times can be better predicted using both past and future values than with just past values. However, longitudinal data like the dental measurement and exercise data are more appropriately modeled using transition models relating present time measurements to past measurements. General conditional models are more appropriate for measurements over clusters like members of the same family, patients of the same provider, and mice in the same litter.

The example analyses demonstrate how to assess nonlinear moderation (modification) effects and compare them to linear moderation effects. These can be based on interaction terms as primary predictors or more generally on geometric combinations consisting of adaptively generated products of powers of distinct primary predictors. For the dental measurement data under AR1 correlations, the linear moderation analysis leads to the conclusion that mean dental measurements do not change over child ages differently for boys and girls. However, the adaptive moderation analysis identifies distinctly different patterns for mean dental measurements over child ages for boy and girls. In this case, moderation can only be identified using an adaptive, nonlinear analysis. EC correlations produce distinctly better LCV scores than AR1 correlations, and the linear moderation effect becomes significant. Thus, alternative correlation structures need to be considered when testing linear moderation effects, or any other fixed effects, in order to draw appropriate conclusions about those effects. However, as for AR1 correlations, the adaptive moderation analysis under EC correlations provides a distinctly better assessment of moderation effects than the linear moderation analysis. Thus, even when linear moderation can be established, adaptive modeling can provide a distinctly better assessment of moderation relationships.

The example analyses also demonstrate how to assess the impact of missingness for incomplete data, including accounting for missingness in LCV scores as well as assessing the effect of missingness predictors on means and variances. Assuming constant variances, conclusions about mean strength for the exercise data are the same when based on LCV scores computed using both matched-set-wise deletion, with all of a subject's measurements allocated to the same fold, and measurement-wise deletion, with each subject's measurements spread out over different folds, indicating that those conclusions are not affected by the presence of missing outcome measurements for some subjects. Furthermore, adaptive constant variances models for mean strength allowing for dependence on how many missing outcome measurements a subject has do not depend on these missingness predictors, further supporting the conclusion that the presence of missing outcome measurements has not affected the results. However, analyses addressing missingness effects on both means and variances identify distinct effects to the number of missing strength measurements not identifiable with constant variances models.

This chapter has also provided formulations for marginal, transition, and general conditional models of possibly incomplete data including likelihoods, ML and GEE estimation, penalized likelihood criteria (PLCs), and likelihood cross-validation (LCV) for marginal and transition models plus pseudolikelihoods, maximum pseudolikelihood estimation, and pseudolikelihood cross-validation (PLCV) for general conditional models. Formulations are provided for LCV and PLCV using matched-set-wise deletion as is appropriate for complete data like the dental measurement data. LCV using measurement-wise deletion, as is appropriate for incomplete data like the exercise data, is also formulated for marginal models. The extension of PLCV scores to measurement-wise deletion does not require a special formulation. Formulations are provided as well for general power transforms of primary predictors with zero or negative values and for cutoffs for a substantial percent decrease (PD) in LCV and PLCV scores.

Adaptive model selection using PLCs can reduce computation times compared to using LCV. However, examples are provided where model selection by LCV distinctly outperforms model selection by AIC, BIC computed using the number of measurements, BIC computed using the number of matched sets, and TIC. These results suggest that the use of PLCs should be avoided except perhaps for large data sets and/or large numbers of primary predictors when time requirements for adaptive modeling with LCV are prohibitive. A formulation is also provided for the PLC called the quasi-likelihood information criterion (QIC) specially created for selection of GEE models. Example analyses using the dental measurements are provided indicating that, in comparison to LCV, QIC does not discriminate well between alternative correlation structures and can produce counterintuitive conclusions about fixed effects. QIC for model selection should be avoided, at least for continuous outcomes and maybe more generally.

See Chap. 5 for details on conducting analyses in SAS of multivariate continuous outcomes as considered in this chapter. See Chaps. 6 and 7 for transformation of outcomes as well as predictors. See Chaps. 10 and 11 for extensions to modeling multivariate discrete outcomes with two or more values. See Chaps. 14 and 15 for extensions to modeling multivariate count/rate outcomes.

References

Aiken, L. S., & West, S. G. (1991). *Multiple regression: Testing and interpreting interactions.* Newbury Park: Sage.

Baron, R. M., & Kenny, D. A. (1986). The moderator-mediator variable distinction in social psychology research: Conceptual, strategic, and statistical considerations. *Journal of Personality & Social Psychology, 51,* 1173–1182.

Brown, H., & Prescott, R. (1999). *Applied mixed models in medicine.* New York: John Wiley & Sons.

Claeskens, G., & Hjort, N. L. (2009). *Model selection and model averaging.* Cambridge: Cambridge University Press.

Diggle, P. J., Heagarty, P., Liang, K.-Y., & Zeger, S. L. (2002). *Analysis of longitudinal data* (2nd ed.). Oxford: Oxford University Press.

Fitzmaurice, G. M., Laird, N. M., & Ware, J. H. (2011). *Applied longitudinal analysis* (2nd ed.). Hoboken, NJ: John Wiley & Sons.

Kleinbaum, D. G., Kupper, L. L., Muller, K. E., & Nizam, A. (1998). *Applied regression analysis and other multivariable methods* (3rd ed.). Belmont, CA: Thomson Brooks/Cole.

Knafl, G. J., & Riegel, B. (2014). What puts heart failure patients at risk for poor medication adherence? *Patient Preference and Adherence, 8,* 1007–1018.

Liang, K.-Y., & Zeger, S. L. (1986). Longitudinal data analysis using generalized linear models. *Biometrika, 73,* 13–22.

Morrison, D. F. (1967). *Multivariate statistical models.* New York: McGraw-Hill.

Pan, W. (2001). Akaike's information criterion in generalized estimating equations. *Biometrics, 57,* 120–125.

Potthoff, R. F., & Roy, S. N. (1964). A generalized multivariate analysis of variance model useful especially for growth curve problems. *Biometrika, 51,* 313–326.

Riegel, B., & Knafl, G. J. (2014). Electronically monitored medication adherence predicts hospitalization in heart failure patients. *Patient Preference and Adherence, 8,* 1–13.

Royston, P., & Sauerbrei, W. (2008). *Multivariable model-building: A practical approach to regression analysis based on fractional polynomials for modelling continuous variables.* Hoboken, NJ: John Wiley & Sons.

SAS Institute (2004). SAS/STAT 9.1 user's guide. Cary, NC: SAS Institute.

Stone, M. (1977). An asymptotic equivalence of choice of model by cross-validation and Akaike's criterion. *Journal of the Royal Statistical Society, Series B, 39,* 44–47.

Verbeke, G., & Molenberghs, G. (2000). *Linear mixed models for longitudinal data.* New York: Springer.

Chapter 5
Adaptive Regression Modeling
of Multivariate Continuous Outcomes in SAS

5.1 Chapter Overview

This chapter provides a description of how to use the genreg macro for adaptive regression modeling in the case of multivariate continuous outcomes treated as multivariate normally distributed. See Khattree and Naik (1999), Littell et al. (2002), and Littell et al. (2006) for details on standard approaches for multivariate normal modeling in SAS. Familiarity with adaptive modeling of univariate continuous outcomes in SAS as described in Chap. 3 is assumed in this chapter. Section 5.2 describes how to load the dental measurement data of Sect. 4.2. Data in wide format are often used in multivariate outcome modeling with outcome measurements under different conditions (for example, ages for the dental measurement data analyzed in Chap. 4) in separate variables (columns) and with one observation (row) per matched set of related outcome measurements (for example, the matched sets of the dental measurement data correspond to dental measurements for different children). However, mixed modeling as used in this chapter to analyze multivariate outcome data requires that the data be converted to long format with all outcome measurements in the same variable, an extra variable to identify the measurement condition, and one observation for each outcome measurement, and so an example of such a conversion is presented. Section 5.3 describes adaptive marginal modeling of means for the dental measurements with parameter estimation based on either maximum likelihood (ML) or generalized estimating equations (GEE) while Sect. 5.4 addresses conditional modeling of those data, including transition and general conditional modeling. Both of these sections provide example residual analyses as well, together with sensitivity analyses to assess the impact of outlying observations. Section 5.5 addresses special issues involved in modeling of the exercise data. Section 5.6 covers adaptive modeling of variances as well as means.

© Springer International Publishing Switzerland 2016
G.J. Knafl, K. Ding, *Adaptive Regression for Modeling Nonlinear Relationships*,
Statistics for Biology and Health, DOI 10.1007/978-3-319-33946-7_5

5.2   Loading the Dental Measurement Data

A data set with dental measurements for 27 children over four ages is analyzed in Chap. 4 (see Sect. 4.2). Assume that this data set has been loaded into the default library (for example, by importing it from a spreadsheet file) under the name dentin. An output title line, selected system options, and labels and formats for the variables can be assigned as in the following code.

```
title "Dental Measurement Data";
options linesize=76 pagesize=53 pageno=1 nodate;
proc format;
  value $gndrfmt "F"="female" "M"="male";
  value nyfmt 0="no" 1="yes";
run;
data dentin;
  set dentin;
  nmiss=nmiss(of dmeas1-dmeas4);
  somemiss=(nmiss>0);
  label subject="Subject Identifier"
        gender="Gender"
        dmeas1="Dental Measurement at Age 8 "
        dmeas2="Dental Measurement at Age 10 "
        dmeas3="Dental Measurement at Age 12 "
        dmeas4="Dental Measurement at Age 14 "
        nmiss="Number of Missing Measurements"
        somemiss="Some Missing Measurements or Not";
  format gender $gndrfmt. somemiss nyfmt.;
run;
```

A character format $gndrfmt is created and assigned to the character variable gender translating its coded values of "F" and "M" to "female" and "male", respectively. These data are in what is called wide or broad format with one observation per matched set, in this case corresponding to a child with identifier in the variable subject, and the associated outcome measurements in separate variables, in this case dmeas1–dmeas4 containing dental measurements at ages 8, 10, 12, and 14 years old. An assessment of missingness is simply accomplished with data in this format including how many measurements are missing as loaded in the variable nmiss using the SAS nmiss function, and whether or not there are any missing measurements as loaded in the indicator variable somemiss. A numeric format nyfmt is created and assigned to the numeric variable somemiss translating its values of 0 and 1 to no and yes, respectively. However, the dental measurement data are complete with no missing measurements for all the children, and so these variables are not needed in this case. They are useful, though, for incomplete data with matched sets having different numbers of associated measurements.

To analyze these data with SAS PROC MIXED and with the genreg macro, they need to be converted to what is called long format with one observation for each measurement. The following code can be used for this purpose. The code creates an array named dmeas from the variables dmeas1–dmeas4, which is used in a do loop to generate variables in long format through the output statement. The outcome variable is named dentmeas and contains dental measurements for each child at each of four ages as specified in the variable age. The character variable gender is replaced by the equivalent numeric indicator variable male for whether the child is a boy or not and this indicator variable is assigned the numeric format nyfmt. The variable agemale is the interaction between the variables age and male, that is, their product. The keep statement is used to remove unneeded variables from the newly created dentdata data set.

```
data dentdata;
  set dentin;
  male=(gender="M");
  array dmeas{4} dmeas1-dmeas4;
  do i=1 to 4;
    age=2*i+6; agemale=age*male; dentmeas=dmeas{i}; output;
  end;
  label male="Male Child or Not"
        age="Age"
        dentmeas="Dental Measurement"
        agemale="Age When the Child is a Male";
  format male nyfmt.;
  keep subject male age dentmeas nmiss somemiss;
run;
```

5.3 Marginal Modeling of Means for the Dental Measurement Data

5.3.1 Marginal Models of Mean Dental Measurement in Age of the Child

Assuming that the genreg macro has been loaded into SAS (see Supplementary Materials), the number of folds can be set using the adaptive model for dentmeas as a function of age under a marginal AR1 model with maximum likelihood (ML) parameter estimates as generated with the following code by varying the value of the macro variable kfold.

```
%let kfold=5;
%genreg(modtype=NORML,datain=dentdata,yvar=dentmeas,
        matchvar=subject,withinvr=age,corrtype=AR1,
        foldcnt=&kfold,expand=y,expxvars=age,
        contract=y);
```

The matchvar parameter specifies the variable whose unique values determine the matched sets, in this case the variable named subject. The withinvr parameter specifies the variable containing values for the repeated measurement conditions within each matched set, in this case the variable named age. The corrtype parameter is used to set the correlation type. The setting "corrtype=AR1" in this case requests an order 1 autoregressive model. The default is "corrtype=IND" for independent data as used in Chap. 2. The option "corrtype=EC" requests exchangeable correlations. The above code is run with the value of the macro variable kfold changed from 5 by multiples of 5 until a local maximum is achieved. This occurs in this case for &kfold=5 (see Sect. 4.5.2), and so subsequent analyses assume that &kfold=5 so that they use 5 folds to compute LCV scores.

As described in Sect. 3.6 for univariate outcomes, the adaptive modeling process can use penalized likelihood criteria (PLCs) in place of LCV scores, which is accomplished using the scretype parameter (with default setting "scretype=LCV"). When "scretype=BIC", Bayesian information criterion (BIC) scores are computed, and by default these BIC scores use the number of measurements. This can be changed to BIC scores using the number of matched sets with the "usenmeas=n" setting, thereby overriding the default setting of "usenmeas=y". Akaike information criterion (AIC) and Takeuchi information criterion (TIC) scores can be requested with the "scretype=AIC" and "scretype=TIC" settings. These PLCs are adjusted from their usual smaller is better form to the larger is better form defined in Sect. 2.10.1.

By default, marginal models use ML parameter estimation. An adaptive AR1 model in age with GEE parameter estimation can be requested as follows.

```
%genreg(modtype=NORML,datain=dentdata,yvar=dentmeas,
        matchvar=subject,withinvr=age,corrtype=AR1,
        foldcnt=&kfold,GEE=y,biasadj=y,spatial=n,
        expand=y,expxvars=age,contract=y);
```

The setting "GEE=y" requests GEE parameter estimation while the default setting "GEE=n" requests ML parameter estimation. By default, correlation and variance estimates are not adjusted for bias. The setting "biasadj=y" requests that correlation and variance estimates be adjusted for bias, as is standard for GEE models. Also by default, AR1 correlations are spatial with distance apart based on actual age values. The setting "spatial=n" requests that standard AR1 correlations be generated with distance apart based on indexes of age values, as is standard for GEE models. Since the dental measurements are equally spaced, these two options are equivalent, but this is not the case for unequally spaced outcome measurements. The setting "corrtype=UN" requests unstructured correlations, that is, with all pairs of distinct outcome measurements having distinct correlation parameters and estimates. However, this option is currently supported only for GEE parameter estimates and not for ML parameter estimates.

5.3.2 Marginal Moderation Models of Mean Dental Measurement in Age and Gender of the Child

An adaptive moderation model for dentmeas in terms of age, male, and the interaction agemale is requested as follows.

```
%genreg(modtype=NORML,datain=dentdata,yvar=dentmeas,
        matchvar=subject,withinvr=age,corrtype=AR1,
        foldcnt=&kfold,expand=y,
        expxvars=age male agemale,contract=y);
```

The associated adaptive main effect model is requested by removing agemale from the expxvars list.

```
%genreg(modtype=NORML,datain=dentdata,yvar=dentmeas,
        matchvar=subject,withinvr=age,corrtype=AR1,
        foldcnt=&kfold,expand=y,expxvars=age male,
        contract=y);
```

An adaptive moderation model based on automatically generated geometric combinations (GCs; defined in Sect. 4.5.4) is requested using the following code. The setting "geomcmbn=y" requests that GCs based on all the expxvars variables be considered in the expansion. The default is "geomcmbn=n", which is why the previous code considers male as having only a covariate effect on the relationship of the mean dental measurements with age.

```
%genreg(modtype=NORML,datain=dentdata,yvar=dentmeas,
        matchvar=subject,withinvr=age,corrtype=AR1,
        foldcnt=&kfold,expand=Y,geomcmbn=y,
        expxvars=age male,contract=y);
```

The first two pages of the output for the above code document a variety of settings for the genreg macro parameters. Table 5.1 contains the part of that output related to the computation of LCV scores. The type of cross-validation is controlled by the measdlte macro parameter. The setting "measdlte=y" requests that LCV scores be computed with measurement-wise deletion (Sect. 4.13). By default, "measdlte=n", as is requested in the above code, meaning that LCV scores are computed with matched-set-wise deletion (Sect. 4.4.1). The requested fold count

Table 5.1 Requested cross-validation settings for the adaptive moderation model for dental measurements in terms of age and the indicator male for the child being a boy

```
cross-validation is matched-set-wise with
     fold count:                                                   5
     initial fold assignment seed:                                 3
     number of empty folds:                                        0
     number of measurements in the smallest nonempty fold:        12
     number of measurements in the largest fold:                  32
     smallest number of matched sets with measurements in a fold:  3
     largest number of matched sets with measurements in a fold:   8
     cutoff for a substantial percent decrease in the
     cross-validation score:                                1.762732%
     degrees of freedom for cutoff:                                1
```

for this analysis is $k = 5$. Matched sets when "measdlte=n" and measurements when "measdlte=y" are randomly assigned to folds. The initial seed for this random assignment can be specified using the initseed macro parameter. Its default value of 3 is used in the above code. In this case, there are no empty folds, with fold sizes varying from 12 measurements for 3 children to 32 measurements for 8 children (and so all 4 measurements for a child in the same fold). The cutoff for a substantial percent decrease (PD) for these data is reported as well and rounds as indicated in Sect. 4.2 to 1.76 %. It is computed using the smallest possible nonzero integer degrees of freedom of $DF = 1$ (this holds in all cases except for multinomial regression as discussed in Sect. 9.8).

The third page of the output describes the base model. Part of that output is provided in Table 5.2. The requested correlation structure is indicated, in this case AR1. A spatial type of autoregression has been requested with correlations determined by actual ages rather than by indexes of ages since the default setting of the spatial macro parameter is "y". The setting "spatial=n" can be used to request a standard autoregression using indexes of the withinvr variable values rather than their actual values. An equivalent model would be generated in this case since the measurements are equally spaced. By default the macro parameter GEE has value "n", meaning generate maximum likelihood (ML) estimates of model parameters as used by PROC MIXED. The setting "GEE=y" requests that model parameters be estimated using generalized estimating equations (GEE) as used by PROC GENMOD. Also provided are the number of matched sets, in this case 27 children, the maximum number of values within the matched sets, in this case 4 for ages of 8, 10, 12, and 14 years, and the total number of observed measurements, in this case 108. The symbol m used in the genreg output denotes the total number of observed measurements for all matched sets (the same as the symbol m(SC) used in the formulations of Chap. 4 and not the same as the symbol m used in those formulations). The lower limit on the correlation parameter in this case is -1 since age has integer values. When the withinvr variable values include non-integer values, the lower limit for AR1 models with "spatial=y" is set to 0 rather than -1 so that correlations are well defined (see Sect. 4.5.1). The base model has constant means with estimated value 24.1 and constant variances with estimate 9.1 and so estimated constant standard deviations 3.0. The estimated within-subject correlation is 0.82.

Table 5.2 The base model for the adaptive moderation analysis of dental measurements in terms of age and the indicator male for the child being a boy

model correlation structure:	AR1
spatial type:	Y
GEE:	N
# of matched sets:	27
maximum # of distinct values within matched sets:	4
m, the number of measurements:	108
lower limit on correlation:	-1

base expectation component

predictor	power	estimate
XINTRCPT	1	24.082827

...

estimated correlation:	0.8248712
MLE of outcome variance:	9.0603893
MLE of outcome standard deviation:	3.0100481
log likelihood:	-247.0784
-2 log likelihood:	494.15676
average log likelihood:	-2.287763
mth root of the likelihood:	0.1014933

...

mth root of the likelihood using deleted predictions:	0.0939084

When "spatial=y" as in this case, this is the correlation for measurements one unit apart, 1 year in this case. The estimated correlation for these data under "spatial=n" would be for 1 index value apart or 2 years, and so its value would be the square of the one reported for "spatial=y". Values are also reported for the log-likelihood $\log(L)$, $-2 \cdot \log(L)$, the average log likelihood $\log(L)/m$, and the mth root of the likelihood $\exp(\log(L)/m) = L^{1/m}$. The LCV score for the base model rounds to 0.09391.

The fourth page of the output (not provided here) describes the macro parameter settings controlling the expansion step. The fifth page describes the expanded model. Table 5.4 contains part of that output. Informally, GCs are generated as follows (see Chap. 20 for the formal process). First the best transforms are identified for each of the variables in the expxvars list. For example, at the first step of the expansion, the best power for age is $age^{2.5}$. Each of these transforms is used as the first term of a GC with the other terms being transforms of the other variables in the expxvars list. For example, the GC generated for age is $XGC\_1 = age^{2.5} \cdot male$. As terms are added to the GC, the powers for previously added terms like $age^{2.5}$ are not adjusted. However, the resulting GC may not be the best choice. Rather than readjusting each of the powers of each of the terms of the generated GC, the whole GC is transformed with a single power. In this case, $age^{2.5} \cdot male$ is raised to the power 1.3 so that is it is equivalent to using the GC $(age^{2.5} \cdot male)^{1.3} = age^{3.25} \cdot male$. If the LCV score for a generated transformed GC improves on the LCV score for its initial single variable transform, then the GC replaces that single

Table 5.3 The expanded model for the adaptive moderation analysis of dental measurements in terms of age and the indicator male for the child being a boy

```
              geometric combination expectation variables:
                    XGC_1    age**(2.5)*male
                    XGC_2    male*age**(6)
                    XGC_3    male*age**(-14)

model correlation structure:                                        AR1
spatial type:                                                         Y
GEE:                                                                  N

                  expanded expectation component

        predictor     power    estimate        score    order

        XINTRCPT        1     18.988357     0.0939084      0
        XGC_1          1.3     0.0011885     0.111065       1
        age            1.5     0.0978036     0.1131745      2
        XGC_2           1     -3.918E-7     0.1137378      3
        XGC_3           1      3.371E12     0.1135572      4
...
mth root of the likelihood using deleted predictions:       0.1135572
```

variable transform. The transform added to the model next at each step of the expansion is the single variable power transform or transformed GC generating the best LCV score over all variables. In this case, the transformed GC $(age^{2.5} \cdot male)^{1.3}$ is added to the model first, followed by the transforms: $age^{1.5}$, $male \cdot age^{6}$, and $male \cdot age^{-14}$. The LCV score for the expanded model rounds to 0.11356. Note that at the fourth step in the expansion, the addition of the transformed GC $male \cdot age^{-14}$ causes the LCV score to decrease. The expansion allows the LCV score to decrease as long as the decrease is not too large as controlled by the expansion stopping tolerance parameter (see Sect. 20.4.5).

The sixth page of the output (not provided here) describes the macro parameter settings controlling the contraction step. The seventh page describes the contracted model. Table 5.3 contains part of that output. The transforms $XGC\_1^{1.3} = (age^{2.5} \cdot male)^{1.3}$ and $XGC\_2 = male \cdot age^{6}$ are removed in that order and then the intercept. Transforms of age and $XGC\_3 = male \cdot age^{-14}$ are left in the model with powers adjusted to 0.19 and -0.15, respectively, so that the final model is based on $age^{0.19}$ and $(male \cdot age^{-14})^{-0.15} = male \cdot age^{2.1}$ without an intercept. The estimated slopes for these two transforms are 14.5 and 0.014. The estimated autocorrelation is 0.78, the estimated standard deviation 2.2, and the LCV score rounds to 0.11467, as reported in Sect. 4.5.4. This is a little larger than the LCV score of 0.11464 for the model generated with the directly specified interaction agemale, which is based on the similar transforms $age^{0.18}$ and $agemale^{2.2}$ without an intercept as reported in Sect. 4.5.3, supporting the validity of the heuristics for generating GCs. Consequently, GCs are used in subsequent moderation analyses.

Models based on standard interactions (i.e., products of untransformed predictors like age·male) can be generated as follows.

```
%genreg(modtype=NORML,datain=dentdata,yvar=dentmeas,
        matchvar=subject,withinvr=age,corrtype=AR1,
        foldcnt=&kfold,expand=Y,geomcmbn=y,
        expxvars=age male,exptrans=n,multtrns=n,
        contract=y,cnretrns=n,condtrns=n,
        procmod=y);
```

The setting "exptrans=n" means do not transform variables in the expxvars list and so also in generated GCs (as opposed to the default setting "exptrans=y" meaning transform variables in the expxvars list and associated GCs). This requires the setting "multtrns=n" indicating that at most one transform of an expxvars variable is to be included in the expanded model (as opposed to the default setting "multtrns=y" meaning allow multiple transforms of variables in the expxvars list). The setting "cnretrns=n" means do not retransform remaining transforms in the model with each contraction (as is done under the default setting "cnretrns=y"). In this case, the expansion first adds in the variable age, then the interaction male·age, and stops. The contraction leaves the expanded model unchanged. Since this would result in a conditional transformation step, possibly changing powers to non-unit values under the default setting "condtrns=y", "condtrns=n" is needed to skip that conditional transformation step. The PROC REG output (generated since "procmod=y"; but not provided here) indicates that both terms of this model are significant ($P < 0.001$).

5.3.3 Residual Analysis of the Adaptive Marginal Moderation Model

Residual analyses can be conducted for marginal models like the model of Table 5.4 as follows.

```
%genreg(modtype=NORML,datain=dentdata,yvar=dentmeas,
        matchvar=subject,withinvr=age,corrtype=AR1,
        foldcnt=&kfold,xintrcpt=n,xvars=age,
        xpowers=0.19,xgcs=male 1 age -14,
        xgcpowrs=-0.15,ranlysis=y);
```

The xgcs macro parameter is used to generate base expectation (x) models with GCs, in this case with the single GC male·age^{-14}. The xgcpowrs macro parameter is used to power transform these GCs, in this case the GC male·age^{-14} is transformed into (male·age$^{-14})^{-0.15}$ = male·age$^{2.1}$. Multiple GCs can be specified by separating

Table 5.4 The contracted model for the adaptive moderation analysis of dental measurements in terms of age and the indicator male for the child being a boy

```
            contracted expectation component

            predictor old power new power    estimate

            age                      1.5    0.19   14.477338
            XGC_3                      1   -0.15    0.0138428

            discarded    old power        score order

                                 .    0.1135572   0
            XGC_1                1.3    0.1144449   1
            XGC_2                  1    0.1138231   2
            XINTRCPT               1    0.1146714   3
...
estimated correlation:                            0.7793193
MLE of outcome variance:                          4.9091404
MLE of outcome standard deviation:                2.215658
...

mth root of the likelihood using deleted predictions:    0.1146714
```

them by colons (:). Each GC consists of pairs of variable names and associated powers. For example, the following two macro parameter settings

```
xgcs=male 1 age -14 : age 4 log_age 2 male,xgcpowrs=-0.15 0.25
```

request the same GC and power as before along with $(age^4 \cdot (\log(age))^2 \cdot male)^{0.25}$ $= age \cdot (\log(age))^{0.5} \cdot male$. Adding in the setting "procmod=y" to the above genreg invocation requests generation of the equivalent model using PROC MIXED. Note that the covariance structure of PROC MIXED is set with the "type=" option of the repeated statement. The choice "type=AR(1)" supported by PROC MIXED uses the indexes of the age values to compute correlations (as for "spatial=n"), not the actual age values as used above. That is the same as the PROC MIXED setting "type=SP(POW)(age)", a spatial autoregression with correlations determined by raising an autocorrelation parameter to powers given by absolute values of differences of age values.

As for the univariate outcome residual analysis reported in Sect. 2.18, scaled residuals (as defined in Sect. 4.3.3) are loaded into the dataout data set under the name stdres (containing standardized residuals for univariate outcomes and scaled residuals for multivariate outcomes), which can be changed with the stdrsvar macro parameter. The associated plot is given in Fig. 5.1. With one distinct exception, the scaled residuals are reasonably close to symmetric, well within ±3, and with similar spread for each predicted value. The exception with scaled residual 4.24 corresponds to the dental measurement for the male child with subject = 20 at 12 years old with value 31 mm compared to much smaller values of 23, 20.5, and 26 mm at

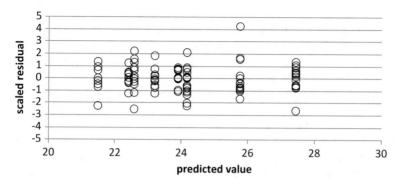

Fig. 5.1 Scaled residual plot for the adaptive marginal order 1 autoregressive model for the dental measurement data

ages 8, 10, and 14 years old. This child's dental measurements fluctuate more than would be expected, resulting in this outlying measurement. EC correlations generate a substantially better model than this one, but the scaled residuals are similar (not displayed here) with the same extreme outlier.

A sensitivity analysis assessing the effect of the extreme outlier on the conclusions can be conducted using the following code.

```
data reduced;
  set dentdata;
  if subject=20 & age=12 then delete;
run;
*  the adaptive model for the reduced data;
%genreg(modtype=NORML,datain=reduced,yvar=dentmeas,
        matchvar=subject,withinvr=age,corrtype=AR1,
        foldcnt=&kfold,measdlte=y,expand=Y,
        geomcmbn=y,expxvars=age male,contract=y,
        ranalysis=y);
*  adaptive model generated with the full data using the reduced data;
%genreg(modtype=NORML,datain=reduced,yvar=dentmeas,
        matchvar=subject,withinvr=age,corrtype=AR1,
        foldcnt=&kfold,measdlte=y,xintrcpt=n,
        xvars=age,xpowers=0.19,xgcs=male 1 age -14,
        xgcpowrs=-0.15);
```

First, the reduced data set is created by making a copy of the dentdata data set and removing the outlier. Then, an adaptive model is generated for the reduced data. It contains the two transforms: $age^{0.18}$ and $(male \cdot age^{0.8})^4$ without an intercept. The power for age has not changed, but the GC now includes age raised to the power $0.8 \cdot 4 = 3.2$ rather than to the power $(-14) \cdot (-0.15) = 2.1$. Next, the model generated for the full data is computed using the reduced data. Since there is now a missing outcome measurement, the LCV scores for these two models are computed with measurement-wise deletion (see Sect. 4.13). due to the setting "measdlte=y". Whether the removal of the outlier has a substantive effect can be addressed with a LCV ratio test. For data with 107 measurements, the cutoff for a substantive PD is 1.78 %. The first model has LCV score 0.14398 and the second 0.14381, and so the PD for the adaptive model generated by the full data is insubstantial at 0.12 %. This indicates that the full-data model is a competitive alternative for the reduced data with the outlier removed, and so the outlier does not have a highly influential effect on conclusions for the dental measurement data.

A residual analysis is requested in the above code (with the setting "ranlysis=y") for the adaptive reduced-data model to assess whether this latter model produces any new outliers. A second outlier is identified with standardized residual 3.30, corresponding to the measurement of 24.5 mm at age 10 years old for the male child with subject $= 24$ having much smaller prior measurement of 17.0 mm at 8 years old and measurements of 26 and 29.5 mm at 12 and 14 years old. A second sensitivity analysis also removing this second outlier generates an adaptive model based on the three transforms: $age^{0.27}$, $(male \cdot age)^{1.8}$, and $(age^{11.1} \cdot male)^{-1}$ without an intercept and no outliers. For data with 106 measurements, the cutoff for a substantive PD is 1.80 %. The measurement-wise LCV score for the adaptive model for the data with the two outliers removed is 0.15255 while the model generated for the full data has LCV score 0.14865 with substantial PD of 2.56 % and the model generated with only the first outlier removed has LCV score 0.14895 with substantial PD 2.36 %. These results indicate that these two outliers combined have a highly influential effect on conclusions for the full dental measurement data.

Under this revised model, the estimated autocorrelation increases to 0.88 (compared to 0.78 for the full data as reported in Sect. 4.5.4) while the estimated variance remains at 2.2. Estimated means are displayed in Fig. 5.2. Compared to Fig. 4.1, the estimated means for male children appear more nonlinear while there is no apparent difference for female children, which is to be expected since the two outliers were for male children)

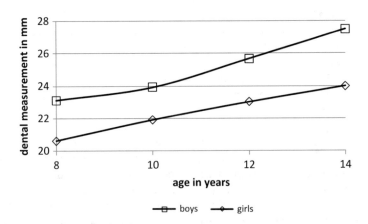

Fig. 5.2 Estimated mean dental measurements based on adaptive marginal AR1 modeling

This sensitivity analysis is based on removal of only outlying measurements. An alternate approach is to remove all observations of matched sets containing any outlying measurements. That seems more appropriate for larger data sets, for which measurements for any matched set are a very small subset of all available measurements.

5.4   Conditional Modeling of Means for the Dental Measurement Data

5.4.1   Transition Models for Mean Dental Measurement

A transition model for mean dental measurements accounting for dependence in terms of the previous measurement can be generated as follows.

```
%genreg(modtype=NORML,datain=dentdata,yvar=dentmeas,
        matchvar=subject,withinvr=age,conditnl=y,
        corrtype=IND,foldcnt=&kfold,expand=y,
        expxvars=age male pre_dentmeas_age_1
                 pre_dentmeas_age_1_miss,
        geomcmbn=y,contract=y);
```

The macro parameter setting "conditnl=y" requests a conditional model requiring the independent correlation structure requested by "corrtype=IND" (which is the default setting and hence not needed). The variables PRE(y,1) and PRE(y,1,$\varnothing$) of Sects. 4.7 and 4.8 are called pre_dentmeas_age_1 and pre_dentmeas_age_1_miss in the above code, and so this is the special case of a transition model. These variables do not need to be computed prior to requesting the model; they are generated automatically with their values determined by their names. The prefix "pre_" denotes a prior dependence predictor. This is followed by the name of the variable whose prior values are to be used in computing the variable, the variable dentmeas in this case, then by the variable whose values are to be used to determine which values are prior, the variable age in this case, and then the indexes for the prior values to be averaged to generate the dependence predictor values, in this case just the first prior value. The variable pre_dentmeas_age_2 has values equal to the second most prior dentmeas value if any while pre_dentmeas_age_1_2 has values equal to the average of the prior two dentmeas values (or just the prior one if that is the only prior measurement). Adding the suffix "_miss" to any one of these variables generates the indicator for that variable having a value of zero due to there being no prior measurements to average. These names can get fairly long, and so it is possible to reduce the length of these names. Assuming a copy of the dentmeas variable has been loaded into the dentdata data set under the name y, the two variables used in the above code can be changed to pre_y_age_1 and pre_y_age_1_m (with "_m" an abbreviation for "_miss"). These names will be used in what follows for brevity. The variables names, like y and age, embedded in dependence predictors, like pre_y_age_1, must not contain underscore (_) characters since these are used to break the dependence predictor names into their components. Variables with names beginning with "pre_" are computed using unweighted averages of prior values. Weighted averages are obtained by using the prefix "wpre_".

The expanded model for the above code has the seven transforms added in the following order: $(age^{1.5} \cdot pre\_y\_age\_1^{3.5})^{0.99}$, $male \cdot age^{2.2}$, $(pre\_y\_age\_1^{-4} \cdot age^{-1})^{0.9}$, $male \cdot pre\_y\_age\_1^{-7}$, $(pre\_y\_age\_1^{3.4} \cdot age)^{2.017}$, $pre\_y\_age\_1^3 \cdot age^{0.1}$, and $male \cdot pre\_y\_age\_1^{1.7} \cdot age^{1.2}$ with LCV score 0.12637. The contraction removes four of these transforms, adjusts the powers generating the transforms $(male \cdot pre\_y\_age\_1^{-7})^{0.7}$, $(pre\_y\_age\_1^{3.4} \cdot age)^2$, $(pre\_y\_age\_1^3 \cdot age^{0.1})^{-2}$, and leaves in the intercept. The LCV score is 0.12813 as reported in Sect. 4.8.1.

A transition model for mean dental measurements accounting for dependence in terms of the average of the up to two previous measurements can be generated as follows.

```
%genreg(modtype=NORML,datain=dentdata,yvar=dentmeas,
        matchvar=subject,withinvr=age,conditnl=y,
        corrtype=IND,foldcnt=&kfold,expand=Y,
        expxvars=age male pre_y_age_1_2
                 pre_y_age_1_2_m,
        geomcmbn=y,contract=Y);
```

The expanded model for the above code has the five transforms added in the following order: $(age^{1.5} \cdot pre\_y\_age\_1\_2^5)^{0.99}$, $male \cdot age^2$, $(male \cdot pre\_y\_age\_1\_2^{1.7} \cdot age^{1.6})^{1.1}$, $(pre\_y\_age\_1\_2^{-3} \cdot age^2)^7$, and $(male \cdot pre\_y\_age\_1\_2^{-1} \cdot age^{-1})^{-1}$. The LCV score is 0.13186. The contraction removes the third transform and adjusts the powers of some of the remaining transforms. The LCV score is 0.13363 as reported in Sect. 4.8.3. This model is used to generate the estimates of Figs. 4.2–4.4.

5.4.2   Residual Analysis of the Adaptive Transition Model

A residual analysis can be generated for this latter transition model as follows.

```
%genreg(modtype=NORML,datain=dentdata,yvar=dentmeas,
        matchvar=subject,withinvr=age,conditnl=Y,
        corrtype=IND,foldcnt=&kfold,
        xgcs=age 1.5 pre_y_age_1_2 5 :
             male 1 age 2 :pre_y_age_1_2 -3 age 2 :
             male 1 pre_y_age_1_2 -1 age -1,
        xgcpowrs=0.99 1.2 7 -1.9,ranlysis=y,
        procmod=y);
```

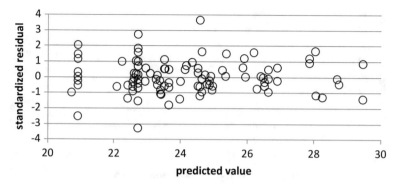

Fig. 5.3 Standardized residual plot for the adaptive transition model for the dental measurement data

The setting "procmod=y" requests that the results be generated for the model by the associated SAS PROC, PROC REG in this case of a transition model. A residual analysis is requested through the "ranlysis=y" option as for marginal models. Since "corrtype=IND" for conditional models, standardized residuals are computed (as in Chap. 2 analyses) rather than scaled residuals as computed for marginal models.

The associated standardized residual plot is displayed in Fig. 5.3. Now there are two extreme outliers. The one with standardized residual greater than 3 corresponds to the same extreme outlier of Fig. 5.1. The one with standardized residual less than -3 corresponds to the measurement of 17.0 mm at age 8 years for the male child with subject $= 24$ and much larger measurements of 24.5, 26, and 29.5 mm at 10, 12, and 14 years old (the same subject but a different measurement identified in the sensitivity analysis as an outlier for the marginal AR1 model).

A sensitivity analysis can be conducted to assess the effect of outliers on transition models, as is conducted for marginal models in Sect. 5.3. For the reduced data with 106 measurements, the cutoff for a substantive PD is 1.80 %. The LCV score (using measurement-wise deletion since now there are some missing measurements) computed for the full-data model applied to these reduced data is 0.14974. The adaptive model generated for the reduced data has LCV score is 0.15795, and so the PD for the full-data model is substantial at 5.20 %. This indicates that results for the full-data analysis are highly influenced by the two outlying measurements. However, there are now no new outliers.

The adaptive model generated for the reduced data includes the four transforms: $(\text{pre\_y\_age\_1\_2}^{6.2} \cdot \text{age}^{0.7})^{0.74}$, $\text{male} \cdot \text{pre\_y\_age\_1\_2\_m} \cdot \text{age}^{2.3}$, $(\text{male} \cdot \text{age}^{2.1} \cdot \text{pre\_y\_age\_1\_2}^{-3})^{3}$, and $(\text{pre\_y\_age\_1\_2}^{-5} \cdot \text{age}^{2.8})^{1.6}$ with an intercept. The estimated standard deviation is 1.5. Estimated mean values are plotted in Fig. 5.4. The estimates for boys still tend to increase with age at given averages of the prior two dental measurements, but with less increase than in Fig. 4.2. There is little difference with age for girls at given averages of the prior two dental measurements.

Whether this relationship is distinctly nonlinear or not can be assessed by comparison to the associated linear relationship model generated using the "exptrans=n", "multtrns=n", "condtrns=n", and "cnretrns=n" options as follows.

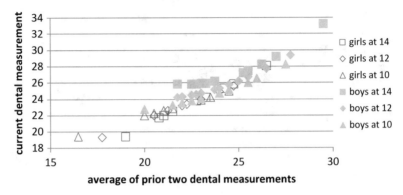

Fig. 5.4 Estimated mean dental measurements based on transition modeling for the dental measurement data with outlying measurements removed

```
%genreg(modtype=NORML,datain=reduced,yvar=dentmeas,
      matchvar=subject,withinvr=age,conditnl=y,
      corrtype=IND,foldcnt=&kfold,expand=Y,
      expxvars=age male pre_y_age_1_2
              pre_y_age_1_2_m,geomcmbn=y,
      exptrans=n,multtrns=n,contract=Y,cnretrns=n,
      condtrns=n);
```

The generated model is based on the untransformed predictors: age·pre_y_age_1_2·male, pre_y_age_1_2, pre_y_age_1_2_m, agemale without an intercept. The LCV score is 0.15288 with substantial PD of 3.21 % compared to the adaptive transition model for these reduced data. Consequently, the patterns described in Fig. 5.4 are distinctly nonlinear.

5.4.3   General Conditional Models for Mean Dental Measurement

General conditional models can be generated similarly to transition models. For example, the variables POST(y,1), POST(y,1,∅), POST(y,1,2), and POST(y,1,2,∅) of Sect. 4.9 are named post_y_age_1, post_y_age_1_m, post_y_age_1_2, and post_y_age_1_2_m. The variables OTHER(y,1), OTHER (y,1,∅), OTHER (y,1,2), and OTHER (y,1,2,∅) of Sect. 4.9 are named other_y_age_1, other_y_age_1_m, other_y_age_1_2, and other_y_age_1_2_m. Pseudolikelihood CV (PLCV) scores for both the transition and general conditional models induced by a marginal model can be generated in the output for marginal models by adding the setting "condscrs=y". The induced transition model is equivalent to the marginal model inducing it, and so its generated PLCV score is the same as the LCV score for the marginal model. Variables with names beginning with "post_" ("other_") are computed using unweighted averages of subsequent (prior and subsequent) values. Weighted averages are obtained by using the prefix "wpost_" ("wother").

5.5 Analyzing the Exercise Data

The exercise data are also available on the Internet (see Supplementary Materials) in wide/broad format and so can be loaded in and converted to long format similarly to the dental measurement data. Missing strength measurements should not be outputted to the long format data set. These are deleted by PROC MIXED, but the genreg macro generates an error message if the yvar variable has missing values. Otherwise, analyses can be conducted using similar code to that presented for analyzing the dental measurement data, except that analyses using measurement-wise deletion are requested using the setting "measdlte=y". Thus, example code for analyzing these data is not presented here. Code to load in and analyze these data is available on the Internet (see Supplementary Materials). For the special cases of transition and general conditional models, "measdlte=y" requires that deleted parameter estimates be computed using pre_, post_, and other_ type predictors recomputed for each complement of each fold. The alternative setting "measdlte=p" requests partial measurement-wise deletion using "pre_", "post_", and "other_" type predictors as computed for the full data to compute measurement-wise deletion parameter estimates to reduce the computations. Since measurements are assigned to the same folds under "measdlte=y" and "measdlte=p", associated LCV scores are comparable.

5.6 Modeling Variances as Well as Means

5.6.1 Marginal Models for Dental Measurements

An adaptive marginal ML-based model for means and variances of the dental measurements using EC correlations can be generated by adding an expvvars list of primary predictors as follows.

```
%genreg(modtype=NORML,datain=dentdata,yvar=dentmeas,
        matchvar=subject,withinvr=age,corrtype=EC,
        foldcnt=&kfold,expand=Y,geomcmbn=y,
        expxvars=age male,expvvars=age male,
        contract=y);
```

The output includes estimated parameter values for the log variance model (not displayed here; see Sect. 3.14 for an example of log variance model output). The generated model has LCV score 0.13570 (as reported in Sect. 4.15.2). The associated GEE-based model with standard bias-adjusted covariance estimates can be generated as follows.

```
%genreg(modtype=NORML,datain=dentdata,yvar=dentmeas,
        matchvar=subject,withinvr=age,corrtype=EC,
        GEE=y,biasadj=y,foldcnt=&kfold,expand=y,geomcmbn=y,
        expxvars=age male,expvvars=age male,
        contract=y);
```

An assessment of the effect of consideration of non-constant variances on the model for the means can be conducted by starting with the model for the means generated with constant variances and adaptively generating a non-constant variances model while holding the model for the means fixed. For the case of ML-based marginal modeling with EC correlations, the model for the means under constant variances is based on the transforms: $age^{0.21}$ and $(age^2 \cdot male)^{0.903}$ without an intercept. An adaptive model for the variances holding this model for the means fixed can be generated as follows.

```
%genreg(modtype=NORML,datain=dentdata,yvar=dentmeas,
        matchvar=subject,withinvr=age,corrtype=EC,
        foldcnt=&kfold,xintrcpt=n,xvars=age,xpowers=0.21,
        xgcs=age 2 male 1,xgcpowrs=0.903,expand=y,geomcmbn=y,
        expvvars=age male,contract=y,nocnxbas=y,
        notrxbas=y);
```

The base model for the means is not changed in the expansion because the expxvars parameter has its default empty setting, but the contraction might change that model. By default, the contraction considers removing next a transform from the model for the means or from the model for the variances. This process is adjusted in the above code to hold the model for the means fixed with the settings "nocnxbas=y", meaning do not contract the base model for the means, and "notrxbas=y", meaning do not transform that base model. Alternately, the "nocnxbas=y" setting can be replaced by the setting "contordr=v", meaning change from the default contraction order (with setting "contordr=."), considering both the mean (or "x") and variance (or "v") components of the model in combination, to the contraction order considering only the variance component of the model. The setting "notrxbas=y" is still needed in case a conditional transformation is invoked to limit its effect to the variance component. As reported in Sect. 4.15.2, the LCV score for the generated model is 0.13528 with insubstantial PD of 0.31 % compared to the model generating means and variances in combination, indicating that the model for the means has not changed substantially with consideration of non-constant variances.

The contraction order for both means and variances can also be changed to contract the means before the variances with the setting "contordr=xv" or to contract the variances before the means with the setting "contordr=vx". The expansion order for means and variances is controlled in the same way with the

Table 5.5 Comparison of alternative expansion and contraction orders for adaptive modeling of both means and variances for dental measurements in terms of age, the indicator male for the child being a boy, and geometric combinations using marginal models with maximum likelihood parameter estimation and exchangeable correlations

Expansion order	Contraction order	Predictors for the means	Predictors for the variances[a]	LCV score	Percent decrease from best LCV score (%)
Means and variances in combination	Means and variances in combination	$age^{0.23}$, age^2 ·male	1, male	0.13570	0.14
Means then variances	Means then variances	$age^{0.23}$, $(age^2$ ·male$)^{1.103}$	1, male	0.13567	0.16
Variances then means	Means then variances	$age^{0.22}$, $(age^{1.5}$ ·male$)^{1.1}$	1, $(male·age^{11})^2$	0.13541	0.35
Means then variances	Variances then means	$age^{0.23}$, $age^{2·}$ male	1, male	0.13570	0.14
Variances then means	Variances then means	$age^{0.23}$, $(age^{1.5}$ ·male$)^{1.6}$	1, $(age^{2.3}$ ·male$)^{-0.3}$	0.13589	0.00

LCV: likelihood cross-validation
[a]The predictor 1 corresponds to including an intercept in the model

expordr parameter with default setting "expordr=." as well as settings "expordr=xv" and "expordr=vx" with the same meanings as for the contordr parameter. A comparison of alternative combinations of these expansion and contraction orders is provided in Table 5.5 for adaptive ML-based modeling with EC correlations. While different models are generated for the cases of Table 5.5, all models have competitive LCV scores. These results indicate that consideration of alternative expansion and contraction orders is not needed for this case, suggesting that this may hold more generally at least for modeling of multivariate continuous outcomes. It also provides support for the effectiveness of the default expansion and contraction orders used in the adaptive modeling process.

5.6.2   Transition Models for Dental Measurements

An adaptive transition model for means and variances can be generated by adding an expvvars list of primary predictors as follows.

```
%genreg(modtype=NORML,datain=dentdata,yvar=dentmeas,
        matchvar=subject,withinvr=age,corrtype=IND,
        conditnl=y,foldcnt=&kfold,expand=Y,geomcmbn=y,
        expxvars=age male pre_y_age_1_2 pre_y_age_1_2_m,
        expvvars=age male pre_y_age_1_2 pre_y_age_1_2_m,
        contract=Y);
```

The generated transition model is shown in Sect. 4.15.2 to provide a distinct improvement over the best constant variances transition model of Sect. 4.8.3. Consequently, a residual analysis as conducted in Sect. 5.4 is needed, but will not be addressed here for brevity (it is left as an exercise). The adaptive transition (and general conditional) modeling process can be applied to a contiguous subset of the withinvr values rather than to all of them. The first and last withinvr values to be modeled are controlled by the winfst and winlst macro parameters. The default values "." for these parameters mean to use the first and last withinvr values, respectively. For example, adding "winfst=2" to the above code requests transition modeling of dentmeas starting at the second withinvr value 10 up to the last value 14. The age 8 values are still used to compute dependence predictors and so affect the results. This can speed up processing when there are many withinvr values.

As mentioned in Sect. 5.4.1, names of conditional variables can be fairly long and so genreg output in some cases may take up more lines than usual. This can be avoided using the condvars macro parameter to create conditional variables with shorter names. For example, the above adaptive transition model for means and variances can alternately be generated as follows.

```
%genreg(modtype=NORML,datain=dentdata,yvar=dentmeas,
        matchvar=subject,withinvr=age,corrtype=IND,
        conditnl=y,foldcnt=&kfold,
        condvars=pre y age 1 2 : pre y age 1 2 m,
        expand=Y,geomcmbn=y,
        expxvars=age male pre_1 pre_2,
        expvvars=age male pre_1 pre_2,contract=Y);
```

The setting for condvars contains one or more conditional variable specifications separated by colons (:). Each specification contains the same components as used to name conditional variables and in the same order, but separated by blanks rather than by underscores (_). The generated names for these variables start with the type (for example, "pre" in the above code), followed by an underscore, and then by an index number starting at 1. For example, the two conditional variables generated by the above code are called pre_1 and pre_2 with pre_1 the same as pre_y_age_1_2 and pre_2 the same as pre_y_age_1_2_m. These names can then be used in defining models as they are used in the above code in the expxvars and expvvars parameter settings. One of the advantages of defining conditional variables through condvars is that the name of variables included in those specifications can contain underscores, which is not allowed with direct naming of conditional variables.

5.6.3   Clock Time Assessments

The adaptive modeling process is not instantaneous. For example, generating the adaptive marginal EC-based model for means and variances requires about 11.7 min of clock time while the generating the adaptive transition model for the means and variances requires about 3.3 min. These are tolerable amounts of time, but times can get much longer as the number of measurements and/or the number of primary expansion predictors increases. The contraction step usually requires most of the time since it involves retransforming remaining transforms with the removal of each transform. For example, the expansion step for the EC-based marginal model requires about 3.2 min or 27 % of the time compared to 1.5 min or 47 % of the time for the transition model. The expanded EC model adds four terms for the means and three terms for the variances (not counting intercepts) for a total of seven terms while the expanded transition model adds five terms for the means and two terms for the variances also for a total of seven. The transition model expansion is more efficient requiring about 0.21 min per expansion transform compared to 0.46 min per expansion transform for the marginal EC model (due to the extra computation to estimate correlations for marginal models not needed for transition models). The contraction time can be reduced using the option "cnretrns=n" to turn off the retransformation (as opposed to the default setting "cnretrns=y" meaning to retransform remaining model transforms with each removal of a transform in the contraction). However, retransformation usually produces distinctly superior models.

In this case, the transition model is computed in about 28 % of the time needed to compute the EC-based marginal model. So for complex analyses involving large numbers of primary predictors and/or large number of measurements, it may be practical to consider only transition models. Also, the clock time to compute the GEE-based marginal model for the means and variances is about 24.7 min or about 2.1 times as long as computing the EC-based marginal model and about 7.5 times as long for the transition model. These timing results together with the fact that in reported analyses the ML-based marginal model has at least a competitive and sometimes a distinctly better LCV score compared to the score of the GEE-based marginal model while the transition model distinctly outperforms the GEE-based marginal model suggest that GEE modeling can reasonably not be considered, at least for multivariate continuous outcomes.

5.7   Practice Exercises

5.1 Using the extended data set of Practice Exercises 3.1–3.4, generate the adaptive model for means in NObnded, SO2index, rain, and GCs in these three predictors with constant variances. Compare the results to those for the second part of Exercise 3.3 to assess what benefits there are in using automatically generated GCs over standard interactions. Conduct a residual analysis for the better of the selected models for the second part of Exercise 3.3 and for Exercise 5.1. If there are any outliers with standardized residuals outside of ± 3, conduct a sensitivity analysis using the reduced data with those outliers removed to compare the model selected for the full data with the associated model selected for the outlier-reduced data. Conduct a residual analysis for the adaptive reduced-data model and iterate this process until no outliers are identified.

5.2 Using the bodyfat data set of Practice Exercises 3.5–3.8, generate the adaptive model for means in height, weight, and GCs in these two predictors with constant variances. Compare the results to those for BMI generated as part of Exercise 3.5. Does consideration of general GCs provide a distinct improvement in predicting bodyfat over using BMI, the standard GC for combining height and weight? Next generate the adaptive model for both means and variances in height, weight, and GCs in these two predictors. Compare this model to the one for means in height, weight, and GCs in these two predictors with constant variances. Are variances distinctly non-constant in height, weight, and GCs?

5.3 Using the dental measurement data, assess the impact of centering age on the adaptive nonlinear moderation analysis for mean dental measurements as a function of age, the indicator variable male, and GCs. Use LCV with matched-set-wise deletion since there are no missing outcome measurements and with 5 folds (see Sect. 4.5.2). Generate models with age replaced by age centered at each integer value between the lowest observed age of 8 and the largest observed age of 14. Which choice generates the best LCV score? Is this a competitive alternative to the nonlinear GC-based moderation model in uncentered age? Does it matter how age is centered in the sense that all centerings generate competitive alternatives or some are distinctly inferior?

5.4 Using the dental measurement data, conduct a residual analysis of the adaptive transition model for the means and variances identified in Sect. 4.15.2 and discussed in Sect. 5.6. Are there any outliers with scaled residuals outside the range of ± 3? If so, conduct a sensitivity analysis to determine if these outliers are highly influential on the conclusions for the full data, removing only any outlying dental measurements. Conduct a residual analysis for the adaptive reduced-data model and iterate this process until no outliers are identified. Use LCV with matched-set-wise deletion when modeling the full data since there are no missing outcome measurements and with 5 folds (see Sect. 4.5.2). Change to measurement-wise deletion with 5 folds for modeling reduced data with outliers removed. Compare results to those for the residual analysis of the constant variances transition model reported in Sect. 5.4.2.

   For Practice Exercises 5.5–5.7, use the Treatment of Lead-Exposed Children (TLC) Study data available on the Internet (see Supplementary Materials). The long format data set is called longtlc. The outcome variable for this data set is called lead and contains blood lead levels in micrograms/dL. The two predictors are succimer, the indicator for being on the chelating agent succimer versus on a placebo, and week with values 0, 1, 4, and 6 weeks into the study. There are 100 subjects in this study, all with the complete set of 4 measurements. Since there are no missing data values, use matched-set-wise deletion to compute LCV scores for all analyses of the full TLC data.

5.5. For the TLC data, use the adaptive model for the mean blood lead level in week with AR1 correlations as a benchmark analysis to set the number of folds for LCV scores. Use ML parameter estimation and constant variances for all analyses of this exercise. Compare this AR1 adaptive model to the adaptive model in week using EC correlations. Use the correlation structure generating the better LCV score in all subsequent marginal models generated for this practice exercise. Compare the adaptive model in week to the linear polynomial model in week and assess whether mean blood lead levels change distinctly nonlinearly or not. Generate the adaptive model in week, succimer, and GCs and assess whether being on succimer vs. a placebo moderates the effect of week on mean blood lead levels.

5.6. For the TLC data, use the number of folds selected in Practice Exercise 5.5 for all analyses of this practice exercise. Also, consider only constant variances models. First, generate the adaptive marginal model for the means using GEE parameter estimation in terms of week, succimer, and GCs and with the correlation structure selected in Practice Exercise 5.5. Compare this model to the associated marginal model using ML parameter estimation generated in Practice Exercise 5.5. Does GEE parameter estimation provide a distinct improvement over ML parameter estimation for modeling the means of these data? Next, generate the adaptive transition model for the means in week, succimer, pre_lead_week_1 (equal to the prior blood lead value for a subject if there is one and 0 if there is not a prior blood lead measurement), pre_lead_week_1_m (the indicator for the prior blood lead measurement for a subject being missing, which only occurs for baseline blood lead measurements at 0 weeks since there are no missing blood lead measurements), and GCs. Does transition modeling of means provide a distinct improvement over marginal modeling of means for these data?

5.7. For the TLC data, use the number of folds selected in Practice Exercise 5.5 for all analyses of this practice exercise. First, generate the adaptive marginal model for both the means and variances in terms of week, succimer, and GCs using ML parameter estimation and with the correlation structure selected in Practice Exercise 5.5. Compare this model to the associated model of Practice Exercise 5.5 to assess whether blood lead levels have distinctly non-constant variances or not. Next, generate the adaptive marginal model for both the means and variances in terms of week, succimer, and GCs using GEE parameter estimation and with the correlation structure selected in Practice Exercise 5.5. Does GEE parameter estimation provide a distinct improvement over ML parameter estimation for these data? Finally, generate the adaptive transition model for both the means and variances in week, succimer, pre_lead_week_1, pre_lead_week_1_m, and GCs. Does transition modeling of means provide a distinct improvement over marginal modeling of means and variances for these data?

References

Khattree, R., & Naik, D. N. (1999). *Applied multivariate statistics with SAS software* (2nd ed.). Cary, NC: SAS Institute.

Littell, R. C., Milliken, G. A., Stroup, R., Wolfinger, R. D., & Schabenberger, O. (2006). *SAS for mixed models* (2nd ed.). Cary, NC: SAS Institute.

Littell, R. C., Stroup, W. W., & Freund, R. J. (2002). *SAS for linear models* (4th ed.). Cary, NC: SAS Institute.

Chapter 6
Adaptive Transformation of Positive Valued Continuous Outcomes

6.1 Chapter Overview

This chapter formulates and demonstrates adaptive transformation of positive valued univariate and multivariate continuous outcomes as well as their predictors. A description of how to conduct adaptive analyses involving transformed outcomes as well their predictors in SAS is provided in Chap. 7.

Section 6.2 provides an overview of outcome power transformation while Sect. 6.3 formulates power transformation of outcomes as well as power-adjusted likelihood cross-validation (LCV) scores for selecting an appropriate power transform for an outcome variable. Sections 6.4–6.7 address the need for power transformation of the previously analyzed univariate death rate outcome of Sect. 2.2, the univariate simulated outcome of Sect. 2.12, the multivariate dental measurement outcome of Sect. 4.2, and the multivariate strength outcome of Sect. 4.12, respectively. Section 6.8 describes the plasma beta-carotene data not previously analyzed to be used in further outcome transformation analyses. Section 6.9 conducts adaptive analyses of the untransformed univariate outcome plasma beta-carotene while Sect. 6.10 addresses the need for transformation of this outcome. Sections 6.11–6.15 provide overviews of the results of the analyses of the five data sets analyzed in the chapter. Formulation sections are not needed to understand analysis sections.

6.2 Transformation of the Outcome Variable

This section addresses the use of Box-Tidwell power transforms y^λ for $\lambda \neq 0$ and $\log(y)$ for $\lambda = 0$ (Box and Tidwell 1962; although they consider these for transforming predictors not outcomes) of a positive valued continuous outcome variable y for real valued powers λ in adaptive modeling of such a transformed outcome in terms of possibly transformed predictors. Carroll and Ruppert (1984)

© Springer International Publishing Switzerland 2016
G.J. Knafl, K. Ding, *Adaptive Regression for Modeling Nonlinear Relationships*,
Statistics for Biology and Health, DOI 10.1007/978-3-319-33946-7_6

also allow for transformation of outcomes and predictors, but with transformation of the predictors that are partially based on theoretical considerations. They use Box-Cox transforms $(y^\lambda - 1)/\lambda$ of the outcome y, which converge to log(y) as λ converges to 0 (Box and Cox 1964). Box-Tidwell transformations are used instead since the case $\lambda = 1$ corresponds exactly to the untransformed outcome y rather than to $y - 1$ as for Box-Cox transforms. Only positive valued outcomes are considered for power transformation. Nonpositive valued outcomes could be shifted by a positive constant to make them positive or an adjustment like the one used in Sect. 4.6.1 for real valued predictors could be considered, but this issue is not addressed here.

For fixed values of λ, means and possibly variances of y^λ (or log(y) when $\lambda = 0$) are adaptively modeled as in prior analyses in terms of available primary predictors using unadjusted LCV scores based on the normal density. Results for these models are then used to compute power-adjusted LCV scores, denoted by LCV(λ), which are maximized to choose an appropriate value for λ. Power-adjusted LCV scores can also be computed for power transformed positive valued multivariate continuous outcomes using marginal models with parameter estimation based on either maximum likelihood (ML) or generalized estimating equations (GEE) or using transition models. General conditional models with parameters estimation based on maximum pseudolikelihood can have power transforms evaluated with power-adjusted pseudolikelihood cross-validation (PLCV). Section 6.3 provides the formulations, which can be skipped to focus on analyses.

6.3   Formulation for Power-Adjusted Likelihoods and LCV Scores

6.3.1   Univariate Outcomes

Assume that y is a positive valued univariate outcome with y^λ normally distributed for some real valued power λ. For $\lambda > 0$, y^λ has positive derivative $\lambda \cdot y^{\lambda-1}$ with respect to y and so is increasing in y. Hence, the distribution function $G(w; \lambda, \boldsymbol{\theta})$ for y satisfies

$$G(w; \lambda, \boldsymbol{\theta}) = P(y \leq w) = \Phi(w^\lambda; \boldsymbol{\theta}),$$

where Φ denotes the univariate normal distribution function with mean and variance determined by a vector of model parameters $\boldsymbol{\theta}$ (and so Φ in general does not correspond to the standard normal distribution function). Consequently, the power-adjusted density function $g(w; \lambda, \boldsymbol{\theta})$ for y satisfies

$$g(w; \lambda, \boldsymbol{\theta}) = \frac{d}{dw} P(y \leq w) = \lambda \cdot w^{\lambda-1} \cdot \phi(w^\lambda; \boldsymbol{\theta}),$$

where ϕ denotes the univariate normal density function (that is, the derivative of Φ). For $\lambda < 0$, y^λ has negative derivative $\lambda \cdot y^{\lambda-1}$ with respect to y and so is decreasing in y. Hence, the distribution function $G(w; \lambda, \boldsymbol{\theta})$ for y satisfies

$$G(w; \lambda, \boldsymbol{\theta}) = P(y \leq w) = 1 - \Phi(w^\lambda; \boldsymbol{\theta})$$

and so

$$g(w; \lambda, \boldsymbol{\theta}) = \frac{d}{dw} P(y \leq w) = -\lambda \cdot w^{\lambda-1} \cdot \phi(w^\lambda; \boldsymbol{\theta}).$$

Consequently, for $\lambda \neq 0$,

$$g(w; \lambda, \boldsymbol{\theta}) = \frac{d}{dw} P(y \leq w) = |\lambda| \cdot w^{\lambda-1} \cdot \phi(w^\lambda; \boldsymbol{\theta}).$$

Similarly, for $\lambda = 0$,

$$g(w; \lambda, \boldsymbol{\theta}) = \frac{d}{dw} P(y \leq w) = w^{-1} \cdot \phi(\log(w); \boldsymbol{\theta})).$$

With the index set $S = \{s : 1 \leq s \leq n\}$ for n univariate subjects (or observations) partitioned as in Sect. 2.5.3 into $k > 1$ disjoint folds $F(h)$ for $h \in H = \{h : 1 \leq h \leq k\}$, the power-adjusted LCV score is defined as

$$\text{LCV}(\lambda) = \prod_{h \in H} \prod_{s \in F(h)} g(y_s; \lambda, \boldsymbol{\theta}(S \backslash F(h); \lambda))^{\frac{1}{n}},$$

where $\boldsymbol{\theta}(S \backslash F(h); \lambda)$ denotes the adaptive estimate of the parameter vector $\boldsymbol{\theta}$ generated using the data in the complement $S \backslash F(h)$ of the fold $F(h)$ and with the outcome y transformed to y^λ (or $\log(y)$ when $\lambda = 0$). The power-adjusted $\text{LCV}(\lambda)$ score is maximized in λ using a grid search to choose an appropriate Box-Tidwell transformation for the outcomes y_s for $s \in S$.

6.3.2   Multivariate Outcomes

Using the complete data notation of Sect. 4.3.1 for brevity (the extension to incomplete data is similar), assume subjects s have associated multivariate outcome vectors $\mathbf{y}_s$ with entries y_{sc} for conditions $c \in C = \{c : 1 \leq c \leq m\}$. Assume also that $y_{sc} > 0$ for all $c \in C$ and $s \in S$. Define $\mathbf{y}_s^\lambda$ to be the vector with entries y_{sc}^λ (or $\log(y_{sc})$ when $\lambda = 0$) for $c \in C$ and $s \in S$ and assume that $\mathbf{y}_s^\lambda$ is multivariate normally distributed for some real valued power λ for $s \in S$.

For $\lambda > 0$, the multivariate distribution function $G(\mathbf{w}; \lambda, \boldsymbol{\theta})$ for $\mathbf{y}_s$ satisfies

$$G(\mathbf{w}; \lambda, \boldsymbol{\theta}) = P(y_{s1} \leq w_1, \cdots, y_{sm} \leq w_m) = \Phi(\mathbf{w}^{\lambda}; \boldsymbol{\theta}),$$

where $\mathbf{w}^{\lambda}$ is the vector $\mathbf{w}$ with its entries power transformed and Φ denotes the multivariate normal distribution function with mean vector and covariance matrix determined by a vector of model parameters $\boldsymbol{\theta}$. Thus, the associated power-adjusted density function $g(\mathbf{w}; \lambda, \boldsymbol{\theta})$ for $\mathbf{y}_s$ satisfies

$$g(\mathbf{w}; \lambda, \boldsymbol{\theta}) = d^m P(y_{s1} \leq w_1, \cdots, y_{sm} \leq w_m)/(dw_1 \cdots dw_m)$$

$$= \left(\prod_{c \in C} \lambda \cdot w_c^{\lambda - 1} \right) \cdot \phi(\mathbf{w}^{\lambda}; \boldsymbol{\theta}),$$

where ϕ denotes the multivariate normal density function (that is, the derivative of Φ). As for univariate outcomes, this extends for $\lambda \neq 0$ to

$$g(\mathbf{w}; \lambda, \boldsymbol{\theta}) = d^m P(y_{s1} \leq w_1, \cdots, y_{sm} \leq w_m)/(dw_1 \cdots dw_m)$$

$$= \left(\prod_{c \in C} |\lambda| \cdot w_c^{\lambda - 1} \right) \cdot \phi(\mathbf{w}^{\lambda}; \boldsymbol{\theta})$$

and for $\lambda = 0$ to

$$g(\mathbf{w}; \lambda, \boldsymbol{\theta}) = d^m P(y_{s1} \leq w_1, \cdots, y_{sm} \leq w_m)/(dw_1 \cdots dw_m)$$

$$= \left(\prod_{c \in C} w_c^{-1} \right) \cdot \phi(\log(\mathbf{w}); \boldsymbol{\theta}).$$

The power-adjusted LCV score is defined as

$$\mathrm{LCV}(\lambda) = \prod_{h \in H} \prod_{s \in F(h)} g(\mathbf{y}_s; \lambda, \boldsymbol{\theta}(S \backslash F(h); \lambda))^{1/m(S)},$$

where $m(S) = m \cdot n$ is the total number of measurements. The power-adjusted $\mathrm{LCV}(\lambda)$ score is maximized in λ using a grid search to choose an appropriate Box-Tidwell transformation for the outcomes $\mathbf{y}_s$ for $s \in S$. Parameters can be estimated with maximum likelihood (ML) or generalized estimating equations (GEE). This formulation is easily extended to allow for different powers λ_c for $c \in C$, but maximizing the power-adjusted LCV score requires a much more complex search. $\mathrm{LCV}(\lambda)$ scores for transition models can be computed using the above formula with the marginal densities $\phi(\mathbf{w}^{\lambda}; \boldsymbol{\theta})$ replaced by the equivalent product of conditional densities for $y^{\#}_{sc}$ (see Sect. 4.7.1) in terms of prior outcome measurements. For general conditional models with parameters estimated with maximum pseudolikelihood (see Sect. 4.9.1), power adjusted $\mathrm{PLCV}(\lambda)$ scores can be computed with the marginal densities $\phi(\mathbf{w}^{\lambda}; \boldsymbol{\theta})$ replaced by products of conditional densities for $y^{\#}_{sc}$ in terms of other outcome measurements.

Table 6.1 Power-adjusted LCV scores over a grid of powers from −2.5 to 2.5 by increments of 0.5 for adaptive modeling of death rates in terms of the bounded nitric oxide pollution index and the annual average precipitation with constant variances

Power λ	5-fold LCV(λ) score
−2.5	0.0000000
−2.0	0.0000010
−1.5	0.0000222
−1.0	0.0004523
−0.5	0.0053592
0.0	0.0056594
0.5	0.0056494
1.0	0.0056386
1.5	0.0055970
2.0	0.0054324
2.5	0.0037541

6.4 Analyses of Transformed Death Rates

Table 6.1 contains power-adjusted LCV(λ) scores over λ varying from −2.5 to 2.5 by increments of 0.5 for death rate as a function of NObnded and rain. Constant variances models are used as justified in Sect. 2.19.2. The maximum is achieved at $\lambda = 0$ with LCV(0) = 0.0056594. A further search over increments of 0.1 around $\lambda = 0$ results in the choice for λ of −0.4 with LCV(−0.4) = 0.0056930. Under this model, the means for $y^{-0.4}$ depend on rain$^{-0.22}$ and NObnded$^{-0.024}$ without an intercept. The LCV(1) score (the same as the power-unadjusted LCV score since $\lambda = 1$) is 0.0056386 (as also reported in Sect. 2.16 and Table 6.1) with insubstantial percent decrease (PD) 0.96 % (that is, less than the cutoff 3.15 % for a substantial PD as reported in Sect. 2.7), indicating that death rate is reasonably treated as untransformed.

6.5 Analyses of the Transformed Simulated Outcome

Using k = 10 folds as justified in Sect. 2.12 and constant variances as justified in Sect. 2.19.3, the maximum value 0.047782 of the power-adjusted LCV(λ) scores over increments of 0.5 for predicting Box-Tidwell transformed ysim of Sect. 2.12 as a function of xsim is achieved at $\lambda = 1$ (and so is the same as its power-unadjusted LCV score reported in Sect. 2.12) as is also the maximum over increments of 0.1 around $\lambda = 1$, as simulated. This result supports the validity of the power-adjusted adaptive modeling process.

6.6 Analyses of Transformed Dental Measurements

The need for transforming the dental measurement outcome dentmeas can be assessed using constant variances (to reduce the computations) and adaptive power-adjusted transition models of dentmeas as a function of age, male, $PRE(ytr(\lambda),1,2)$, $PRE(ytr(\lambda),1,2,\varnothing)$, and GCs (since that choice generates the best untransformed constant variances model). Transformed dentmeas is denoted by $ytr(\lambda)$. The use of $PRE(ytr(\lambda),1)$ is more appropriate than the use of $PRE(y,1)$, where y denotes untransformed dentmeas, since then dependence predictors for transformed outcomes are based on prior values of those transformed outcomes and not on prior values of the common untransformed outcome. Matched-set-wise deletion is used since there are no missing measurements with $k = 5$ folds (Sect. 4.5.2).

Varying the powers λ from -2.5 to 2.5 by increments of 0.5, the best $LCV(\lambda)$ score of 0.13568 is achieved at $\lambda = 1.5$. A further search over increments of 0.1 around $\lambda = 1.5$ results in the choice for λ of 1.1 with $LCV(1.1)$ score 0.13634. The PD for the $\lambda = 1$ model with $LCV(1) = 0.13363$ (as also reported in Sect. 4.8.3) is substantial at 1.98 % (that is, greater than the cutoff 1.76 % reported in Sect. 4.2), indicating that transformation of dentmeas, even with a small change from the power 1, can provide a distinct improvement at least under constant variances. The model generated for $\lambda = 1$ based on $PRE(y,1)$ but with dentmeas transformed by $\lambda = 1.1$ has $LCV(1.1)$ score 0.13367 with substantial PD 1.96 % compared the model generated for $\lambda = 1.1$. When $PRE(y,1)$ is changed to $PRE(try(1.1),1)$, the $LCV(1.1)$ score is even smaller at 0.13227. Consequently, even though the power has changed from 1 by the small amount of 0.1, there is a substantial change in the model for the means.

The associated adaptive non-constant variances model with $\lambda = 1.1$ has $LCV(1.1)$ score 0.14830, which is a substantial improvement on the associated untransformed model with LCV score 0.14264 (as reported in Sect. 4.15.2) with PD 3.82 %. This power transformed transition model has means based on the four transforms: $(male \cdot age^2)^{1.2}$, male· $PRE(ytr(1.1),1,2)^{1.7}$, $(PRE(ytr(1.1),1,2)^4 \cdot age^{0.3})^{1.03}$, and $PRE(ytr(1.1),1,2)^{-3}$ with an intercept and variances based on the two transforms: $PRE(ytr(1.1),1,2)^{1.7}$ and $(male \cdot PRE(ytr(1.1,1,2) \cdot age)^{0.1}$ also with an intercept.

Estimated means for this model are displayed in Fig. 6.1. Means increase with increasing average of the prior two transformed dental measurements, they are at higher levels as boys age, and there is not too much difference as girls age. A comparison to Fig. 4.2 indicates that there are no longer any counterintuitive low values for girls. Estimated standard deviations for this model are displayed in Fig. 6.2. Standard deviations decrease with increasing average of the prior two transformed dental measurements and at lower levels for girls than for boys. The pattern for girls does not depend on age since age is only included in the model for the variances interacting with the indicator male. However, the pattern for boys suggests that it changes little with age for boys as well.

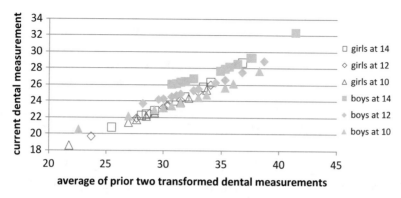

Fig. 6.1 Estimated mean dental measurements based on non-constant variances transition modeling

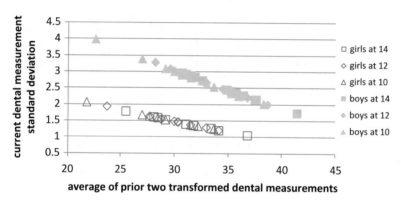

Fig. 6.2 Estimated dental measurement standard deviations based on non-constant variances transition modeling

6.7 Analyses of Transformed Strength Measurements

Adaptive transition models for means and variances of strength outperform associated non-constant variances marginal models, and so non-constant transition models are a natural choice for assessing the need for transformation of the strength measurements. Specifically, models with means and variances depending on time, incrwgts, PRE(tr(y),1), and PRE(tr(y),1,∅) are considered. Measurement-wise deletion is used to compute LCV(λ) scores since there are missing measurements with k = 15 folds (Sect. 4.12). However, generating adaptive models of this kind can be time-consuming, so a search is used that reduces the number of powers λ to be considered and that identifies a local maximum starting from $\lambda = 1$.

As reported in Sect. 4.15.4, LCV(1) equals 0.19089. LCV(1.5) has the smaller value 0.18810 while LCV(0.5) has the larger value 0.19165. LCV(0) equals 0.17257, and so $\lambda = 0.5$ is a local maximum over ±0.5. LCV(0.4) has the smaller value 0.18862 while LCV(0.6) has the larger value 0.19348. LCV(0.7) equals 0.19078, and so $\lambda = 0.6$ is a local maximum over ± 0.1 and is used in subsequent analyses. The PD for the LCV(1) scores compared to the LCV(0.6) score is substantial at 1.34 % (that is, greater than the cutoff 0.80 % reported in Sect. 4.12), indicating that transformation of the strength measurements provides a substantial benefit.

Under the selected model for transformed strength, the means are based on the five transforms: $\mathrm{PRE(ytr(0.6), 1)}^{4.21}$, $(\mathrm{time}^{0.04} \cdot \mathrm{PRE(ytr(0.6), 1)}^{-11})^{16}$, $(\mathrm{incrwgts} \cdot \mathrm{PRE(ytr(0.6), 1)}^{-38})^{1.1}$, $\mathrm{PRE(ytr(0.6), 1)}^{-4}$, and $(\mathrm{time}^{-2.5} \cdot \mathrm{PRE(ytr(0.6), 1)}^{10})^{1.1}$ with an intercept while the variances are based on the three transforms: $\mathrm{time}^{-0.06}$, time^{-8}, and $(\mathrm{incrwgts} \cdot \mathrm{PRE(ytr(0.6), 1)}^{10.1})^{1.02}$ with an intercept. The effect of incrwgts on the means as determined by the transform $(\mathrm{incrwgts} \cdot \mathrm{PRE(ytr(0.6), 1)}^{-38})^{1.1}$ is to increase the mean transformed strength by an estimated amount 0.056 for the small value 13.2 for PRE(ytr(0.6),1) and by smaller amounts as PRE(ytr(0.6),1) increases up to essentially no increase by the high value 15.0 for PRE(ytr(0.6),1). These results suggest that increasing the weights over time has more of an impact when the prior strength measurement is smaller (but increases of 0.056 or less may not be meaningful improvements). The effect of incrwgts on the variances as determined by the transform $(\mathrm{incrwgts} \cdot \mathrm{PRE(ytr(0.6), 1)}^{10.1})^{1.02}$ is to decrease the transformed strength standard deviations by an estimated multiple of 0.91 for the small value 13.2 for PRE(ytr(0.6),1) and by smaller multiples as PRE(ytr(0.6),1) increases up to a multiple of 0.69 for the high value 15.0 for PRE(ytr(0.6),1). These results suggest that increasing the weights over time decreases the transformed strength standard deviations with more of a decrease for larger prior outcome measurements.

6.8   The Plasma Beta-Carotene Data

A data set on positive plasma levels of beta-carotene (Nierenberg et al. 1989) in ng/ml and loaded into the variable betaplasma for 314 subjects is available on the Internet (see Supplementary Materials). There is one other subject in the original data set, but that subject's beta-carotene plasma level equals 0 and has been excluded so that the analyses address positive beta-carotene plasma levels. There are a variety of predictors in the data set but the analyses only address the variable fiber with values grams of fiber consumed in a day and the indicator variable oftvituse for fairly often vitamin use versus not often or no vitamin use. The cutoff for a substantial PD in the LCV scores is 0.61 %.

6.9   Analyses of Untransformed Plasma Beta-Carotene Levels

The adaptive analysis of the untransformed outcome variable betaplasma as a function of fiber with constant variances is used to set the number k of folds (Sect. 2.8). The first local maximum in the LCV scores is achieved at k = 10 and so that is used in subsequent analyses. The 10-fold LCV score, which equals the 10-fold LCV(1) score, is 0.0013355. The model for the means is based on the single transform $fiber^{3.9}$ with an intercept. The adaptive model for the means of betaplasma in terms of fiber, oftvituse, and GCs with constant variances is based on the three transforms: $(oftvituse \cdot fiber^3)^{1.6}$, oftvituse, and $fiber^{0.27}$ without an intercept and with LCV score 0.0013941. The adaptive additive model for the means of betaplasma in terms of fiber and oftvituse with constant variances is based on the two transforms: $fiber^{3.9}$ and oftvituse with an intercept and LCV score 0.0013654. The PD in the LCV scores is substantial at 2.06 %, indicating that oftvituse distinctly moderates the effect of fiber on betaplasma when the variances are treated as constant.

Using non-constant variances models, the adaptive model for the means and variances of betaplasma in terms of fiber, oftvituse, and GCs has means based on the single transform: $(fiber^{-6} \cdot oftvituse)^{-0.2}$ with an intercept, variances based on the two transforms: $(fiber^2 \cdot oftvituse)^{0.6}$ and $fiber^{-0.07}$ without an intercept, and LCV score 0.0014988. The PD in the LCV scores for the associated constant variances model is substantial at 6.94 %, indicating that the variances for betaplasma are distinctly non-constant. The adaptive additive model for the means and variances of betaplasma in terms of fiber and oftvituse has means based on the two transforms:oftvituse and $fiber^{0.1}$ without an intercept, variances based on the two transforms:oftvituse and $fiber^7$ with an intercept, and LCV score 0.0014214. The PD in the LCV scores is substantial at 5.16 %, indicating that oftvituse also distinctly moderates the effect of fiber on betaplasma when the variances are treated as non-constant.

Figure 6.3 displays the normal (probability) plot for the standardized residuals of the GC-based non-constant variances model for untransformed betaplasma with the best LCV score. It is distinctly nonlinear and the associated Shapiro-Wilk test for normality is highly significant $(P < 0.001)$. Consequently, the assumption of normality is very questionable for these data, suggesting consideration of transformations of betaplasma.

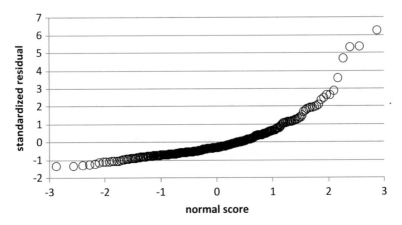

Fig. 6.3 Normal plot generated by the standardized residuals for the adaptive model of the untransformed plasma beta-carotene levels as a function of grams of fiber in the diet, fairly often vitamin use, and geometric combinations in these two predictors with non-constant variances

6.10   Analyses of Transformed Plasma Beta-Carotene Levels

A grid search using constant variances models based on fiber over powers λ varying from -2.5 to 2.5 by increments of 0.5 has best 10-fold LCV(λ) score 0.0023326 achieved at $\lambda = 0$. A further search over increments of 0.1 around $\lambda = 0$ results again in the choice for λ of 0. Under this model, the means for log(betaplasma) depend on the two transforms: $fiber^{3.9}$ and $fiber^{0.03}$ without an intercept. The PD for the LCV(1) scores compared to the LCV(0) score is very substantial at $42.75\ \%$, indicating that transforming betaplasma provides a very distinct improvement. The model for log(betaplasma) linear in fiber has LCV(0) score 0.0023108 with substantial PD $0.93\ \%$. Consequently, there is a distinct benefit to transforming both the outcome betaplasma and the predictor fiber.

The adaptive model for the means of log(betaplasma) in terms of fiber, oftvituse, and GCs with constant variances is based on the two transforms: $(fiber^{2.9} \cdot oftvituse)^{0.7}$ and $fiber^{24.1}$ without an intercept and LCV(0) score 0.0023830. The adaptive additive model for the means of log(betaplasma) in terms of fiber and oftvituse with constant variances is based on the three transforms: $fiber^{5.9}$, oftvituse, and $fiber^{0.05}$ without an intercept and LCV(0) score 0.0023713. The PD in the power-adjusted LCV scores is insubstantial at $0.49\ \%$, indicating that oftvituse does not distinctly moderate the effect of fiber on log(betaplasma). However, the PD for the model based on only fiber compared to the additive model in fiber and oftvituse is substantial at $1.63\ \%$, indicating that there is a distinct covariate effect to oftvituse on log(betaplasma). The adaptive model for the means and variances of log(betaplasma) in terms of fiber, oftvituse, and GCs has LCV(0) score 0.0023789. Since this is smaller than the score for the associated

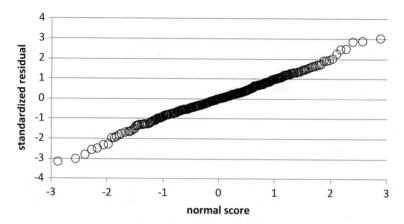

Fig. 6.4 Normal plot generated by the standardized residuals for the adaptive model of the natural log transformed plasma beta-carotene levels as a function of grams of fiber in the diet, fairly often vitamin use, and geometric combinations in these two predictors with constant variances

constant variances model, log(betaplasma) is reasonably considered to have constant variances.

The adaptive additive constant variances model is a competitive alternative to the adaptive GC-based constant variances model. It can be considered simpler in the sense that it has no interaction terms. However, it can also be considered more complex since it is based on three transforms without an intercept compared to two transforms without an intercept. Residual analyses for these models indicate that under the additive model the Shapiro-Wilk test for normality of the standardized residuals is significant ($P = 0.050$) while it is nonsignificant ($P = 0.190$) for the GC-based model. Consequently, the latter model seems preferable. Figure 6.4 displays the normal plot for the standardized residuals of this GC-based model. The nearly linear pattern of this plot, combined with a nonsignificant Shapiro-Wilk test, indicate that the assumption of normality is reasonable for these data. These results indicate that power transforming outcomes can resolve both non-normality and non-constant variances for untransformed outcomes, at least in some cases, so that standard assumptions of normality with constant variances are reasonable for those transformed outcomes.

6.11   Overview of Analyses of Death Rates

Using constant variances models for death rate in terms of NObnded and rain, the best power for transforming death rate is -0.4 (this and the following results reported in Sect. 6.4). However, the associated model for untransformed death rate is a competitive alternative, and so the univariate death rate outcome is reasonably modeled without transformation.

6.12   Overview of Analyses of the Simulated Outcome

Using constant variances models for ysim in terms of xsim, the best power for transforming ysim is 1, as simulated (Sect. 6.5). This result supports the validity of the power-adjusted adaptive modeling process.

6.13   Overview of Analyses of Dental Measurements

Using constant variances transition models for dentmeas in terms of age and male, the best power for transforming dentmeas is 1.1 (this and the following results reported in Sect. 6.6). The associated model for untransformed dentmeas generates a substantial PD in the power-adjusted LCV scores, and so there is a distinct benefit to power transformation of this multivariate dental measurement outcome. Consideration of non-constant variances transition models for power transformed dentmeas provides a substantial improvement over constant variances transition models. Estimated means and standard deviations for the selected non-constant variances transition model are displayed in Figs. 6.1 and 6.2.

6.14   Overview of Analyses of Strength Measurements

Using transition models for strength means and variances in terms of time, incrwgts, PRE(tr(y),1), and PRE(tr(y),1,$\emptyset$), the best power for transforming strength is 0.6 (this and the following results reported in Sect. 6.7). The associated model for untransformed strength generates a substantial PD in the power-adjusted LCV scores, and so there is a distinct benefit to power transformation of this multivariate strength outcome. Under this power-adjusted model, increasing the weights over time has more of an impact on mean strength when the prior strength measurement is smaller, but estimated increases may not be meaningful improvements. Increasing the weights over time also decreases the transformed strength standard deviations with more of a decrease for larger prior outcome measurements.

6.15   Overview of Analyses of Plasma Beta-Carotene Levels

For the plasma beta-carotene data (Sect. 6.8), analyses use k $=$ 10 folds (this and the following results reported in Sect. 6.9). The adaptive GC-based model for untransformed betaplasma in fiber and oftvituse with constant variances outperforms the associated adaptive additive model. The adaptive GC-based model in fiber and oftvituse with non-constant variances outperforms the associated adaptive constant variances model and the associated additive non-constant variances model. The standardized residuals for this model are distinctly nonnormal; see Fig. 6.3 for the normal plot.

Using constant variances models for transformed betaplasma in terms of fiber, the best power for transforming betaplasma is 0 (corresponding to the natural log transform; this and the following results reported in Sect. 6.10). The associated model for untransformed betaplasma generates a substantial PD in the power-adjusted LCV scores, and so there is a distinct benefit to power transformation of this univariate plasma beta-carotene outcome. Moreover, log(betaplasma) is distinctly nonlinear in fiber. These results provide an example where there is a distinct benefit to transforming both the outcome and its predictor.

The adaptive additive constant variances model in fiber and oftvituse is a parsimonious, competitive alternative to the associated GC-based model and provides a substantial improvement over the model in fiber by itself (Sect. 6.10). Consideration of transformed betaplasma changes the conclusion about moderation of the effect of fiber by oftvituse compared to using untransformed betaplasma.

The adaptive GC-based non-constant variances model for log(betaplasma) generates a smaller LCV(0) score than the associated GC-based constant variances model, indicating that log(betaplasma) is reasonably treated as having constant variances (this and the following results reported in Sect. 6.10).The standardized residuals for this latter model are reasonably close to normal; see Fig. 6.4 for the normal plot. Consequently, power transforming outcomes can resolve both non-normality and non-constant variances for the untransformed outcome, at least in some cases, so that standard assumptions of normality with constant variances are reasonable for those transformed outcomes.

6.16 Chapter Summary

This chapter has presented a series of analyses of the death rate and simulated data with univariate outcomes analyzed in Chaps. 2–3, the dental measurement and exercise data with multivariate outcomes analyzed in Chaps. 4–5, and the univariate outcome of the plasma beta-carotene data not considered before. These analyses demonstrate adaptive regression modeling involving transformation of positive valued univariate and multivariate continuous outcomes as well as their predictors using fractional polynomials. The chapter also provides the formulation for power-adjusted LCV scores for selecting appropriate power transforms for such outcomes.

Analyzing an untransformed outcome can be a reasonable alternative to transforming that outcome. For example, the univariate death rate and simulated outcomes analyzed without transformation in Chaps. 2–3 are reasonably modeled without transformation. The death rate outcome is best modeled after transforming it with the power −0.4, but the power 1 provides a competitive alternative. The simulated outcome is best modeled without transformation as simulated, supporting the validity of the power-adjusted adaptive modeling process.

On the other hand, transforming the outcome can provide a distinct improvement over not transforming it. For example, transformation of the multivariate dental measurement and strength outcomes analyzed without transformation in Chaps. 4–5 provide distinct improvements over not transforming them. The dental measurement outcome is best modeled after transforming it with the power 1.1, indicating that even small changes from not transforming an outcome with associated power 1 can provide distinct improvements. The strength outcome is best modeled after transforming it with the power 0.6, which provides a distinct improvement over the power 1.

Analyses are also reported for the plasma beta-carotene data not analyzed before. The univariate plasma beta-carotene outcome is best modeled in terms of the grams of fiber per week after transforming it with the power 0, that is, with the natural log transform, and this provides a distinct improvement over not transforming it. This is an example of the benefit to outcome transformation for univariate outcomes (the other two univariate outcomes considered in this chapter do not require transformation). Moreover, the model for transformed plasma beta-carotene is distinctly nonlinear in the predictor grams of fiber per week, providing an example with benefits to nonlinear transformation of both the outcome and the predictor. Using untransformed plasma beta-carotene, the indicator for fairly often vitamin use, distinctly moderates the effect of grams of fiber per day. This conclusion no longer holds for transformed plasma beta-carotene, indicating the need for consideration of outcome transformation to correctly identify effects on outcomes. Using untransformed plasma beta-carotene, the usual assumptions of normality and constant variances do not hold, but transformed plasma beta-carotene is reasonably considered to be close to normal and to having constant variances. Power transforming outcomes can resolve both non-normality and non-constant variances for the untransformed outcome, at least in some cases, so that standard assumptions of normality with constant variances are reasonable for those transformed outcomes.

See Chap. 7 for details on conducting analyses in SAS like those presented in this chapter. Power transformation is only considered for continuous outcomes. Transformation of dichotomous and polytomous outcomes as addressed in Part II would only change the labels for their values. Fractional polynomial transforms of count outcomes as addressed in Part III would generate non-integer valued outcomes in most cases, which cannot be modeled using Poisson regression. Only integer valued powers would generate integer valued outcomes, and these do not seem important enough to address.

References

Box, G. E. P., & Cox, D. R. (1964). An analysis of transformations. *Journal of the Royal Statistical Society, Series B, 26*, 211–252.

Box, G. E. P., & Tidwell, P. W. (1962). Transformation of the independent variables. *Technometrics, 4*, 531–550.

Carroll, R. J., & Ruppert, D. (1984). Power transformations when fitting theoretical models to data. *Journal of the American Statistical Association, 79*, 321–328.

Nierenberg, D. W., Stukel, T. A., Baron, J. A., Dain, B. J., & Greenberg, E. R. (1989). Determinants of plasma levels of beta-carotene and retinol. *American Journal of Epidemiology, 130*, 511–521.

Chapter 7
Adaptive Transformation of Positive Valued Continuous Outcomes in SAS

7.1 Chapter Overview

This chapter describes how to use the ypower macro for adaptive regression modeling accounting for fractional polynomial transformation of positive valued univariate and multivariate continuous outcomes as well as their predictors as also covered in Chap. 6. See Supplementary Materials for a more complete description of this macro. SAS supports Box-Cox (Box and Cox 1964) transformation of outcome variables using PROC TRANSREG (SAS Institute 2004), but not Box-Tidwell transforms.

Example code and output are provided for analyzing the univariate outcome plasma beta-carotene levels for 314 subjects in terms of their fiber intake and vitamin usage and the multivariate outcome dental measurements for 27 children in terms of their age and gender. Section 7.2 covers loading in the plasma beta-carotene data, Sect. 7.3 transformation of the univariate outcome plasma beta-carotene levels, and Sect. 7.4 transformation of the multivariate outcome dental measurements, including transition models in Sect. 7.4.1 and marginal models in Sect. 7.4.2. Practice exercises are also provided for conducting analyses similar to those presented in Chaps. 6 and 7.

7.2 Loading in the Plasma Beta-Carotene Data

A data set on plasma beta-carotene levels is analyzed in Chap. 6 (see Sects. 6.8–6.10). Assume that the full plasma beta-carotene data have been loaded into the default library (for example, by importing it from a spreadsheet file) under the name plasma.

© Springer International Publishing Switzerland 2016
G.J. Knafl, K. Ding, *Adaptive Regression for Modeling Nonlinear Relationships*,
Statistics for Biology and Health, DOI 10.1007/978-3-319-33946-7_7

An output title line, selected system options, and labels for the variables can be assigned with the following code.

```
title "Plasma Beta-Carotene Data";
options linesize=76 pagesize=53 pageno=1 nodate;
proc format;
  value vitfmt 1="often" 2="not often" 3="no";
  value nyfmt 0="no" 1="yes";
run;
data plasma;
  set plasma;
  oftvituse=(vituse=1);
  label fiber="Grams of Fiber Consumed per Day" vituse="Vitamin Use"
        betaplasma="Plasma Beta-Carotene in ng/ml"
        oftvituse="Often Vitamin Use vs. Not Often or No Vitamin Use"
  format vituse vitfmt. oftvituse nyfmt.;
run;
```

The variable vituse contains vitamin usage coded into the three levels of the vitfmt format. This is recoded into the indicator oftvituse for fairly often vitamin use versus not often or no vitamin use. There are 315 observations in the plasma data set, but one observation has a zero betaplasma value. Consequently, the posplasma data set with this one observation excluded and created with the following code is used in analyses.

```
data posplasma;
  set plasma;
  if betaplasma>0;
run;
```

7.3 Adaptive Transformation of Plasma Beta-Carotene Levels

Assuming the ypower and genreg macros have been loaded, power-adjusted LCV scores LVC(λ) (as defined in Sect. 6.3) for adaptive modeling of transformed betaplasma as a function of fiber for powers λ ranging from -2.5 to 2.5 by steps of size 0.5 are generated as follows using $k = 10$ folds (Sect. 6.9).

Table 7.1 Power-adjusted LCV scores over a grid of powers from −2.5 to 2.5 by increments of 0.5 for adaptive modeling of plasma beta-carotene levels in terms of grams of fiber consumed per day with constant variances

Power for Transforming betaplasma	Power-Adjusted LCV Score
-2.5	0.0000287
-2.0	0.0002480
-1.5	0.0007106
-1.0	0.0013406
-0.5	0.0020148
0.0	0.0023326
0.5	0.0020263
1.0	0.0013355
1.5	0.0007013
2.0	0.0003090
2.5	0.0001285

```
%ypower(datain=posplasma,yvar=betaplasma,foldcnt=10,yfst=-2.5,ycnt=11,
    ystp=0.5,expand=y,expxvars=fiber,contract=y);
```

The datain, yvar, foldcnt, expand, expxvars, and contract macro parameters have the same meanings as for the genreg macro. The yfst, ycnt, and ystp macro parameters are used respectively to set the first power to consider, how many powers to generate, and the step size or increment for consecutive powers. The ypower macro invokes the genreg macro once for each of the requested transformed outcomes betaplasma$^\lambda$ (or log(betaplasma) when $\lambda = 0$) to generate a constant variances fractional polynomial model for its means in terms of fiber, compute its power-adjusted LCV(λ) score, store this score into a data set called scoreout, and then print out all the requested scores. The name of the scoreout data set can be changed with the ypower macro parameter scoreout.

Table 7.1 contains the output for the above call to ypower. The maximum LCV(λ) score of 0.0023326 (as also reported in Sect. 6.10) is achieved at $\lambda = 0$, corresponding to the transform log(betaplasma). The format for these LCV(λ) scores is controlled by the ypower scorefmt parameter. Its value should be a valid SAS w.d format where w is the width and d the number of decimal places. The default value as used above is "10.7".

Given that the maximum in this case is achieved at $\lambda = 0$, a grid search around $\lambda = 0$ with increments of 0.1 can be requested by changing the above code to include "yfst=−0.4", "ycnt=9", and "ystp=0.1". The best score is still achieved at $\lambda = 0$. Once the power $\lambda = 0$ has been identified as generating the best LCV(λ) score over multiples of 0.1, the fractional polynomial model for the selected natural log transformation of betaplasma can be generated as follows.

```
%ypower(datain=posplasma,yvar=betaplasma,foldcnt=10,yfst=0,expand=y,
        expxvars=fiber,contract=y,noglog=n,nogprint=n);
```

There is no need for the ycnt parameter since its default setting is 1. By default, the ypower macro turns off the log and print output of the genreg macro to limit the amount of output. In the above code, the setting "noglog=n" requests that ypower have genreg display the analysis steps in the SAS log window while "nogprint=n" requests that ypower have genreg display results in the SAS output window. In versions 9.3 and later, this requires that the SAS command "ods listing;" be executed earlier. Usually, these settings would only be used when ypower generates a single model.

The genreg output in this case indicates that the means of log(betaplasma) are modeled in terms of the two transforms: $fiber^{3.9}$ and $fiber^{0.03}$ without an intercept. This model and its LCV(λ) score can be generated directly using the following code.

```
%ypower(datain=posplasma,yvar=betaplasma,foldcnt=10,yfst=0,
        xintrcpt=n,xvars=fiber fiber,xpowers=3.9 0.03,
        noglog=n,nogprint=n);
```

Most of the genreg parameters are supported by ypower (like the xintrcpt, xvars, and xpowers parameters used in the above code) so that general adaptive modeling of transformed outcomes is possible. These parameters usually have the same meaning as for the genreg macro but there are exceptions. For example, the ypower parameters yvar and ytransvr replace the genreg parameter yvar. The yvar variable specifies the name of the variable in the datain data set loaded with the untransformed outcome values. This is used to create the variable loaded with the transformed outcome values having name specified by the ytransvr parameter with default setting "ytr". The ypower dataout parameter has the same meaning as the genreg macro parameter but some of that data set's variables are loaded by genreg and some by ypower. For example, the ytransvr variable is loaded into the dataout data set by ypower.

The ypower parameters yhatvar and ytrhatvr specify names for the variables to be loaded in the dataout data set with predicted values for the untransformed and transformed outcome, respectively. The genreg macro loads the ytrhatvr variable through its yhatvar parameter. The ypower macro uses this variable to create and load its yhatvar variable with the inverse transform of the ytrhatvr variable based on the power 1/λ (or the exponential function for $\lambda = 0$). When $\lambda \neq 0$, even though the transformed outcome has all positive values, predicted values for the transformed outcome can sometimes be nonpositive. In such cases, the negative values are replaced by the smallest positive predicted value (or set to missing if all predicted values are nonpositive) before computing the inverse transform. This adjustment is not needed for $\lambda = 0$.

Unit lower and upper bounds on the transformed predicted values (that is, ± one estimated standard deviation) are loaded into the dataout data set using the names of the ypower parameters loytrerrvr and upytrerrvr. These are loaded by genreg using its loerrvar and uperrvar parameters. These lower and upper bound variables are used by ypower to create lower and upper bounds on the untransformed predicted values through the associated inverse transform. For $\lambda \neq 0$, when there are nonpositive bounds on the transformed predicted values, these bounds are adjusted before inverse transforming them as described above for nonpositive predicted values.

Some genreg parameters are not supported since they not needed. For example, there is no need for a modtype parameter since outcome transformation requires "modtype=norml".

Several data sets are created by ypower and/or genreg in the default library. The dataout data set is created in part by genreg and in part by ypower. The scoreout data set with LCV(λ) scores for all requested λ is created by ypower. Data sets created by genreg include the xmodlout and vmodlout data sets describing the generated transforms for the means and the variances, respectively, and the xcmbnout and vcmbnout data sets describing any generated geometric combinations (GCs) for the means and the variances, respectively. The data sets generated by genreg are created for every requested power λ, but ypower only keeps the data sets generated for the power λ with the best LCV(λ) score.

Once a choice for the power λ has been identified, further analysis can be conducted with that power fixed. For example, the adaptive non-constant variances model for log(betaplasma) in terms of fiber, oftvituse, and GCs can be generated as follows using parameters with the same meanings as for genreg.

```
%ypower(datain=posplasma,yvar=betaplasma,foldcnt=10,yfst=0,expand=y,
        expxvars=fiber vituse,expvvars=fiber vituse,geomcmbn=y,contract=y,
        noglog=n,nogprint=n);
```

7.4   Adaptive Transformation of Dental Measurements

7.4.1   Using Transition Models

Power-adjusted LCV(λ) scores for powers λ varying from -2.5 to 2.5 by increments of 0.5 for adaptive constant variances transition models for transformed dentmeas, denoted ytr(λ), as a function of age, male, PRE(ytr(λ),1,2) (pre_ytr_age_1_2 in the code), PRE(ytr(λ),1,2,$\varnothing$) (pre_ytr_age_1_2_m in the code), and GCs can be generated as follows with $k = 5$ folds (Sect. 4.5.2).

```
%ypower(datain=dentdata,yvar=dentmeas,matchvar=subject,withinvr=age,
        corrtype=IND,conditnl=y,foldcnt=5,yfst=-2.5,ycnt=11,ystp=0.5,
        expand=y,expxvars=age male pre_ytr_age_1_2 pre_ytr_age_1_2_m,
        geomcmbn=y,contract=y);
```

The matchvar, withinvr, corrtype, and conditnl macro parameters are used to generate conditional models in the same way as for genreg. The ypower macro creates the variable called ytr with the current transformation of the yvar variable. The name of this variable can be changed using the ytransvr macro parameter. These are transition models based on averages of the prior two transformed outcome measurements. Note that since a copy of dentmeas named y is in the datain data set, if the above code is changed to use the variables pre_y_age_1_2 and pre_y_age_1_2_m, all transformed outcomes are modeled in terms of averages of the untransformed outcome. It is more appropriate to use pre_ytr_age_1_2 and pre_ytr_age_1_2_m so that these predictors are based on the current transformed outcome. As reported in Sect. 6.6, the best $LCV(\lambda)$ of 0.13568 is generated for $\lambda = 1.5$. A grid search around $\lambda = 1.5$ with increments of 0.1 is requested by changing the above code to include "yfst=1.1", "ycnt=9", and "ystp=0.1". As reported in Sect. 6.6, this results in the selection of $\lambda = 1.1$ with $LCV(1.1) = 0.13634$. Since $LCV(1)$ is 0.13363, the percent (PD) for $\lambda = 1$ is substantial at 1.98 % (that is, larger than the cutoff 1.76 % for the data), indicating that transforming dentmeas provides a distinct improvement over using ntransformed dentmeas using constant variances transition models.

7.4.2   Using Marginal Models

Marginal models can have their outcomes transformed as well. The adaptive constant variances marginal model with exchangeable correlation (EC) structure (since it distinctly outperforms AR1 correlations; Sect. 4.8.2) and maximum likelihood (ML) parameter estimation for dentmeas transformed using $\lambda = 1.1$ as chosen for transition models is generated as follows.

```
%ypower(datain=dentdata,yvar=dentmeas,matchvar=subject,withinvr=age,
        corrtype=EC,foldcnt=5,yfst=1.1,expand=y,expxvars=age male,
        geomcmbn=y,contract=y);
```

The $LCV(1.1)$ score is 0.12965 with substantial PD 4.91 % compared to the transition model of Sect. 7.4.1, indicating as for untransformed dentmeas that transition modeling distinctly outperforms marginal modeling. However, there might be a benefit to using a different power than the one identified for transition modeling. Power-adjusted $LCV(\lambda)$ scores for powers λ varying from -2.5 to 2.5 by increments of 0.5 for adaptive constant variances marginal ML-based models with EC correlations for dentmeas as a function of age, male, and GCs can be generated as follows.

```
%ypower(datain=dentdata,yvar=dentmeas,matchvar=subject,withinvr=age,
        corrtype=EC,foldcnt=5,yfst=-2.5,ycnt=11,ystp=0.5,expand=y,
        expxvars=age male,geomcmbn=y,contract=y);
```

The best LCV(λ) of 0.13414 is generated for $\lambda = 0.5$. A grid search around $\lambda = 0.5$ with increments of 0.1 is requested by changing the above code to include "yfst=0.9", "ycnt=9", and "ystp=0.1". This results in the selection of $\lambda = 0.5$. The PD for $\lambda = 1$ with LCV(1) = 0.12975 is substantial at 7.15 %, indicating that there is a distinct benefit to square root transformation of dentmeas using ML-based marginal models with EC correlations and constant variances. Moreover, the appropriate power for marginal modeling is different from the one for transition modeling. In this case, the power-adjusted LCV score is improved sufficiently that the marginal model becomes a competitive alternative with PD 1.61 % compared to the transition model of Sect 7.4.1.

Using $\lambda = 0.5$, EC correlations, and ML parameter estimation, the adaptive non-constant variances marginal model in age, male, and GCs is generated as follows.

```
%ypower(datain=dentdata,yvar=dentmeas,matchvar=subject,withinvr=age,
        corrtype=EC,foldcnt=5,yfst=0.5,expand=y,expxvars=age male,
        expxvars=age male,geomcmbn=y,contract=y,noglog=n,nogprint=n);
```

The LCV(0.5) score is 0.13925 with substantial PD 6.10 % compared to the power-adjusted non-constant variances transition model with LCV(1.1) 0.14830 as reported in Sect. 6.6. Consequently, transition modeling distinctly outperforms marginal modeling as long as sufficiently general models are considered.

7.5 Practice Exercises

For Practice Exercise 7.1, use the body fat data set available on the Internet (see Supplementary Materials) used in Practice Exercises 3.5–3.8 and 5.2. The outcome variable for this data set is called bodyfat and contains body fat values in gm/cm^3 for 252 men. One of the men has a zero body fat value, so the load code for these data on the Internet also creates the data set posbodyfat with this observation dropped. Use the posbodyfat data set for Practice Exercise 7.1. Only the predictor BMI is considered in Practice Exercise 7.1.

7.1. Conduct an assessment of how possibly transformed positive valued body fat depends on BMI. Use the number of folds determined for Practice Exercise 3.5. First, generate power-adjusted LCV scores for powers −2.5 to 2.5 by increments of 0.5. Next, search over increments of 0.1 around the power with the best power-adjusted LCV score in the first search. Generate the model for the best power-adjusted LCV score for this second search. Is the model with power 1 a competitive alternative or is there a distinct benefit to transformation of body fat? Note that the cutoff for a substantial PD in this case is 0.76 % because there is one less observation.

For Practice Exercises 7.2–7.3, use the Treatment of Lead-Exposed Children (TLC) Study data available on the Internet (see Supplementary Materials) used in Practice Exercises 5.5–5.7. The long format data set is called longtlc. The outcome variable for this data set is called lead and contains blood lead levels in micrograms/dL. The two predictors are succimer, the indicator for being on the chelating agent succimer versus on a placebo, and week with values 0, 1, 4, and 6 weeks into the study. There are 100 subjects in this study, all with the complete set of 4 measurements. Since there are no missing data values, use matched-set-wise deletion in these practice exercises to compute power-adjusted LCV scores with the number of folds selected in Practice Exercise 5.5.

7.2. For the TLC data, conduct an assessment of the need for transformation of the outcome variable lead. To limit the amount of computations, consider only adaptive marginal models with ML parameter estimation; means depending on week, succimer, and GCs; constant variances; and the correlation structure selected in Practice Exercise 5.5. Use the ypower macro to generate such models for Box-Tidwell transforms of lead for powers 0–2 by increments of 0.5. If the best score is achieved at 0 (2) generate models for smaller (larger) multiples of 0.5 until a local maximum occurs, otherwise use the best score in between these two values. Let λ^* denote the local max over multiples of 0.5. If LCV($\lambda^*-0.5$) is larger (smaller) than LCV($\lambda^*+0.5$), search between $\lambda^*-0.4$ and $\lambda^*-0.1$ ($\lambda^*+0.1$ and $\lambda^*+0.4$) by increments of 0.1. If a local maximum is achieved stop the search, otherwise continue the search on the other side of λ^*. Let λ^{**} denote the local maximum within ± 0.1 identified by this search. Compare the power-adjusted LCV(λ^{**}) score to LCV(1) to assess the need for power transformation of lead. Describe the model generated for λ^{**}.

7.3. For the TLC data, use the power λ^{**} selected in Practice Exercise 7.2 for marginal models to generate the adaptive constant variances transition model with means depending on week, succimer, pre_ytr_week_1, pre_ytr_week_1_m, and GCs. Compare this model to the one identified in Practice Exercise 7.2. Next assess whether improvements are possible using powers around λ^{**}. To do this, first compute transition models at $\lambda^{**}-0.1$ and $\lambda^{**}+0.1$. If LCV(λ^{**}) is a local maximum, stop the search. Otherwise, if LCV ($\lambda^{**}-0.1$) is larger (smaller) than LCV($\lambda^{**}+0.1$), compute LCV($\lambda^{**}-0.2$) (LCV($\lambda^{**}+0.2$)), then smaller (larger) multiples of 0.1 until a local maximum λ^{***} is identified. Compare results for the transition model generated with λ^{***} to the one generated with λ^{**}. If the model for λ^{***} is better, compare it to the marginal model based on λ^{**}. Is constant variances marginal or transition modeling better for analyzing possibly transformed lead? Using the better of these two modeling approaches with the associated best power, assess the need for non-constant variances using the same predictors for the variances as for the means.

References

Box, G. E. P., & Cox, D. R. (1964). An analysis of transformations. *Journal of the Royal Statistical Society, Series B, 26*, 211–252.

SAS Institute (2004). *SAS/STAT 9.1 user's guide*. Cary, NC: SAS Institute.

Part II
Adaptive Logistic Regression Modeling

Chapter 8
Adaptive Logistic Regression Modeling of Univariate Dichotomous and Polytomous Outcomes

8.1 Chapter Overview

This chapter formulates and demonstrates adaptive fractional polynomial modeling of univariate dichotomous and polytomous outcomes with two or more values and with either unit dispersions as in standard logistic regression modeling or with non-unit (constant or non-constant) dispersions. A description of how to generate these models in SAS is provided in Chap. 9. A familiarity with logistic regression modeling is assumed, for example, as treated in Hosmer et al. (2013) or Kleinbaum and Klein (2010). A data set with a univariate dichotomous outcome is described in Sect. 8.2. The formulation for logistic regression modeling of dichotomous outcomes is provided in Sect. 8.3 followed by unit dispersions analyses in Sects. 8.4–8.6 of the dichotomous outcome of Sect. 8.2. Then, the formulation for logistic regression modeling of univariate polytomous outcomes is provided in Sect. 8.7 followed by a description of a data set with a polytomous outcome in Sect. 8.8 and unit dispersions analyses of that outcome in Sects. 8.9–8.11. Section 8.12 addresses the proportion of correct deleted predictions (PCDP), an alternative cross-validation criterion for assessing logistic regression models. Section 8.13 generalizes the formulations to modeling of dispersions as well as means and conducts such analyses for the dichotomous outcome of Sect. 8.2 (see Sect. 9.12 for a polytomous outcome example). Sections 8.14–8.15 provide overviews of the results of analysis of dichotomous and polytomous mercury levels, respectively. Formulations can be skipped to focus on analyses.

© Springer International Publishing Switzerland 2016
G.J. Knafl, K. Ding, *Adaptive Regression for Modeling Nonlinear Relationships*,
Statistics for Biology and Health, DOI 10.1007/978-3-319-33946-7_8

8.2   The Mercury Level Data

A data set on mercury levels for $n = 169$ largemouth bass caught in one of two rivers (Lumber and Waccamaw) in North Carolina is available on the Internet (see Supplementary Materials). These data are analyzed here to demonstrate how to conduct logistic regression analyses that account for nonlinearity in predictor variables. The variable mercury in ppm (parts per million) is used to compute dichotomous and polytomous outcomes for these analyses. As a start, the dichotomous merchigh variable categorizes mercury levels into high (mercury level >1.0 ppm) with value 1 and low (mercury level ≤ 1.0 ppm) with value 0. A total of 80 (or 47.3 %) of the fish have a high mercury level, and so the cutoff (1.0 ppm) for this variable is close to the median mercury level. It is also the Federal Drug Administration limit for human consumption (http://www.fda.gov/OHRMS/ DOCKETS/ac/02/briefing/3872_Advisory%207.pdf, accessed 6/18/16). The possible predictor variables are weight (in kg), length (in cm), and river ($0 =$ Lumber, $1 =$ Waccamaw). The station along the river where the fish were caught is also available in the original data set, but is not considered here. All reported logistic regression analyses use nonzero intercept models, thereby always estimating the logit or log odds when the predictor value is 0 rather than allowing that logit to sometimes be treated as equal to 0. The cutoff for a substantial percent decrease (PD) in LCV scores for these data with 169 measurements is 1.13 % (using the formula of Sect. 4.4.2).

8.3   Multiple Logistic Regression Modeling of Dichotomous Outcomes

8.3.1   Multiple Logistic Regression Model Formulation

The observed data for logistic (or binomial) regression models to be considered in Sects. 8.4–8.6 consist of observations $O_s = (y_s, \mathbf{x}_s)$ for subjects $s \in S = \{s: 1 \leq s \leq n\}$ where each outcome measurement y_s has two possible values coded as 0 and 1 (as for merchigh) and $\mathbf{x}_s$ is a $r \times 1$ column vector of r predictor values x_{sj} (including unit predictor values if an intercept is included in the model) with indexes $j \in J = \{j \ : \ 1 \leq j \leq r\}$. The mean or expected value μ_s for y_s satisfies $\mu_s = Ey_s = P(y_s = 1|\mathbf{x}_s)$ for $s \in S$. In other words, the conditional mean for the dichotomous outcome y_s is the probability that it takes on the value 1. With the logit (or log odds) function defined as $\text{logit}(u) = \log(u/(1-u))$ for $0 < u < 1$, model the logit of the mean as $\text{logit}(\mu_s) = \mathbf{x}_s^T \cdot \boldsymbol{\beta}$ for a $r \times 1$ vector $\boldsymbol{\beta}$ of coefficients. Solving for μ_s gives $\mu_s = \exp(\mathbf{x}_s^T \cdot \boldsymbol{\beta})/(1 + \exp(\mathbf{x}_s^T \cdot \boldsymbol{\beta}))$. The odds ratio (OR) for $y_s = 1$ under a unit change in a predictor value x_{sj} and adjusted for the other predictor values $x_{sj'}$ for $j' \neq j$ (if any) is computed as $OR = \exp(\beta_j)$. The conditional variance for y_s is $\sigma_s^2 = \mu_s \cdot (1 - \mu_s)$.

The likelihood term L_s for the s_{th} subject is based on the Bernoulli distribution and satisfies

$$\ell_s = \log(L_s) = y_s \cdot \log(\mu_s) + (1 - y_s) \cdot \log(1 - \mu_s).$$

The likelihood $L(S; \boldsymbol{\beta})$ is the product of the individual likelihood terms L_s over $s \in S$ and satisfies

$$\ell(S; \boldsymbol{\beta}) = \log(L(S; \boldsymbol{\beta})) = \sum_{s \in S} \ell_s.$$

The maximum likelihood estimate $\boldsymbol{\beta}(S)$ of $\boldsymbol{\beta}$ is computed by solving the estimating equations $\partial \ell(S; \boldsymbol{\beta}) / \partial \boldsymbol{\beta} = \mathbf{0}$ obtained by differentiating $\ell(S; \boldsymbol{\beta})$ with respect to $\boldsymbol{\beta}$, where $\mathbf{0}$ denotes the zero vector. For simplicity of notation, parameter estimates $\boldsymbol{\beta}(S)$ are denoted as functions of indexes for the data used in their computation without hat ($^\wedge$) symbols. With this notation, the LCV formulation of Sect. 2.5.3 extends to the logistic regression context. For $s \in S$, the estimated value for the mean μ_s is $\mu_s(S) = \exp(\mathbf{x}_s^T \cdot \boldsymbol{\beta}(S)) / (1 + \exp(\mathbf{x}_s^T \cdot \boldsymbol{\beta}(S)))$ and the corresponding residual is $e_s(S) = y_s - \mu_s(S)$ (with only two possible values of $1 - \mu_s(S)$ when $y_s = 1$ and $-\mu_s(S)$ when $y_s = 0$). The estimated value for the variance σ_s^2 is $\sigma_s^2(S) = \mu_s(S) \cdot (1 - \mu_s(S))$. The standardized or Pearson residual $\text{stde}_s(S) = e_s(S)/\sigma_s(S)$ is obtained by standardizing the residual by dividing by the estimated standard deviation.

The predictor vectors $\mathbf{x}_s$ can be based on fractional polynomial transforms of primary predictors as considered in analyses reported in Chaps. 2 and 4. Adaptive fractional polynomial models can also be selected using the adaptive modeling process controlled by LCV scores as in Chaps. 2 and 4, but with the LCV scores computed for the logistic regression case.

8.3.2   Odds Ratio Function Formulation

When a predictor value $x_{sj} = u_{sj}^P$ is a power transform of a primary predictor value u_{sj} (assuming that u_{sj}^P is well-defined), the exponent $\exp(\beta_j)$ of the associated slope β_j represents the OR for $y_s = 1$ under a unit change in the predictor value x_{sj} adjusted for the other predictor values $x_{sj'}$ for $j' \neq j$ (if any). However, there are problems with this definition of the OR in general. First, if one of the other predictors $x_{sj'} = u_{sj'}^{P'}$ is a transform of the same primary predictor (for example, two transforms of weight for the mercury level data) so that $u_{sj'} = u_{sj}$, the values of all the other transforms do not remain constant when the value of x_{sj} changes by one unit. Second, it seems more appropriate to account for effects on the odds of changes in the primary predictor value u_{sj}, not changes in its transformed value. For example, how the odds for a high mercury level over 1.0 ppm change with changes in weight of the fish seems more important than how the odds change with unit changes in some power transform weight^p of weight with $p \neq 1$ (for example, $p = -0.5$ as selected in Sect. 8.4). In the fractional polynomial context, the OR can be generalized to account for changes in the primary predictor and for all transforms of that primary predictor in the model.

For standard logistic regression with each predictor untransformed and none of them transforms of the other predictors, the log(OR) for a predictor is its associated slope. When the predictor is continuous, that slope is also the derivative of the logit function with respect to the predictor and so is the instantaneous rate of change of the log odds for $y_s = 1$ in that predictor as well as the change in the log odds due to a unit change in the predictor. In the fractional polynomial context, the log(OR(u)) for a primary predictor u can be generalized to the first derivative function of the logit function with respect to that primary predictor. Each transform of that primary predictor in the fractional polynomial is simply differentiated (for example, the derivative of $u_{sj}^p \cdot \beta_j$ with respect to u_{sj} is $p \cdot u_{sj}^{p-1} \cdot \beta_j$; see Sect. 9.3 for an example). The derivative function of the logit function is exponentiated to obtain the odds ratio function OR(u) representing the exponentiated instantaneous rate of change in the log odds for $y_s = 1$ at each value of the primary predictor u, adjusting for the values of all the other distinct primary predictors for the model (if any). In the case where there is a single primary predictor u, the odds under a change Δu in u can be approximated using a Taylor expansion of logit(u) as

$$\text{odds}(u + \Delta u) = \exp(\text{logit}(u + \Delta u)) \approx \exp(\text{logit}(u) + \partial \text{logit}(u)/\partial u \cdot \Delta u)$$

$$= \text{odds}(u) \cdot \text{OR}(u)^{\Delta u}.$$

Assuming this approximation holds for a unit increase $\Delta u = 1$, the above relationship means that under a unit increase from a given value u of the primary predictor, the odds at $u + 1$ are approximately equal to the odds ratio OR(u) at u multiplied by the odds at u. A similar interpretation holds when adjusting for values of other primary predictors. Reported analyses use this approach to simplify the interpretation of generated OR functions.

8.4 Dichotomous Mercury Level as a Function of Weight

The adaptive model for merchig as a function of weight is used as a benchmark analysis for setting the number k of folds (see Sect. 2.8). The first local maximum in the LCV score is attained at $k = 15$, and so this value is used in subsequent analyses of this outcome. This adaptively chosen model is based on the single power transform weight$^{-0.5}$ (all models for means reported in this chapter have intercepts) with 15-fold LCV score 0.56081. The estimated slope for this weight transform is negative so that the logits and hence the probabilities for a high mercury level under this model increase with weight as would be expected. The same model is selected at $k = 20$

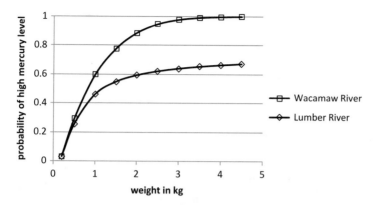

Fig. 8.1 Estimated probability of a high mercury level over 1.0 ppm as a function of weight moderated by river for fish caught in the Lumber and Waccamaw Rivers based on adaptive logistic regression modeling

while the model based on the single power transform weight$^{-0.4}$ is selected at k = 5 and k = 10, and so the adaptive model in this case is relatively robust to the choice of k. The model linear in weight has LCV score 0.54346 with PD of 3.09 % compared to the adaptive model and so substantial (that is, larger than the cutoff 1.13 % for the data). Consequently, the logits for merchigh are distinctly nonlinear in weight.

How merchigh depends on weight might change with the river in which the fish were caught (an issue called moderation or modification; see Sect. 4.5.3). This can be addressed with the adaptive model based on weight, river, and geometric combinations (GCs) in these two predictors (see Sect. 4.5.4 for the definition of GCs). The generated model is based on the two transforms: weight$^{-0.8}$ and $(\text{river} \cdot \text{weight}^{-2})^{-0.8}$ with LCV score 0.57192. The model based on weight and river without GCs is the same as the model based on weight alone with LCV score 0.56081 and substantial PD 1.94 %. Thus, the dependence of merchigh on weight is different for the two rivers. Estimated probabilities generated by the GC-based model are plotted in Fig. 8.1. The probability of a mercury level over 1.0 ppm increases as the weight of the fish increases from approximately 0.2 kg to 4.5 kg, starting at about the same near zero value for the two rivers, but to a distinctly higher level for fish caught in the Waccamaw River.

8.5 Dichotomous Mercury Level as a Function of Length

The adaptive model for merchigh as a function of length is based on the single power transform length$^{0.5}$ with LCV score 0.59140. The model linear in length has LCV score 0.59136 with insubstantial PD of 0.01 % compared to the adaptive model. Thus, the logits for merchigh are reasonably close to linear in length. The adaptive model based on length, river, and possible GCs in these two predictors

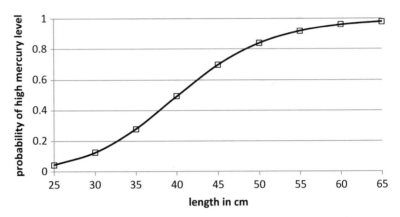

Fig. 8.2 Estimated probability of a high mercury level over 1.0 ppm as a function of length for fish caught in the Lumber and Waccamaw Rivers based on adaptive logistic regression modeling

depends only on length and is the same model as generated for length by itself. Consequently, the dependence of the logits for merchigh on length is reasonably treated as the same for the two rivers. Estimated probabilities generated by this latter model for a high level of mercury are plotted in Fig. 8.2. The probability of fish having a mercury level over 1.0 ppm increases in an s-shaped pattern as their lengths increase from approximately 25 cm to 65 cm, and this is the same for fish caught in the two rivers.

For the linear model in length, the odds ratio (OR), for a unit change in length, is estimated by exponentiating the estimated slope for length. Since the relationship is linear, the slope for length is also the derivative of the logit function with respect to length at each of its values. For nonlinear models in length, the OR is no longer a constant but is the function of length obtained by first differentiating the relationship between the logits for merchigh and length with respect to length and then exponentiating. The estimated OR function for the adaptive model in length is plotted in Fig. 8.3. The OR decreases from about 1.25 at a length of 25 cm to about 1.15 at a length of 65 cm. The values of the function represent the exponentiated instantaneous rates of change in the log odds for a high mercury level of over 1.0 ppm at different lengths and can be used to approximate the proportional change in the odds with a unit increase in length (see Sect. 8.3). For example, under a unit increase in length the odds for a high mercury level are approximately 1.25 units larger than the odds at length 25 cm, approximately 1.2 units larger at length 38 cm, and approximately 1.15 units at length 65 cm. For the linear model in length, the estimated constant OR is 1.20 with 95 % confidence interval 1.13 to 1.27. The fact that all the values of the estimated OR function of Fig. 8.3 lie within this confidence interval provides support for the conclusion that the OR for merchigh is constant in length, further supporting the earlier conclusion that the logits for merchigh are close to linear in length.

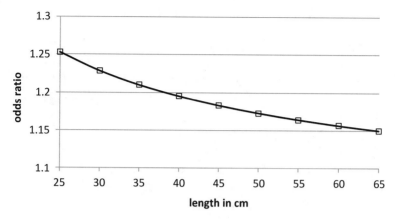

Fig. 8.3 Estimated odds ratio function for a high mercury level over 1.0 ppm as a function of length for fish caught in the Lumber and Waccamaw Rivers based on adaptive logistic regression modeling

8.6   Dichotomous Mercury Level as a Function of Weight and Length

The adaptive additive model in weight and length is based on two transforms: $\text{length}^{0.9}$ and $\text{weight}^{0.3}$ with LCV score 0.60382. The best singleton predictor model is the one for length with LCV score 0.59140 and substantial PD of 2.06 %, and so weight explains aspects of merchigh not explained by length alone. The linear model in weight and length has LCV score 0.60244 with insubstantial PD of 0.23 %. Thus, after controlling for the nearly linear effect to length, the distinct nonlinear effect to weight by itself becomes reasonably close to linear. The adaptive model in weight and length and possible GCs is based on the three transforms: $\text{length}^{1.5}$, $(\text{weight}^{0.3} \cdot \text{length}^{-0.4})^{10}$, and $\text{weight}^{2.5}$ along with an intercept and improved LCV score 0.61585. The PD for the additive model is substantial at 1.95 % indicating that the logits for merchigh are reasonably considered to change differently in weight (length) for different values of length (weight). The adaptive model in weight, length, and river with GCs is based on the four transforms: $\text{length}^{0.5}$, $(\text{river} \cdot \text{weight}^{-2} \cdot \text{length})^{0.5}$, $(\text{river} \cdot \text{weight}^{0.7} \cdot \text{length}^{-0.3})^{3.4}$, and $(\text{length}^{0.5} \cdot \text{weight}^{-0.2})^{3}$ with improved LCV score 0.64474. This is a substantial improvement over the GC-based model in weight and length with substantial PD 4.48 %. Consequently, the dependence of mean merchigh on weight and length in combination is reasonably considered to be different for the two rivers.

Figure 8.4 displays estimated probabilities for the Lumber and Waccamaw Rivers of a high mercury level over 1.0 ppm as a function of weight for the relatively low length of 30 cm generated by the model based on river, weight, length, and GCs with the best overall LCV score. The range of weight values is based on observed weight values for fish close to 30 cm in length. The probability of a high mercury level decreases with increasing weight of fish caught in the Lumber

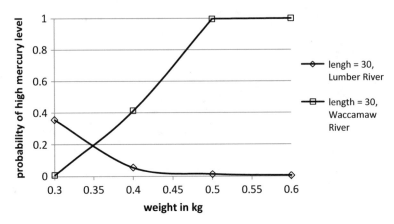

Fig. 8.4 Estimated probability of a high mercury level over 1.0 ppm as a function of weight for fish caught in the Lumber and Waccamaw Rivers for length 30 cm based on adaptive logistic regression modeling

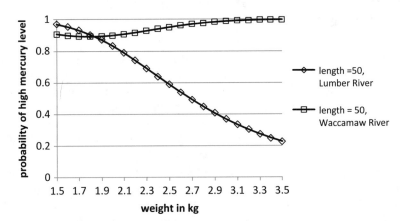

Fig. 8.5 Estimated probability of a high mercury level over 1.0 ppm as a function of weight for fish caught in the Lumber and Waccamaw Rivers for length 50 cm based on adaptive logistic regression modeling

River to essentially zero by 0.5 kg and increases for fish caught in the Waccamaw River and to essentially 1 by 0.5 kg. Figure 8.5 displays estimated probabilities of the same kind, but for the relatively high length of 50 cm. As before, the range of weight values is based on observed weight values for fish, but now when close to 50 cm in length. The probability of a high mercury level is relatively high for low weights of fish caught in both rivers, but a little lower for fish caught in the Waccamaw River. It then decreases with increasing weight of fish caught in the Lumber River and increases somewhat for fish caught in the Waccamaw River. For fish caught in the Wacammaw River having the relatively high length of 50 cm, the probability of having a high mercury level >1 ppm is quite high at 0.89 or higher and this holds as well for larger lengths (not plotted in the figures).

8.7 Multiple Logistic Regression Modeling of Polytomous Outcomes

Outcomes with more than two but a finite number of values are called polytomous (or polychotomous). The outcome values are assumed here to be coded as numeric values, but those values can be nominal (that is, numeric in name only) or ordinal (that is, truly numeric and ordered). Outcomes with nominal values can only be appropriately analyzed with multinomial regression using generalized logits relative to one reference outcome value for each of the other outcome values. Outcomes with ordinal values can be appropriately analyzed with multinomial regression or with ordinal regression using cumulative logits for the cumulative probabilities for the outcome values in order (except for the last outcome value with cumulative probability 1). For multinomial regression, each generalized logit has its own separate set of coefficients for the predictors of the model including the intercepts of the model corresponding to the unit predictor (that is, with constant value 1). For ordinal regression, each cumulative logit has its own separate intercept coefficient along with the same slope coefficients for the other predictors of the model. Since these slope coefficients are the same, they generate a common proportional odds ratio. Multinomial regression is formulated in Sect. 8.7.1 and ordinal regression in Sect. 8.7.2 (but these can be skipped to focus on analyses).

8.7.1 Multinomial Regression

Extending the notation of Sect. 8.3, assume that the outcome measurements y_s can have integer values $v = 0, 1, \cdots, K$ where $K > 1$ (the case $K = 1$ is the same as the dichotomous outcome case of Sect. 8.3). For $0 \leq v \leq K$, let y_{sv} be the indicator for $y_s = v$. Conditioned on the observed predictor vector $\mathbf{x}_s$, the mean or expected value μ_{sv} for y_{sv} satisfies $\mu_{sv} = Ey_{sv} = P(y_s = v|\mathbf{x}_s)$ for $s \in S$. Using generalized logits, model $\mathrm{glogit}(\mu_{sv}) = \log(\mu_{sv}/\mu_{s0}) = \mathbf{x}_s^T \cdot \boldsymbol{\beta}_v$ for $1 \leq v \leq K$ (and so with $v = 0$ as the reference value) and K r $\times 1$ vectors $\boldsymbol{\beta}_v$ of coefficients. The odds ratio OR for $y_s = v$ versus $y_s = 0$ under a unit change in a predictor value x_{sj} adjusted for the other predictor values $x_{sj'}$ for $j' \neq j$ (if any) is computed as $\mathrm{OR} = \exp(\beta_{vj})$. Solving for μ_{sv} gives

$$\mu_{sv} = \frac{\exp(\mathbf{x}_s^T \cdot \boldsymbol{\beta}_v)}{1 + \exp(\mathbf{x}_s^T \cdot \boldsymbol{\beta}_1) + \cdots + \exp(\mathbf{x}_s^T \cdot \boldsymbol{\beta}_K)}$$

for $1 \leq v \leq K$ and, for $v = 0$, $\mu_{s0} = 1/(1 + \exp(\mathbf{x}_s^T \cdot \boldsymbol{\beta}_1) + \cdots + \exp(\mathbf{x}_s^T \cdot \boldsymbol{\beta}_K))$. The conditional variance for y_{sv} is $\sigma_{sv}^2 = \mu_{sv} \cdot (1 - \mu_{sv})$.

The likelihood term L_s for the sth subject is based on the categorical distribution and satisfies

$$\ell_s = \log(L_s) = y_{s0} \cdot \log(\mu_{s0}) + \cdots + y_{sK} \cdot \log(\mu_{sK}).$$

With $\boldsymbol{\theta} = (\boldsymbol{\beta}_1^T, \cdots, \boldsymbol{\beta}_K^T)^T$, the likelihood $L(S;\boldsymbol{\theta})$ is the product of the likelihood terms L_s over $s \in S$ and satisfies

$$\ell(S; \boldsymbol{\theta}) = \log(L(S; \boldsymbol{\theta})) = \sum_{s \in S} \ell_s.$$

The maximum likelihood estimate $\boldsymbol{\theta}(S)$ of $\boldsymbol{\theta}$ is computed by solving the estimating equations $\partial \ell(S; \boldsymbol{\theta})/\partial \boldsymbol{\theta} = \mathbf{0}$ obtained by differentiating $\ell(S; \boldsymbol{\theta})$ with respect to $\boldsymbol{\theta}$, where $\mathbf{0}$ denotes the zero vector. For simplicity of notation, parameter estimates $\boldsymbol{\theta}(S)$ are denoted as functions of indexes for the data used in their computation without hat (^) symbols. With this notation, the LCV formulation of Sect. 8.3 extends to the multinomial regression context.

For $s \in S$, the estimated value for the mean μ_{sv} for $1 \le v \le K$ is

$$\mu_{sv}(S) = \frac{\exp\left(\mathbf{x}_s^T \cdot \boldsymbol{\beta}_v(S)\right)}{1 + \exp\left(\mathbf{x}_s^T \cdot \boldsymbol{\beta}_1(S)\right) + \cdots + \exp\left(\mathbf{x}_s^T \cdot \boldsymbol{\beta}_K(S)\right)},$$

while for $v = 0$, $\mu_{s0}(S) = 1/(1 + \exp(\mathbf{x}_s^T \cdot \boldsymbol{\beta}_1(S) + \cdots + \exp(\mathbf{x}_s^T \cdot \boldsymbol{\beta}_K(S))$.

The estimated values for the variances σ_{sv}^2 are $\sigma_{sv}^2(S) = \mu_{sv}(S) \cdot (1 - \mu_{sv}(S))$. The residuals are $e_{sv}(S) = y_{sv} - \mu_{sv}(S)$ and are combined into the K-dimensional vectors $\mathbf{e}_s(S)$. The covariance matrix $\boldsymbol{\Sigma}_s(S)$ for $\mathbf{e}_s(S)$ satisfies $\boldsymbol{\Sigma}_s(S) = \text{diag}(\mu_s(S)) - \mu_s(S) \cdot \mu_s(S)^T$ (see, for example, Eq. (A.13.15), Bickel and Doksum 1977) where $\mu_s(S)$ is the K-dimensional vector with entries $\mu_{sv}(S)$ for $1 \le v \le K$ and $\text{diag}(\mu_s(S))$ is the diagonal matrix with diagonal entries $\mu_{sv}(S)$. As in Sect. 4.3.3, scaled residual vectors $\mathbf{sclde}_s(S)$ can then be computed as $\mathbf{sclde}_s(S) = (\mathbf{U}_s^T(S))^{-1} \cdot \mathbf{e}_s(S)$ where $\mathbf{U}_s(S)$ is the square root of the covariance matrix $\boldsymbol{\Sigma}_s(S)$ determined by its Cholesky decomposition. The entries of $\mathbf{sclde}_s(S)$ can be combined over all s and analyzed in combination as for independent data.

The predictor vectors $\mathbf{x}_s$ can be based on fractional polynomial transforms of primary predictors as considered in analyses reported in Sects. 8.4–8.6. Adaptive fractional polynomial models can also be selected using the adaptive modeling process controlled by LCV scores as used in Sects. 8.4–8.6, but with LCV scores computed for the multinomial regression case. The normalizing constant used in the LCV formulation of Sect. 2.5.3 for continuous univariate outcomes is the number n of subjects, which is also appropriate to use for dichotomous outcomes. For polytomous outcomes, each subject's outcome value is determined by the K indicators y_{sv} for $1 \le v \le K$, and so the normalizing constant is changed to the effective number $n \cdot K$ of measurements. As in Sect. 8.3, OR functions for fractional polynomial models can be computed by exponentiating derivatives of generalized logit functions in primary predictors. In this case, there are multiple OR functions for $1 \leq v \leq K$.

8.7.2 Ordinal Regression

The model of Sect. 8.7.1 applies to any polytomous outcome whether the values are nominal or ordinal. When the outcome is ordinal, an alternate model can be considered based on cumulative logits under the proportional odds assumption as formulated in this section. Since the outcome values are ordinal, they can be ordered either from lowest to highest or from highest to lowest.

Assume that unit predictor values are not included in the predictor vectors $\mathbf{x}_s$. Conditioned on the random predictor vector having the observed value $\mathbf{x}_s$, denote the cumulative probabilities as $P_{sv} = P(y_s \leq v | \mathbf{x}_s)$ for $s \in S$. Using cumulative logits, model $\text{logit}(P_{sv}) = \alpha_v + \mathbf{x}_s^T \cdot \boldsymbol{\beta}$ for $0 \leq v \leq K - 1$ where the α_v are K intercept parameters and $\boldsymbol{\beta}$ is a $r \times 1$ vector of coefficients. Solving for P_{sv} gives

$$P_{sv} = \frac{\exp(\alpha_v + \mathbf{x}_s^T \cdot \boldsymbol{\beta})}{1 + \exp(\alpha_v + \mathbf{x}_s^T \cdot \boldsymbol{\beta})}$$

for $0 \leq v \leq K - 1$ while $P_{sK} = 1$. Since P_{sv} are cumulative probabilities, they must increase with v. It is straightforward to show that $\exp(\alpha + \mathbf{x}_s^T \cdot \boldsymbol{\beta})/(1 + \exp(\alpha + \mathbf{x}_s^T \cdot \boldsymbol{\beta}))$ is increasing in α, and so α_v is constrained to be strictly increasing in v (so P_{sv} differ). The odds ratio (OR) for $y_s \leq v$ versus $y_s > v$ under a unit change in a predictor value x_{sj} and adjusted for the other predictor values $x_{sj'}$ for $j' \neq j$ (if any) is computed as $\text{OR} = \exp(\beta_j)$. Since these ORs are constant in v, this is called proportional odds. With $\boldsymbol{\theta} = (\alpha_0, \cdots, \alpha_{K-1}, \boldsymbol{\beta}^T)^T$, the maximum likelihood and LCV formulations of Sect. 8.7.1 extend to the ordinal regression context.

For $s \in S$, the estimated value for P_{sv} with $0 \leq v \leq K - 1$ is

$$P_{sv}(S) = \frac{\exp\left(\alpha_v(S) + \mathbf{x}_s^T \cdot \boldsymbol{\beta}(S)\right)}{1 + \exp\left(\alpha_v(S) + \mathbf{x}_s^T \cdot \boldsymbol{\beta}(S)\right)}.$$

Since $\mu_{s0} = P_{s0}$ and $\mu_{sv} = P_{sv} - P_{sv-1}$ for $1 \leq v \leq K - 1$, they are estimated as $\mu_{s0}(S) = P_{s0}(S)$, $\mu_{sv}(S) = P_{sv}(S) - P_{sv-1}(S)$ for $1 \leq v \leq K - 1$ while $\mu_{sK}(S) = 1 - (\mu_{s0}(S) + \cdots + \mu_{sK-1}(S))$. The variances σ_{sv}^2 are estimated as $\sigma_{sv}^2(S) = \mu_{sv}(S) \cdot (1 - \mu_{sv}(S))$. The residuals are $e_{sv}(S) = y_{sv} - \mu_{sv}(S)$ and are combined into the K-dimensional vectors $\mathbf{e}_s(S)$. As in Sect. 8.7.1, scaled residual vectors $\mathbf{sclde}_s(S)$ can then be computed as $\mathbf{sclde}_s(S) = (\mathbf{U}_s^T(S))^{-1} \cdot \mathbf{e}_s(S)$ where $\mathbf{U}_s(S)$ is the square root of the covariance matrix $\Sigma_s(S) = \text{diag}(\mu_s(S)) - \mu_s(S) \cdot \mu_s(S)^T$. The entries of **sclde**$_s$(S) can be combined over all s and analyzed in combination as for independent data.

The predictor vectors x_s can be based on fractional polynomial transforms of primary predictors as considered in analyses of Sects. 8.4–8.6. Adaptive fractional polynomial models can also be selected using the adaptive modeling process controlled by LCV scores as in Sects. 8.4–8.6, but with LCV scores computed for the ordinal regression case normalized by the n·K effective measurements. As in Sect. 8.3, OR functions for fractional polynomial models can be computed by exponentiating derivatives of cumulative logit functions in primary predictors, but now there is only one OR function for all $0 \leq v \leq K - 1$.

8.8   Mercury Level Categorized into Three Ordinal Levels

A variable called merclevel exists in the mercury data set with values categorizing mercury levels into the three levels of high (mercury > 1.3 ppm) with value 2, medium (0.72 ppm $<$ mercury ≤ 1.3 ppm) with value 1, and low (mercury ≤ 0.72 ppm) with value 0. A total of 61 (or 36.1 %) of the fish had a high mercury level, 52 (or 30.8 %) had a medium mercury level, and 56 (33.1 %) had a low mercury level, and so the cutoffs (0.72 and 1.3 ppm) for this variable are close to splitting the mercury levels into tertiles. The cutoff for a substantial PD in the LCV scores for these data with $169 \cdot 2 = 338$ effective measurements is 0.57 %.

8.9   Polytomous Mercury Level as a Function of Weight

The adaptive ordinal regression model for merclevel as a function of weight is used as a benchmark analysis for setting the number k of folds. For k $= 5$, the generated model is based on the single transform weight$^{0.1}$ with LCV score 0.61864. The model generated for k $= 10$ is also based on weight$^{0.1}$ while the model for k $= 15$ is based on weight$^{0.2}$, but both with smaller LCV scores. Since k $= 5$ generates the largest LCV score, it is used in subsequent analyses of merclevel. The model linear in weight has LCV score 0.61172 with substantial PD of 1.12 % compared to the adaptive model, and so the logits for merclevel are distinctly nonlinear in weight. The adaptive multinomial regression model for merclevel as a function of weight is based on the single transform weight$^{-0.1}$ but has smaller LCV score 0.61709, and so there is no benefit to the more complex multinomial model over the simpler ordinal regression model. Consequently, only ordinal regression models are considered in subsequent analyses of merclevel.

It is possible that the dependence of merclevel on weight changes with the river in which the fish were caught. This can be addressed with the adaptive model based

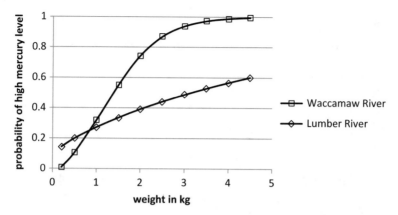

Fig. 8.6 Estimated probability of a high mercury level over 1.3 ppm as a function of weight moderated by river for fish caught in the Lumber and Waccamaw Rivers based on adaptive ordinal regression modeling

on weight, river, and possible GCs in these two predictors. The generated model is based on the three transforms $weight^{0.4}$, $(river \cdot weight^{1.7})^{0.7}$, and $river \cdot weight^{-1.1}$. The LCV score is 0.63458. The generated additive model for weight and river without GCs is the same as the model based on weight alone with LCV score 0.61864 and substantial PD 2.51 %. Thus, the dependence of the logits for merclevel on weight is different for the two rivers. Estimated probabilities, as generated by the GC-based model, for a high level of mercury are plotted in Fig. 8.6. The probability of fish having a mercury level over 1.3 ppm is somewhat higher for fish caught in the Lumber River than in the Waccamaw River at a low weight of about 0.2 kg for fish in the Lumber River, increases as weights increase to 4.5 kg, but to higher levels for fish caught in the Waccamaw River. Plots for probabilities for a low and for a low or medium mercury level are not provided but they decrease with increased weight, to lower levels for fish caught in the Waccamaw River than in the Lumber River, and with lower values for a low than for a low or medium mercury level.

8.10 Polytomous Mercury Level as a Function of Length

The adaptive model for merclevel as a function of length is based on the single power transform $length^{2.5}$ with LCV score 0.64103. The model linear in length has LCV score 0.63993 with insubstantial PD of 0.17 % compared to the adaptive model. Thus, cumulative logits for merclevel are reasonably close to linear in length. The adaptive model based on length, river, and possible GCs in these two predictors depends only on length, and so the dependence of the cumulative logits for merclevel on length is reasonably treated as the same for the two rivers.

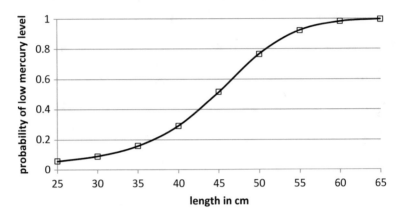

Fig. 8.7 Estimated probability of a high mercury level over 1.3 ppm as a function of length for fish caught in the Lumber and Waccamaw Rivers based on adaptive ordinal regression modeling

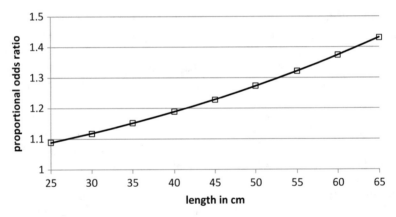

Fig. 8.8 Estimated proportional odds ratio function for cumulative mercury level of high over 1.3 ppm and of medium or high over 0.72 ppm as a function of length for fish caught in the Lumber and Waccamaw Rivers based on adaptive ordinal regression modeling

Estimated probabilities for the model in length for a high level of mercury are plotted in Fig. 8.7. The probability of fish having a mercury level over 1.3 ppm increases in an s-shaped pattern as their lengths increase from approximately 25 cm to 65 cm and is the same for fish caught in the two rivers.

Using the adaptive model in length with mercury levels ordered from high to low, the estimated proportional OR function is plotted in Fig. 8.8. The OR increases nearly linearly from 1.08 at a length of 25 cm to 1.43 at a length of 65 cm. For this model, the value of the proportional OR function at a given length represents the approximate proportional change, with a unit increase in length, in the odds for a higher mercury level (that is, a high level or a medium to high level) versus a lower mercury level (that is, a low to medium level or a low level). In this case, the OR is always greater than 1, and so the odds for a higher versus lower mercury level increase with an increase in length. Since the OR function increases, the increase in odds for a higher versus lower mercury level with an increase in length is greater starting at larger lengths. For example, with a unit increase in length, the odds for a higher versus lower mercury level are approximately 1.08 times what they are at 25 cm and approximately 1.43 times what they are at 65 cm.

8.11 Polytomous Mercury Level as a Function of Weight and Length

The adaptive additive model in weight and length is based on the two transforms: $\text{length}^{3.1}$ and $\text{weight}^{1.1}$ with LCV score 0.64583. The best singleton predictor model is the one for length with LCV score 0.64103 and substantial PD of 0.74 %, and so weight explains aspects of merclevel not explained by length alone. The linear model in weight and length has LCV score 0.63981 with substantial PD of 0.93 %. Consequently, the additive model in both length and weight is distinctly nonlinear, in contrast to the analyses of merchigh reported in Sect. 8.6. The adaptive model in weight and length and possible GCs is based on the three transform: $(\text{weight}^6 \cdot \text{length}^{-20})^{2.3}$, $(\text{weight} \cdot \text{length}^{-0.5})^{1.8}$, and $(\text{weight}^{-11} \cdot \text{length}^3)^{1.56}$ with LCV score 0.66452. The PD for the additive model is substantial at 2.81 %, indicating that the effects of these two variables on merclevel distinctly interact with each other. The adaptive model in weight, length, and river along with possible GCs is based on the six transforms: $(\text{length}^{2.5} \cdot \text{weight}^{-0.24})^{0.9}$, $(\text{weight}^6 \cdot \text{length}^{-20})^{3.1}$, $(\text{river} \cdot \text{weight}^{-1.2} \cdot \text{length})^{1.41}$, $(\text{length}^{2.5} \cdot \text{river} \cdot \text{weight}^{0.8})^{-0.81}$, $(\text{length}^{1.5} \cdot \text{weight}^{-0.6})^2$, and $\text{length}^{1.26}$ with improved LCV score 0.67602. The PD for the model not considering river is substantial at 1.70 %, and so the effects of length and weight are substantially different for the two rivers.

Figure 8.9 displays estimated probabilities for the Lumber and Waccamaw Rivers of a high mercury level over 1.3 ppm as a function of weight for the relatively low length of 30 cm generated by the model based on river, weight, length, and GCs with the best overall LCV score. The range of weight values is based on observed weight values for fish close to 30 cm in length. The probability of a high mercury level decreases with increasing weight of fish caught in the Lumber River and increases for fish caught in the Waccamaw River. Figure 8.10 displays estimated probabilities of the same kind, but for the relatively high length of 50 cm. As before, the range of weight values is based on observed weight values for fish, but now when close to 50 cm in length. The probability of a high mercury level increases with increasing weight of fish caught in both rivers, but starting at a lower level for fish caught in the Waccamaw River at lower weights and becoming somewhat higher for weights larger than 1.9 kg.

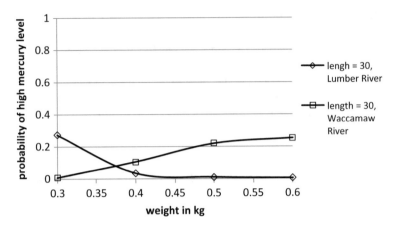

Fig. 8.9 Estimated probability of a high mercury level over 1.3 ppm as a function of weight for fish caught in the Lumber and Waccamaw Rivers for length 30 cm based on adaptive ordinal regression modeling

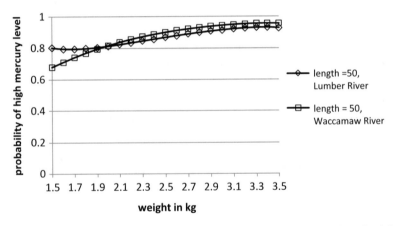

Fig. 8.10 Estimated probability of a high mercury level over 1.3 ppm as a function of weight for fish caught in the Lumber and Waccamaw Rivers for length 50 cm based on adaptive ordinal regression modeling

8.12 Proportion of Correct Deleted Predictions

Logistic regression models of all types (that is, for dichotomous outcomes and for polytomous outcomes modeled with multinomial or ordinal regression) generate estimates of the probability of an outcome having each of the possible outcome values under alternative settings of predictor vectors. These in turn generate predictions of the outcome values for the observations. An observation's predicted outcome value (using maximum likelihood estimation) is the outcome value with the largest estimated probability under the predictor vector for that observation. This is a correct prediction when the predicted outcome value is the actual outcome value for the observation. For a given fold assignment, deleted predicted values can be computed for observations in each fold using predicted probabilities computed from the observations in the complement of the fold. The proportion of correct deleted predictions (PCDP) over all folds can be used as a model selection score. For example, Efron (1983) uses the leave-one-out (LOO) PCDP score for selecting logistic regression models for dichotomous outcomes. The LOO PCDP score can be computed from the estimated LOO predicted probabilities generated by PROC LOGISTIC with the "predprobs = (crossvalidate)" option of the output statement (but only for dichotomous outcomes). More general k-fold PCDP scores are computed by the genreg macro for logistic regression models of all types and can be used in place of LCV scores to generate adaptive logistic regression model. A formulation is provided in Sect. 8.12.1 (which can be skipped) and example analyses of merchigh and merclevel using PCDP scores in Sects. 8.12.2 and 8.12.3.

8.12.1 Formulation

Let $\mu_{sv}(S)$ be the estimated probability for each subject (or observation) $s \in S = \{s : 1 \leq s \leq n\}$ and for each outcome value v with $0 \leq v \leq K$ under any type of logistic regression model for any number $K + 1 \geq 2$ of outcome values. Under maximum likelihood estimation, the predicted value for each subject $s \in S$ is given by $y_s(S) = v(s)$ where $\mu_{sv(s)}(S) = \max_{0 \leq v' \leq K}(\mu_{sv'}(S))$, that is, $y_s(S)$ is the outcome value with the largest predicted probability for the subject. When ties occur for the largest predicted value, genreg uses the smallest such outcome value to simplify computations compared to randomly selecting between ties. Partition S into $k > 1$ disjoint folds $F(h)$, $h \in H = \{h : 1 \leq h \leq k\}$. The k-fold proportion of correct deleted predictions is given by

$$PCDP = \frac{1}{n} \sum_{h \in H} \sum_{s \in F(h)} \delta(y_s, y_s(S \backslash F(h))),$$

where $\delta(y_s, y_s(S \backslash F(h)))$ is the indicator for $y_s = y_s(S \backslash F(h))$, that is, it equals 1 when $y_s = y_s(S \backslash F(h,))$ and 0 otherwise. LOO PCDP scores correspond to the case where each subject s is in its own fold. Otherwise, random fold assignment is used (as in Sect. 2.5.3). Since larger PCDP scores indicate better models, PCDP scores can be used in place of LCV scores to control the adaptive modeling process.

8.12.2 Example Analyses of Dichotomous Mercury Level

The adaptive unit dispersions model for merchigh in terms of weight, length, river, and GCs based on LCV scores is described in Sect. 8.6. It has the largest LCV score of 0.64474 for prior models of merchigh and PCDP score 0.79882 (135/169 correctly predicted merchigh values; both types of scores are generated by genreg for logistic regression models). The associated adaptive model based on PCDP scores includes the two transforms for the means: $(\text{weight}^{-1} \cdot \text{length}^{-2.1})^{1.1}$ and $(\text{length}^{-2} \cdot \text{weight}^{0.9})^2$ with lower PCDP score 0.78107 (132/169 correctly predicted merchigh values) and LCV score 0.56584. The PD in the LCV scores for the PCDP-based model is substantial at 12.24 %. In this case, the LCV-based model outperforms the PCDP-based model on the basis of both PCDP and LCV scores and leads to a different conclusion about the impact of river. These results indicate that PCDP scores can generate distinctly inferior adaptive models for dichotomous outcomes. The adaptive modeling process may not be appropriate for use with PCDP scores for such outcomes. Also, since likelihoods are the basis for parameter estimation in the logistic regression context, the use of LCV scores for model selection reflects the parameter estimation more closely and so seems more appropriate.

8.12.3   Example Analyses of Polytomous Mercury Level

The adaptive unit dispersions model for merclevel in terms of weight, length, river, and GCs based on LCV scores is described in Sect. 8.11. It has the largest LCV score of 0.67602 for prior models of merclevel and PCDP score 0.66272 (112/169 correctly predicted merclevel values). The associated adaptive model based on PCDP scores has PCDP score 0.62722 (106/169 correctly predicted merclevel values) and LCV score 0.64885. The PD in the LCV scores for the PCDP-based model is substantial at 4.02 %. Once again, the LCV-based model outperforms the PCDP-based model on the basis of both PCDP and LCV scores. These results indicate that PCDP scores can generate distinctly inferior adaptive models for polytomous outcomes. Since this also is the case for dichotomous outcomes (Sect. 8.12.2), the use of PCDP scores is not recommended for adaptive modeling.

8.13   Modeling Dispersions as Well as Means

This section provides formulations (which can be skipped) and example analyses for logistic regression modeling of dispersions along with means. Sections 8.13.1 and 8.13.2 provide formulations for the dichotomous and polytomous outcome cases, respectively. Section 8.13.3 provides example adaptive analyses of means and dispersions for the dichotomous merchigh outcome variable. See Sect. 9.12 for an example analysis of means and dispersions for the polytomous outcome merclevel.

8.13.1   Formulation for Dichotomous Outcomes

For standard logistic regression models, outcome measurements y_s are dichotomous with values 0 and 1, means $\mu_s = P(y_s = 1)$, and variances $V(\mu_s) = \mu_s \cdot (1 - \mu_s)$. Consequently, variances are functions of the means and not separate parameters as for the normal distribution. The deviance terms are defined as (McCullagh and Nelder 1999)

$$d(y_s; \mu_s) = 2 \cdot \left[y_s \cdot \log\left(\frac{y_s}{\mu_s}\right) + (1 - y_s) \cdot \log\left(\frac{1 - y_s}{1 - \mu_s}\right) \right],$$

where $0 \cdot \log(0)$ is set equal to 0. Dispersion parameters ϕ_s can be incorporated into the logistic model through the extended quasi-likelihood terms QL_s^+ (McCullagh and Nelder 1999) satisfying

$$\ell_s^+ = \log(QL_s^+) = -\frac{1}{2} \cdot d(y_s; \mu_s)/\phi_s - \frac{1}{2} \cdot \log(\phi_s).$$

Let $\boldsymbol{\theta}$ denote the vector of all the parameters determining μ_s and ϕ_s for $s \in S$. Then, the extended quasi-likelihood $QL^+(S; \boldsymbol{\theta})$ satisfies

$$\ell^+(S; \boldsymbol{\theta}) = \log\left(QL^+(S; \boldsymbol{\theta})\right) = \sum_{s \in S} \ell_s^+ = \sum_{s \in S} \left((\ell_s - a_s)/\phi_s - \frac{1}{2} \cdot \log(\phi_s) \right),$$

where $\ell_s = y_s \cdot \log(\mu_s) + (1 - y_s) \cdot \log(1 - \mu_s)$ are the usual log likelihood terms and

$$a_s = y_s \cdot \log(y_s) + (1 - y_s) \cdot \log(1 - y_s) = 0$$

for $s \in S$. Extended variances σ_s^2 incorporating the dispersions can then be defined as $\sigma_s^2 = \phi_s \cdot V(\mu_s)$.

Assume as in Sect. 8.3 that $\text{logit}(\mu_s) = \mathbf{x}_s^T \cdot \boldsymbol{\beta}$. When $\phi_s = \phi$ are constant, $\boldsymbol{\theta} = (\boldsymbol{\beta}^T, \phi)^T$, and maximizing $\ell^+(S; \boldsymbol{\theta})$ in $\boldsymbol{\theta}$ generates the same estimates $\boldsymbol{\beta}(S)$ as maximum likelihood estimation of $\boldsymbol{\beta}$ under the unit dispersions logistic regression model. The maximum extended quasi-likelihood estimate $\phi(S)$ of ϕ then satisfies $\phi(S) = \sum_{s \in S} d(y_s; \mu_s(S))/n$ where $\mu_s(S)$ are the estimates of μ_s determined by $\boldsymbol{\beta}(S)$. More generally, model the log of the dispersions ϕ_s as a function of selected predictor variables and associated coefficients (in the same way as variances are modeled in Sect. 2.19.1). Specifically, let $\log(\phi_s) = \mathbf{v}_s^T \cdot \boldsymbol{\gamma}$ where, for $s \in S$, $\mathbf{v}_s$ is a $q \times 1$ column vector of q predictor values v_{sj} (including unit predictor values if an intercept is to be included) with indexes $j \in Q = \{j : 1 \leq j \leq q\}$ and $\boldsymbol{\gamma}$ is the associated $q \times 1$ column vector of coefficients. The $(r + q) \times 1$ parameter vector

$\boldsymbol{\theta} = (\boldsymbol{\beta}^T, \boldsymbol{\gamma}^T)^T$ is estimated through maximum extended quasi-likelihood estimation. Alternative models can be compared with extended quasi-likelihood cross-valida-tion (QLCV$^+$) scores computed as LCV scores are computed in Sect. 8.3, but using extended quasi-likelihoods rather than likelihoods and maximum extended quasi-likelihood estimates of $\boldsymbol{\theta}$ rather than maximum likelihood estimates. The adaptive modeling process can be extended to search through models for the means and dispersions in combination (see Chap. 20).

As in Sect. 8.3, for $s \in S$, the estimated value for the mean μ_s is

$$\mu_s(S) = \frac{\exp(\mathbf{x}_s^T \cdot \boldsymbol{\beta}(S))}{1 + \exp(\mathbf{x}_s^T \cdot \boldsymbol{\beta}(S))}$$

and the corresponding residual is $e_s(S) = y_s - \mu_s(S)$. The estimated value of the associated dispersion ϕ_s is $\phi_s(S) = \exp(\mathbf{v}_s^T \cdot \boldsymbol{\gamma}(S))$, and the estimated value for the extended variance σ_s^2 is $\sigma_s^2(S) = \phi_s(S) \cdot V(\mu_s(S))$. The standardized or Pearson residual $\text{stde}_s(S) = e_s(S)/\sigma_s(S)$ is obtained by standardizing the residual by divid-ing by the estimated extended standard deviation.

8.13.2   Formulation for Polytomous Outcomes

Using the notation of Sect. 8.7.1, for outcome measurements y_s with integer values $v = 0, 1, \cdots, K$, the deviance terms are defined as (McCullagh and Nelder 1999)

$$d(y_s; \mu_{s0}, \cdots, \mu_{sK}) = 2 \cdot \left[y_{s0} \cdot \log\left(\frac{y_{s0}}{\mu_{s0}}\right) + \cdots + y_{sK} \cdot \log\left(\frac{y_{sK}}{\mu_{sK}}\right) \right].$$

Dispersion parameters ϕ_s (and so the same for all $1 \leq v \leq K$) can be incorporated into the model through the extended quasi-likelihood terms QL_s^+ satisfying

$$\ell_s^+ = \log(QL_s^+) = -\frac{1}{2} \cdot d(y_s; \mu_{s0}, \cdots, \mu_{sK})/\phi_s - \frac{1}{2} \cdot \log(\phi_s).$$

Let $\boldsymbol{\theta}$ denote the vector of all the parameters determining $\mu_{s0}, \cdots, \mu_{sK}$ and ϕ_s for $s \in S$. Then, the extended quasi-likelihood $QL^+(S; \boldsymbol{\theta})$ satisfies

$$\ell^+(S; \boldsymbol{\theta}) = \log\left(QL^+(S; \boldsymbol{\theta})\right) = \sum_{s \in S} \ell_s^+ = \sum_{s \in S} \left((\ell_s - a_s)/\phi_s - \frac{1}{2} \cdot \log(\phi_s) \right),$$

where $\ell_s = y_{s0} \cdot \log(\mu_{s0}) + \cdots + y_{sK} \cdot \log(\mu_{sK})$ are the log likelihood terms and $a_s = y_{s0} \cdot \log(y_{s0}) + \cdots + y_{sK} \cdot \log(y_{sK}) = 0$ for $s \in S$. Extended variances σ_{sv}^2 can be defined that incorporate the dispersions as $\sigma_{sv}^2 = \phi_s \cdot V(\mu_{sv})$.

Assume as in Sect. 8.7.1 that $\mathrm{glogit}(\mu_{sv}) = \log(\mu_{sv}/\mu_{s0}) = \mathbf{x}_s^T \cdot \boldsymbol{\beta}_v$ for $1 \le v \le K$. When $\phi_s = \phi$ are constant, $\boldsymbol{\theta} = (\boldsymbol{\beta}_1^T, \cdots, \boldsymbol{\beta}_K^T, \phi)^T$, and maximizing $\ell^+(S; \boldsymbol{\theta})$ in $\boldsymbol{\theta}$ generates the same estimates $\boldsymbol{\beta}_1(S), \cdots, \boldsymbol{\beta}_K(S)$ as generated by maximum likelihood estimation of $\boldsymbol{\beta}_1, \cdots, \boldsymbol{\beta}_K$ under the unit dispersions multinomial regression model. The maximum extended quasi-likelihood estimate $\phi(S)$ of ϕ then satisfies

$$\phi(S) = \frac{1}{n} \sum_{s \in S} d\left(y_s; \mu_{s0}(S), \cdots, \mu_{sK}(S)\right),$$

where $\mu_{s0}(S), \cdots, \mu_{sK}(S)$ are the estimates of $\mu_{s0}, \cdots, \mu_{sK}$ determined by $\boldsymbol{\beta}_1(S), \cdots, \boldsymbol{\beta}_K(S)$. More generally, model the log of the dispersions ϕ_s as a function of selected predictor variables and associated coefficients (as in Sect. 8.13.1). Specifically, let $\log(\phi_s) = \mathbf{v}_s^T \cdot \boldsymbol{\gamma}$ where, for $s \in S$, $\mathbf{v}_s$ is a $q \times 1$ column vector of q predictor values v_{sj} (including unit predictor values if an intercept is to be included) with indexes $j \in Q = \{j : 1 \le j \le q\}$ and $\boldsymbol{\gamma}$ is the associated $q \times 1$ column vector of coefficients. The $(r \cdot K + q) \times 1$ parameter vector $\boldsymbol{\theta} = (\boldsymbol{\beta}_1^T, \cdots, \boldsymbol{\beta}_K^T, \boldsymbol{\gamma}^T)^T$ is estimated through maximum extended quasi-likelihood estimation. Alternative models can be compared with QLCV^+ scores computed as LCV scores are computed in Sect. 8.3, but using extended quasi-likelihoods rather than likelihoods and maximum extended quasi-likelihood estimates of $\boldsymbol{\theta}$ rather than maximum likelihood estimates. The adaptive modeling process can be extended to search through models for the means and dispersions in combination (see Chap. 20).

As in Sect. 8.7.1, for $s \in S$, the estimated value for the mean μ_{sv} is

$$\mu_{sv}(S) = \frac{\exp\left(\mathbf{x}_s^T \cdot \boldsymbol{\beta}_v(S)\right)}{1 + \exp\left(\mathbf{x}_s^T \cdot \boldsymbol{\beta}_1(S)\right) + \cdots + \exp\left(\mathbf{x}_s^T \cdot \boldsymbol{\beta}_K(S)\right)}$$

for $1 \le v \le K$ while, for $v = 0$,

$$\mu_{s0}(S) = \frac{1}{\left(1 + \exp\left(\mathbf{x}_s^T \cdot \boldsymbol{\beta}_1(S) + \cdots + \exp(\mathbf{x}_s^T \cdot \boldsymbol{\beta}_K(S))\right)\right.}$$

The corresponding residuals are $e_{sv}(S) = y_{sv} - \mu_{sv}(S)$. The estimated value of the associated dispersion ϕ_s is $\phi_s(S) = \exp(\mathbf{v}_s^T \cdot \boldsymbol{\gamma}(S))$, and the estimated values for the extended variances σ_{sv}^2 are $\sigma_{sv}^2(S) = \phi_s(S) \cdot V(\mu_{sv}(S))$. The extended covariance matrix $\boldsymbol{\Sigma}_s(S)$ for $\mathbf{e}_s(S)$ satisfies

$$\boldsymbol{\Sigma}_s(S) = \phi_s(S) \cdot (\mathrm{diag}(\boldsymbol{\mu}_s(S)) - \boldsymbol{\mu}_s(S) \cdot \boldsymbol{\mu}_s(S)^T)$$

where $\boldsymbol{\mu}_s(S)$ is the K-dimensional vector with entries $\mu_{sv}(S)$ for $1 \le v \le K$. As in Sect. 8.7.1, scaled residual vectors $\mathbf{sclde}_s(S)$ can then be computed as $\mathbf{sclde}_s(S) = (\mathbf{U}_s^T(S))^{-1} \cdot \mathbf{e}_s(S)$ where $\mathbf{U}_s(S)$ is the square root of the covariance matrix $\Sigma_s(S)$ determined by its Cholesky decomposition. The entries of $\mathbf{sclde}_s(S)$ can be combined over all s and analyzed in combination as for independent data.

The ordinal regression model of Sect. 8.7.2 can be extended using a similar formulation. In that case, the parameter vector $\boldsymbol{\theta} = (\alpha_0, \cdots, \alpha_{K-1}, \boldsymbol{\beta}^T, \boldsymbol{\gamma}^T)^T$ is $(K + r + q) \times 1$. Residuals and scaled residuals can be defined that account for extended variances but with $0 \leq v \leq K - 1$ since the case $v = K$ is determined from the other values (instead of $v = 0$ as for multinomial regression).

8.13.3 Analysis of Dichotomous Mercury Level Means and Dispersions

The adaptive modeling process can be applied to model both the means and the dispersions of merchigh in combination. As for other analyses, models for logits of means are not allowed to have zero intercepts, but models for log dispersions are allowed to have zero intercepts (since they correspond to unit dispersions). When this process is applied using the singleton predictor length for both means and dispersions (using length since it is the better singleton predictor for merchigh means), the generated model has extended quasi-likelihood cross-validation (QLCV$^+$) score 0.64457. The adaptive model with unit dispersions has QLCV$^+$ score 0.59140 (the same as its LCV score as reported in Sect. 8.5) and so with substantial PD of 8.25 %. Consequently, non-unit dispersions models provide a distinct improvement over unit dispersions models for merchigh as a function of length. The means in this model are now based on the transform length$^{4.2}$. The dispersions of this model depend on the single transform length$^{6.6}$ with an intercept. The model with both means and dispersions based on untransformed length has QLCV$^+$ score 0.58575 with substantial PD of 9.13 %, indicating that log dispersions for merchigh are distinctly nonlinear in length in contrast to prior results for the logits of the means. Also, after adjusting for non-unit dispersions, the means now depend on the nonlinear transform length$^{4.2}$ rather than on length$^{0.5}$ as was the case for unit dispersions. Whether this is a distinct change can be assessed using the adaptive model for the dispersions in length with the model for the logits of the means fixed and based on length$^{0.5}$. The generated model for the dispersions is again based on the single transform length$^{6.6}$ with an intercept, but the QLCV$^+$ score is 0.61097 with substantial PD of 5.21 %, indicating that the dependence of the logits of the means are distinctly changed by consideration of non-unit dispersions based on length.

Estimated probabilities for a high mercury level based on the adaptive model for the means and dispersions in combination are plotted in Fig. 8.11. They increase in an s-shaped pattern from about 0.13 at 25 cm to essentially 1 by 65 cm. Estimated dispersions for this model are plotted in Fig. 8.12. They decrease in an inverse s-shaped pattern from about 1.9 at 25 cm to essentially 0 by 65 cm. Similar analyses

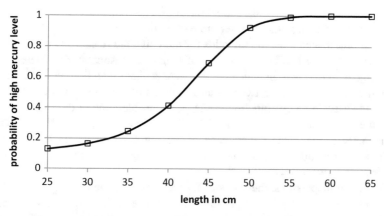

Fig. 8.11 Estimated probabilities for a high mercury level over 1.0 ppm as a function of length for fish caught in the Lumber and Waccamaw Rivers based on adaptive logistic regression modeling of both means and dispersions

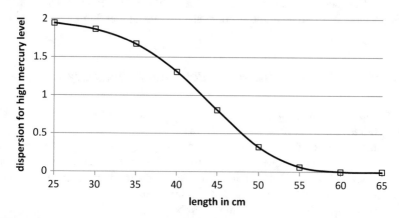

Fig. 8.12 Estimated dispersions for a high mercury level over 1.0 ppm as a function of length for fish caught in the Lumber and Waccamaw Rivers based on adaptive logistic regression modeling of both means and dispersions

can be conducted accounting for non-unit dispersions for merchigh and for merclevel in terms of river, weight, and length, either separately or in combination, and with or without GCs. These are not considered here for brevity (but see Sect. 9.12 for an example merclevel analysis).

8.14 Overview of Analyses of Dichotomous Mercury Levels

1. For the dichotomous mercury levels (Sect. 8.2), analyses use $k = 15$ folds (Sect. 8.4).
2. Using unit dispersions, the log odds for merchigh are distinctly nonlinear in weight of the fish and the effect of weight is moderated by the river, in which the

fish were caught (Sect. 8.4). Probabilities of a high mercury level over 1.0 ppm as a function of weight and river are plotted in Fig. 8.1.

3. Using unit dispersions, the log odds for merchigh are reasonably close to linear in length of the fish and the effect of length is reasonably considered not to change with the river, in which the fish were caught (Sect. 8.5). Probabilities of a high mercury level over 1.0 ppm as a function of length are plotted in Fig. 8.2 and the associated OR function in Fig. 8.3. Consideration of dispersions as well as means depending on length of the fish distinctly improved the model and distinctly changed the dependence of the log odds on length (Sect. 8.13.3). Revised probabilities as a function of length are plotted in Fig. 8.11 and the associated dispersions in Fig. 8.12.

4. Using unit dispersions, the log odds for merchigh change in complex ways with weight and length of the fish and the river, in which the fish were caught (Sect. 8.6). Probabilities of a high mercury level over 1.0 ppm as a function of weight and river for alternative length values are plotted in Figs. 8.4 and 8.5. The model generated with LCV scores outperformed the associated model generated with PCDP scores on the basis of both the LCV and PCDP scores (Sect. 8.12.2). See Sect. 9.6 for an example residual analysis using merchigh.

8.15   Overview of Analyses of Polytomous Mercury Levels

1. For the polytomous mercury levels (Sect. 8.8), analyses use $k = 5$ folds (Sect. 8.9).

2. Ordinal regression is more appropriate for analyzing polytomous mercury levels and so is used in subsequent analyses (this and the following results reported in Sect. 8.9). Using unit dispersions, the log odds for merclevel are distinctly nonlinear in weight of the fish and the effect of weight is moderated by the river, in which the fish were caught. Probabilities as a function of weight and river are plotted in Fig. 8.6.

3. Using unit dispersions, the log odds for merclevel are reasonably close to linear in length of the fish and the effect of length is reasonably considered not to change with the river, in which the fish were caught (Sect. 8.10). Probabilities of a high mercury level over 1.3 ppm as a function of length are plotted in Fig. 8.7 and the associated proportional OR function in Fig. 8.8.

4. Using unit dispersions, the log odds for merclevel change in complex ways with weight and length of the fish and the river, in which the fish were caught (Sect. 8.11). Probabilities of a high mercury level over 1.3 ppm as a function of weight and river for alternative length values are plotted in Figs. 8.9 and 8.10. The model generated with LCV scores outperformed the associated model generated with PCDP scores on the basis of both the LCV and PCDP scores (Sect. 8.12.3). See Sect. 9.10 for an example residual analysis using merclevel. See Sect. 9.12 for an analysis of dispersions as well as means for merclevel.

8.16   Chapter Summary

This chapter presents a series of analyses of the mercury level data. These analyses address how mercury level categorized as low and high (with cutoff 1.0 ppm near its median) and as low, medium, and high (with cutoffs 0.72 ppm and 1.3 ppm near its tertiles) for n = 169 largemouth bass caught in the Lumber and Waccamaw Rivers of North Carolina depend on weight, length, and river.

Using unit dispersions models for mercury in fish categorized into the two levels of high and low, the log odds depend distinctly nonlinearly on the weight of the fish, and this relationship changes with the river in which the fish were caught, a moderation effect. On the other hand, the relationship with the length of the fish is reasonably close to linear and reasonably considered not to change with river. The log odds depend on both weight and length in combination using an additive model. This relationship is reasonably close to linear in both variables, and so also controlling for length alters the relationship in terms of weight from distinctly nonlinear to reasonably close to linear. The model in weight, length, and geometric combinations (GCs) in these two predictors provides a substantial improvement over the additive model in weight and length, indicating that the effects of weight and length distinctly interact. Moreover, river moderates this relationship in weight and length. The adaptive model with both means and dispersions depending on length provides a distinct improvement over the associated unit dispersions model. Under this model, the log dispersions are distinctly nonlinear in the length of the fish. Moreover, the dependence of the log odds on length identified with unit dispersions is substantially changed by consideration of non-unit dispersions from close to linear to distinctly nonlinear. Consequently, dispersion modeling can have a substantial impact on the model for the means and so is important to consider. Analyses allowing for means and dispersions to depend on combinations of weight, length, river, and GCs are left as practice exercises (see Chap. 9).

Using unit dispersions models for mercury in fish categorized into the three ordered levels of high, medium, and low, the log proportional odds (using ordinal regression, which is preferable for these data to multinomial regression) depend distinctly nonlinearly on the weight of the fish, and this relationship changes with the river in which the fish were caught. On the other hand, the relationship with the length of the fish is reasonably close to linear and reasonably considered not to change with the river. The log proportional odds depend on both weight and length in combination using an additive model. This relationship is distinctly nonlinear in contrast to results for mercury categorized into two levels. The model in weight, length, and geometric combinations (GCs) in these two predictors provides a substantial improvement over the additive model in weight and length, indicating that the effects of weight and length distinctly interact. Moreover, river moderates this relationship in weight and length, indicating that the log proportional odds change with weight and length differently for the two rivers. Adaptive modeling of the means and dispersions for this ordinal outcome are not addressed in this chapter. Chapter 9 provides an adaptive analysis of its means and dispersions in terms of the length, river and GCs. Analyses allowing for its means and dispersions to depend on combinations of weight, length, river and GCs are left as practice exercises (see Chap. 9).

The proportion of correct deleted predictions (PCDP) is an alternate criterion for comparing and evaluating logistic regression models. However, adaptive modeling based on LCV scores can outperform adaptive modeling based on PCDP scores on the basis of both the LCV and PCDP scores. Consequently, adaptive modeling based on PCDP scores is not recommended.

These analyses demonstrate adaptive logistic regression modeling using fractional polynomials, including modeling of dichotomous outcomes, extensions to adaptive multinomial and ordinal regression for polytomous outcomes, and how to model dispersions as well as means. The chapter also provides formulations for these alternative regression models; for associated k-fold LCV scores for unit dispersions models; for the PCDP model selection criterion; for extended quasi-likelihood cross-validation ($QLCV^+$) scores for non-unit dispersions models based on extended quasi-likelihoods; for odds ratio (OR) functions generalizing the OR used in standard logistic regression; and for residuals and standardized (or Pearson) residuals. The example analyses demonstrate assessing whether the log odds for an outcome are nonlinear in individual predictors, whether those relationships are better addressed with multiple predictors in combination compared to using singleton predictors, whether those relationships are additive in predictors, whether the predictors interact using GCs, whether ordinal polytomous outcomes are better modeled with ordinal or multinomial regression, and whether there is a benefit to considering non-unit dispersions. Example residual analyses are not reported in this chapter. See Chap. 9 for a description of how to conduct analyses of univariate dichotomous and polytomous outcomes in SAS including residual analyses.

References

Bickel, P. J., & Doksum, K. A. (1977). *Mathematical statistics: Basic ideas and selected topics.* San Francisco: Holden-Day.

Efron, B. (1983). Estimating the error rate of a prediction rule: Improvement on cross-validation. *Journal of the American Statistical Association, 78,* 316–331.

Hosmer, D. W., Lemeshow, S., & Sturdivant, R. X. (2013). *Applied logistic regression* (3rd ed.). New York: Wiley.

Kleinbaum, D. G., & Klein, M. (2010). *Logistic regression: A self-learning text* (3rd ed.). New York: Springer.

McCullagh, P., & Nelder, J. A. (1999). *Generalized linear models* (2nd ed.). Boca Raton, FL: Chapman & Hall/CRC.

Chapter 9
Adaptive Logistic Regression Modeling of Univariate Dichotomous and Polytomous Outcomes in SAS

9.1 Chapter Overview

This chapter describes how to use the genreg macro for adaptive logistic regression modeling as described in Chap. 8 and its generated output in the special case of univariate dichotomous and polytomous outcomes. Familiarity with the use of the genreg macro as presented in Chap. 3 is assumed. See Supplementary Materials for a more complete description of this macro. See Allison (2012), SAS Institute (1995), Stokes et al. (2012), and Zelterman (2002) for details on standard approaches for logistic regression modeling in SAS. Section 9.2 provides a description of the mercury data analyzed in Chap. 8. Section 9.3 provides code for modeling means for mercury in fish categorized into the two levels of high and low in terms of weight of the fish, Sect. 9.3 in terms of length of the fish, and Sect. 9.6 in terms of weight and length of the fish and river in which the fish were caught. Residual analyses based on continuous predictors, like weight and length, of dichotomous and polytomous outcomes are better conducted using grouped data. Section 9.4 provides a formulation for grouped-data residual analyses based on continuous predictors of dichotomous outcomes (which can be skipped) while Sect. 9.5 provides an example grouped-data residual analysis. Section 9.7 provides code for analyzing means for mercury categorized into the three levels of high, medium, and low in terms of weight, length, and river. Section 9.8 provides a formulation for grouped-data residual analyses based on continuous predictors of polytomous outcomes (which can be skipped) while Sect. 9.9 provides an example grouped-data residual analysis for the polytomous mercury level outcome. Section 9.10 provides code for modeling means and dispersions of mercury in fish categorized into the two levels of high and low while Sect. 9.11 provides code for modeling means and dispersions of mercury in fish categorized into the three levels of high, medium, and low.

© Springer International Publishing Switzerland 2016
G.J. Knafl, K. Ding, *Adaptive Regression for Modeling Nonlinear Relationships*,
Statistics for Biology and Health, DOI 10.1007/978-3-319-33946-7_9

9.2   Loading in the Mercury Level Data

Analyses are conducted in Chap. 8 of categorized mercury levels for $n = 169$ largemouth bass caught in one of two rivers (Lumber and Waccamaw) in North Carolina (see Sects. 8.2 and 8.8). Assume that these mercury level data have been loaded into the default library (for example, by importing them from a spreadsheet file) under the name mercury. An output title line, selected system options, labels for the variables, and formats for values of selected variables can be assigned as follows.

```
title1 "Mercury Level Data";
options nodate pageno=1 pagesize=53 linesize=76;
%let merccut=1.0; %let mlocut=0.72; %let mhicut=1.3;
proc format;
 value rvrfmt 0="0:Lumber" 1="1:Waccamaw";
 value mlvl1fmt 0="0:low" 1="1:high";
 value mlvl2fmt 0="0:low" 1="1:medium" 2="2:high";
run;
data mercury;
 set mercury;
 *  convert from grams to kilograms;
 weight=weight/1000;
 merchigh=(mercury>&merccut);
 if mercury<=&mlocut then merclevel=0;
 else if mercury<=&mhicut then merclevel=1;
 else merclevel=2;
 label river="River"
       station="Station Number"
       length="Length (cm)"
       weight="Weight (kg)"
       mercury="Mercury Concentration (ppm)"
       merchigh="High Mercury Level > &merccut"
       merclevel="Mercury Level";
 format river rvrfmt. merchigh mlvl1fmt. merclevel mlvl2fmt.;
run;
```

The merccut macro variable is used to compute the dichotomous outcome merchigh with values 0 (mercury ≤ 1.0 ppm (parts per million)) and 1 (mercury >1.0 ppm) while the macro variables mlocut and mhicut are used to compute the polytomous outcome variable merclevel with the three ordered values low (mercury ≤ 0.72 ppm), medium (0.72 ppm $<$ mercury ≤ 1.0 ppm), and high (mercury ≤ 1.3 ppm). The value for merccut is chosen to be close to the median for mercury levels while the values for mlocut and mhicut are chosen to be close to the tertiles. These are set with macro variables so that the values for these cutoffs can be simply changed if desired. Formats are created with PROC FORMAT for the values of the river, merchigh, and merclevel variables and assigned with the format statement in the data step. Weights in the input data file are in grams and are converted to kilograms so that their range of values can be more simply displayed in generated plots. The cutoff for a substantial percent decrease (PD) for analyses of merchigh with 169 measurements is 1.13 % (as reported in Sect. 8.2) while it is 0.57 % for analyses of merclevel with $169 \cdot 2 = 338$ effective measurements (as reported in Sect. 8.8).

9.3   Modeling Means for Merchigh Based on Weight

Assuming that the genreg macro has been loaded into SAS (see Supplementary Materials), an adaptive model for merchigh as a function of weight can be generated as follows.

```
%genreg(modtype=logis,datain=mercury,yvar=merchigh,
        vintrcpt=n,foldcnt=15,expand=y,expxvars=weight,
        contract=y,nocnxint=y);
```

The parameter setting "modtype=logis" requests a logistic regression model. The datain parameter specifies the input data set, in this case the mercury data set. The yvar parameter specifies the dichotomous or polytomous outcome variable, in this case the dichotomous outcome variable named merchigh. The yvar variable in this case has numeric values, but it can have character values instead. The base models for both the means and dispersions by default are both the constant, intercept-only model. The option "vintrcpt=n" requests a unit dispersions model (more precisely, the equivalent zero log dispersions model is requested). The parameter setting "foldcnt=15" (as justified in Sect. 8.4) requests that 15-fold LCV scores be computed for models. This setting generates the first local maximum in LCV scores for this analysis, and so $k = 15$ is used in all subsequent analyses of merchigh. The parameter setting "expand=y" requests that the base model be expanded. The model for the means is expanded by adding in transforms of primary predictor variables listed in the setting for the expxvars parameter. In this case, only weight is considered for expansion. The model for the dispersions is not changed since the expvvars macro parameter has its default empty setting. The parameter setting "contract=y" requests that the expanded model be contracted. The setting "nocnxint=y" requests that the contraction not remove the intercept for the model for the means. The default setting "nocnxint=n" is a reasonable option for "modtype=norml", but is not considered in all reported analyses of Chaps. 8 and 9. This way, the logit, or log odds, when a predictor variable has value 0 is always estimated rather than allowing it sometimes to be zero. Parameters like xintrcpt, xvars, expxvars, and nocnxint are used to control settings for the mean, expectation or "x" component of the model while corresponding parameters like vintrcpt, vvars,

Table 9.1 Expanded model for a high mercury level over 1.0 ppm (merchigh) as a function of the weight of the fish

```
                   expanded logit expectation component

      parameter estimates for logits relative to smallest merchigh=0

         predictor      power    merchigh=1        score    order

         XINTRCPT           1    3.0746531    0.4973167        0
         weight          -0.5    -2.860968    0.5608136        1

                   expanded log dispersion component

         predictor      power    estimate          score    order

         VZERO              1            0    0.4973167        0
...
proportion of correct deleted predictions:                0.6745562
...
mth root of likelihood using deleted predictions:         0.5608136
```

expvvars, and nocnvint are used to control the variance/dispersion or "v" component of the model (see Sects. 9.11 and 9.12).

The base model is generated first, in this case the model with constant means (since the default settings of "xintrcpt=y" and "xvars=" are used), unit dispersions, and LCV score 0.49732. This is expanded by adding in the single transform weight$^{-0.5}$ for the means with associated LCV score 0.56081, and the contraction leaves this expanded model unchanged. Table 9.1 contains part of the output describing the expanded model. The component of the model for the logits of the expectations or means (called the logit expectation component in the output) is described first. It is based on an intercept parameter (denoted as XINTRCPT) and the transform of the primary predictor weight raised to the power −0.5. The order that terms are added into the model is indicated in the output. The intercept has order 0 indicating it was in the base model while the single transform for weight has order 1 since it is the first and only term added into the model. By default, the smaller of the two outcome values is used as the reference value. The larger value can be used as the reference value by requesting "refyval=max" (as opposed to the default setting "refyval=min"). Estimates of coefficients are reported for the non-reference value, in this case merchigh $= 1$ (that is, mercury >1.0 ppm), and so the estimated relationship is

$$\text{logit}\left(P\left(\text{merchigh} = 1 \middle| \text{weight}\right)\right) = 3.0746531 - 2.860968 \cdot \text{weight}^{-0.5}.$$

Since the power and the slope are both negative, the logits, and so also the probabilities for a high level of mercury >1.0 ppm, increase as expected with weight. The component of the model for the log of the dispersions is described next.

It is based on a zero intercept parameter (denoted as VZERO) as requested by the "vintrcpt=n" option and no other transforms since the vvars and expvvars macro parameters have their empty default settings. Its order is 0 since it is in the base model. In general, transforms for the log of the dispersions can be added into the model along with transforms for the logits of the expectations or means in intermingled order. Several values describing the model are generated last. Of these, only the proportion of correct deleted predictions (PCDP; see Sect. 8.12) and the LCV score are included in Table 9.1, both rounded to 7 digits. The number of character positions and hence digits for PCDP and LCV scores can be changed with the screchrs macro parameter from its default value of 9.

The estimated slope for weight$^{-0.5}$ generates the estimated OR $=$ $\exp(-2.860968) = 0.057$, representing the proportional change in odds for merchigh $= 1$ with a unit change in weight$^{-0.5}$. However, how the odds change with weight rather than with the generated transform for weight seems more meaningful. This can be estimated (see Sect. 8.3) by first differentiating the logit function with respect to weight giving

$$\partial \text{logit}(P(\text{merchigh} = 1|\text{weight}))/\partial(\text{weight}) = -0.5 \cdot (-2.860968) \cdot \text{weight}^{-0.5-1}$$
$$= 1.430484 \cdot \text{weight}^{-1.5}.$$

Exponentiating then gives the odds ratio function

$$\text{OR}(\text{weight}) = \exp(1.430484 \cdot \text{weight}^{-1.5}).$$

This function is plotted in Fig. 9.1. Starting at an arbitrary value w for weight, the odds with a unit increase, and so to w + 1, are approximately equal to the value of the odds ratio function OR(w) at w times the odds at w. Alternately, the odds change proportionally with unit increases by the amount of the OR function at any

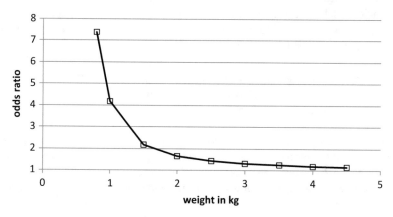

Fig. 9.1 Odds ratio function for a high mercury level over 1.0 ppm (merchigh) as a function of the weight of the fish

given value for weight. In this case, the OR function is always greater than 1, indicating that the odds for a high mercury level over 1.0 ppm increase proportionally with increases in weight. However, they increase by lower proportional amounts for larger weights. ORs for weights lower than 1 are not displayed in Fig. 9.1 since the OR increases to essentially infinity as weights decrease to their lowest observed value.

The linear polynomial model in weight can be generated as follows using the xvars parameter.

```
%genreg(modtype=logis,datain=mercury,yvar=merchigh,
        xvars=weight,foldcnt=15,vintrcpt=n,procmod=y);
```

The setting "procmod=y" requests that an equivalent model be generated through the appropriate standard SAS PROC, PROC LOGISTIC in this case. Using the PROC LOGISTIC output, the slope for weight is significant at $P < 0.001$ with estimated value 1.2305 generating an estimated OR = 3.4 with 95 % confidence interval 2.1–5.7. The LCV score is 0.54346 with substantial PD of 3.09 % (that is, greater than the cutoff of 1.13 % for the data) compared to the adaptively generated model in weight (as also reported in Sect. 8.4). Consequently, the estimated OR results for the linear model are misleading in this case. Proportional changes (ORs) in the odds under the adaptive model can be distinctly larger for small weights than the upper bound of 5.7 for the linear model and distinctly lower for large weights than the lower bound of 2.1 for that model. This provides further support for the distinct nonlinearity of the logits for merchigh in weight.

Since the adaptive model has an intercept and the transform of weight with power -0.5, which is one of the recommended degree 1 powers (see Sect. 2.12), there is no need for a comparison of the adaptive model to models based on recommended degree 1 powers. However, such comparisons can be informative in general and can be conducted using the RA1compare macro (see Sect. 3.8) and the RA2compare macro (see Sect. 3.9). For example, a comparison of the adaptive monotonic model in weight (in this case, the same model as the one generated without restricting to a single transform) can be compared to the degree 1 recommended fractional power transforms as follows.

```
%RA1compare(modtype=logis,datain=mercury,yvar=merchigh,
            xvar=weight,vintrcpt=n,foldcnt=15,
            scorefmt=7.5,nocnxint=y);
```

The "nocnxint=y" setting is needed to guarantee that the adaptive model generated by RA1compare has a non-zero intercept for its logit expectation component. The scorefmt option requests that LCV scores be reported by RA1compare formatted into 7 character positions and rounded to 5 decimal digits as reported in Chaps. 8 and 9. The recommended degree 1 power generating the best score is -0.5 and so is the same as the adaptive monotonic model with LCV score 0.56018, as also reported in Sect. 8.4.

An assessment of the recommended degree 2 powers can be obtained by changing "RA1compare" in the above code to "RA2compare" with the same parameter settings. The two recommended powers -2 and -1 combine to generate the best LCV score of 0.55775 among recommended degree 2 powers, which is smaller than the LCV score for the recommended degree 1 power -0.5. Consequently, recommended degree 2 models are not needed in this case.

An adaptive model in weight, river, and GCs in these two predictors can be generated as follows.

```
%genreg(modtype=logis,datain=mercury,yvar=merchigh,
        vintrcpt=n,foldcnt=15,expand=y,
        expxvars=weight river,geomcmbn=y,contract=y,
        nocnxint=y);
```

GCs are requested with the "geomcmbn=y" setting. The default setting "geomcmbn=n" is used to generate an additive model in weight and river. The expanded model (output not shown) is based on the four transforms: $\text{weight}^{-0.5}$, $(\text{river} \cdot \text{weight}^2)^{0.8}$, $\text{river} \cdot \text{weight}^{-2}$, and river with LCV score 0.57179. This is contracted to the model based on the two transforms: $\text{weight}^{-0.8}$, and $(\text{river} \cdot \text{weight}^{-2})^{-0.8}$ with improved LCV score 0.57192 (as reported in Sect. 8.4).

9.4 Modeling Means for Merchigh Based on Length

Analyses of merchigh as a function of length can be generated similarly to analyses of weight as in Sect. 9.3 with the predictor weight changed to length. Results of these analyses are reported in Sect. 8.5. The adaptively generated model is based on $\text{length}^{0.5}$. Estimated probabilities for this model are displayed in Fig. 8.2 and the estimated OR function in Fig. 8.3. This relationship does not change with the type of river, which is justified by the results generated by the follow code.

```
%genreg(modtype=logis,datain=mercury,yvar=merchigh,
        vintrcpt=n,foldcnt=15,expand=y,
        expxvars=length river,geomcmbn=y,contract=y,
        nocnxint=y);
```

The expanded model for the means is based on three transforms: $\text{length}^{0.5}$, $(\text{river} \cdot \text{length}^3)^2$, and river with LCV score 0.58903. The contraction removes the last two transforms and leaves the first transform unchanged, and so results in the same model as generated for length alone with larger LCV score of 0.59140.

Residual analyses can be conducted for adaptive logistic regression models. The genreg macro generates standardized or Pearson residuals for these models as defined in Sect. 8.3. These are loaded into a variable named stdres in a data set

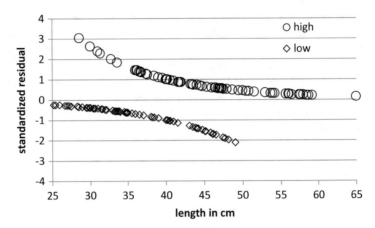

Fig. 9.2 Standardized residuals versus lengths for the adaptive model of a high mercury level over 1.0 ppm as a function of the length of the fish with observed values of low at most 1.0 ppm and of high over 1.0 ppm

called dataout (along with a variety of other generated variables; see Supplementary Materials). The name of the variable can be changed with the stdrsvar parameter and the name of the data set with the dataout parameter. Using the adaptive model in length, the plot of the standardized residuals versus length is displayed in Fig. 9.2, distinguishing between observations with low and high observed values for merchigh. For fish with low observed mercury levels at most 1.0 ppm, the standardized residuals are all negative and decrease from −0.23 to −2.11 while, for fish with high observed mercury levels over 1.0 ppm, the standardized residuals are all positive and decrease from 3.05 to 0.14. A residual assessment based on the residuals of Fig. 9.2 is not very meaningful. This is the case for models based on ungrouped continuous predictor variables like length. The length variable values need to be grouped in order to conduct a more meaningful residual assessment.

9.5   Grouped Residuals for Univariate Dichotomous Outcomes

This section provides a formulation (which can be skipped) for conducting residual analyses of grouped data for univariate dichotomous outcomes. This is similar to what is called events/trials format by PROC LOGISTIC (SAS Institute 2004; Stokes et al. 2012).

Using the notation of Sect. 8.3, suppose the indexes $s \in S$ for the n observations have been partitioned into G nonempty, disjoint subsets S_g for $1 \le g \le G$. For $1 \le g \le G$, let $\mathbf{x}_g$ denote the average of the predictor vectors $\mathbf{x}_s$ over $s \in S_g$, n_{gv} the number of observations with indexes $s \in S_g$ with $y_s = v$ for $v = 0$ and 1, and $n_g = n_{g0} + n_{g1}$ the number of observations with indexes $s \in S_g$. The grouped data consist of observations $O_g = (n_{g0}, n_{g1}, \mathbf{x}_g)$ for $1 \leq g \leq G$. Let μ_g denote the common mean for all observations y_s with $s \in S_g$, and model $\text{logit}(\mu_g) = \mathbf{x}_g^T \cdot \boldsymbol{\beta}$ for a $r \times 1$ vector $\boldsymbol{\beta}$ of coefficients. The likelihood term L_g for the gth group satisfies

$$\ell_g = \log(L_g) = n_{g1} \cdot \log(\mu_g) + n_{g0} \cdot \log(1 - \mu_g).$$

The likelihood $L(S; \boldsymbol{\beta})$ is the product of the individual likelihood terms L_g over $1 \leq g \leq G$ and satisfies

$$\ell(S; \boldsymbol{\beta}) = \log(L(S; \boldsymbol{\beta})) = \sum_{1 \leq g \leq G} \ell_g.$$

The maximum likelihood estimate $\boldsymbol{\beta}(S)$ of $\boldsymbol{\beta}$ is computed by solving the estimating equations $\partial \ell(S; \boldsymbol{\beta})/\partial \boldsymbol{\beta} = \mathbf{0}$ obtained by differentiating $\ell(S; \boldsymbol{\beta})$ with respect to $\boldsymbol{\beta}$, where $\mathbf{0}$ denotes the zero vector. For $1 \leq g \leq G$, the estimated value for the mean μ_g is

$$\mu_g(S) = \frac{\exp(\mathbf{x}_g^T \cdot \boldsymbol{\beta}(S))}{1 + \exp(\mathbf{x}_g^T \cdot \boldsymbol{\beta}(S))}.$$

The random variable n_{g1} is binomially distributed with estimated mean $n_g \cdot \mu_g(S)$ and so its associated residual is naturally defined as $e_g(S) = n_{g1} - n_g \cdot \mu_g(S)$, that is, as the difference between its observed value and its estimated mean. The estimated value for the variance σ_g^2 is $\sigma_g^2(S) = n_g \cdot \mu_g(S) \cdot (1 - \mu_g(S))$. The standardized or Pearson residual $\text{stde}_g(S) = e_g(S)/\sigma_g(S)$ is obtained by standardizing the residual by dividing by the estimated standard deviation. These are all the residuals generated by PROC LOGISTIC for data in events/trials format. However, observations are inputted to genreg in ungrouped format and only logically, not physically grouped, and so residuals are assigned to each ungrouped observation as generated through the grouping. Specifically, each observation y_s with $s \in S_g$ is assigned the residual $e_s(S) = e_g(S)$ and standardized residual $\text{stde}_s(S) = \text{stde}_g(S)$. Note that for a group of size 1, when the only $y_s = 1$, the associated residual is $1 - \mu_s(S)$ and, when the only $y_s = 0$, the associated residual is $-\mu_s(S)$, and these are the same as for ungrouped data.

Each observation can also be assigned a likelihood term using estimated values determined from the grouped data. These likelihood terms can then be evaluated at parameter estimates generated from fold complements and used to generate LCV scores for grouped data models. The observation index set S is partitioned into the $k > 1$ disjoint folds $F(h)$ for $h \in H = \{h : 1 \leq h \leq k\}$ as usual. The groups used to compute parameter estimates for a fold complement $S \backslash F(h)$ are the intersections $(S \backslash F(h)) \cap S_g$ for $1 \leq g \leq G$. In other words, group assignments are not changed, but only observations in each group that are also in a fold complement are used to generate grouped estimates for that fold complement.

Grouped modeling of univariate dichotomous outcomes extends readily to include modeling of dispersions as well as means using extended quasi-likelihoods based on binomial likelihoods. The extension is similar to the extension in Sect. 8.13.1 for ungrouped univariate dichotomous outcomes.

9.6 Grouped Residual Analysis of Merchigh as a Function of Length

Adaptive grouping of length values can be requested as follows.

```
%let wndwval=0.07;
%genreg(modtype=logis,datain=mercury,yvar=merchigh,
        vintrcpt=n,foldcnt=15,regroup=y,
        grpvars=length,window=&wndwval,expand=y,
        expxvars=length,contract=y,nocnxint=y);
```

The setting "regroup=y" requests that observed values of the grpvars variables, only the length variable in this case, be grouped into subsets with relative distances within the proportion designated by the window parameter setting, in this case 0.07. The lowest length value is used to start the grouping, it is grouped with all other length values having proportional distance within the window value of 0.07, then the lowest remaining ungrouped value is used to generate the next group, and the process continues until all length values are in a group. The grouping process can be applied to more than one grouping variable. The model can be adaptively generated using the current grouping, as in this case, or it can be fixed at the adaptive model generated with the ungrouped data. The LCV score is computed for ungrouped outcome values using estimates based on the generated grouping and so can be compared to choose the setting of the window parameter. The choice of 0.07 maximizes the LCV score over window values with multiples of 0.01 from 0.01 to 0.10 generated by varying the value for the wndwval macro variable in the above code. The LCV score is 0.60101. The PD for the adaptive model based on the ungrouped data is substantial at 1.60 %, indicating that grouping has distinctly improved the model. A total of 10 groups are generated with from 1 to 41 observations per group (as reported in the output). Regenerating the adaptive model for each grouping can generate different power transforms than for the ungrouped data. The model for the "window=0.07" grouping is based on the single transform $length^{-0.5}$ compared to $length^{0.5}$ for the ungrouped data. However, the linear model in grouped lengths has LCV score 0.60031 with insubstantial PD of 0.12 %, indicating that, while the generated power is further from the power 1 for the linear model, the adaptive model is still reasonably close to linear (as reported for the ungrouped data in Sect. 8.5), but in grouped lengths.

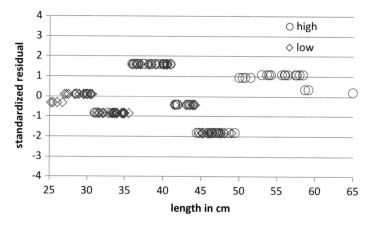

Fig. 9.3 Standardized residuals versus lengths for the adaptive model of mercury level as a function of grouped length values with observed values of low at most 1.0 ppm and of high over 1.0 ppm

The plot of the standardized residuals versus lengths for the grouped data model is displayed in Fig. 9.3, distinguishing between low and high observed values for merchigh. These are all well within ±3 (and actually within ±2), and so there are no outliers. They are also relatively symmetric about 0 except for observations with relatively high lengths over 50 cm. All fish with such large lengths have high mercury levels over 1.0 ppm, suggesting that the probability may be constant once the length gets large enough. This also suggests considering models based on lengths bounded above somewhere around 50 cm, but that is not considered here. The benefit of conducting a grouped versus an ungrouped residual analysis can be seen by comparing Fig. 9.3 with Fig. 9.2.

The dataout data set contains the variable grpindex with integer values indicating the assigned group for each observation. The name of this variable can be changed with the gpindvar macro parameter. For large data sets and/or large numbers of grouping variables, the grouping computations can take a long time to complete. To speed up computations, a previously generated grouping can be reused by setting "pregrpd=y", indicating that the data have been pregrouped. The gpindvar variable must exist in the datain data set and be loaded with integer values indicating the assigned group for each observation. This can be generated by a prior call to the genreg macro. That prior call can request "grponly=y" so that only the groups are computed and not any models. Alternately, the groups can be generated with other approaches like the clustering methods of PROC CLUSTER and PROC FASTCLUS.

9.7 Modeling Means for Merchigh Based on Weight and Length

An adaptive additive model in weight and length can be generated as follows.

```
%genreg(modtype=logis,datain=mercury,yvar=merchigh,
        vintrcpt=n,foldcnt=15,expand=y,
        expxvars=weight length,contract=y,
        nocnxint=y);
```

GCs based on weight and length are also considered when the "geomcmbn=y" setting is added the above code. The linear additive model in weight and length is generated as follows.

```
%genreg(modtype=logis,datain=mercury,yvar=merchigh,
        vintrcpt=n,foldcnt=15,xvars=weight length);
```

The adaptive model in weight, length, and river possibly with GCs based on any two or all three of these variables is generated as follows.

```
%genreg(modtype=logis,datain=mercury,yvar=merchigh,
        vintrcpt=n,foldcnt=15,expand=y,
        expxvars=weight length river,geomcmbn=y,
        contract=y,nocnxint=y);
```

Results for these analyses are reported in Sect. 8.6.

9.8 Modeling Means for Merclevel Based on Weight and Length

The genreg macro can also be used to model means for polytomous outcomes. When "modtype=logis", the number of unique values for the outcome variable, as determined by the setting of the yvar macro parameter, determines how that outcome is modeled. When there are exactly two unique outcome values, standard logistic regression models are generated. Otherwise, multinomial regression models based on generalized logits are generated. In both these cases, the reference outcome value is the smallest such value, but this can be changed to the largest outcome value by requesting "refyval=max". The macro parameter refyval can also be set to an integer, for example, "refyval=2" means use the second smallest outcome value as the reference value. When there are more than two unique outcome values and they are ordinal, an ordinal regression model based on cumulative logits with proportional odds can be generated by requesting "propodds=y".

By default, cumulative logits are generated in increasing order of the outcome values with the probability for the largest outcome value computed from probabilities for the other outcome values. This can be changed to cumulative logits in the reverse, decreasing order with probabilities for the smallest outcome value computed from probabilities for the other outcome values by requesting "rvrsordr=y". For example, the OR function of Fig. 8.6 is based on the model with cumulative logits in decreasing order.

An adaptive multinomial regression model for the means of merclevel as a function of weight can be generated as follows using 5 folds as justified in Sect. 8.9 and the default setting "propodds=n".

```
%genreg(modtype=logis,datain=mercury,yvar=merclevel,
        vintrcpt=n,foldcnt=5,expand=y,
        expxvars=weight,contract=y,nocnxint=y);
```

Since the removal of one term from a multinomial regression model for the means of merclevel results in the removal of two parameters corresponding to slopes for the generalized logits for a low level and for a low to medium level, LCV ratio tests comparing multinomial regression models for mean merclevel are more appropriately based on two degrees of freedom (DF) than on one DF (and in general, on DF equal to 1 less than the number of unique outcome values), and so the adaptive modeling process adjusts for this. On the other hand, removal of one term from the dispersions model for multinomial regression results in removal of only one parameter, and so the adaptive modeling process uses DF = 1 for those adjustments.

Since merclevel is ordinal, an alternative adaptive ordinal regression model (but with LCV ratio tests based on DF = 1) can be requested by adding in the setting "propodds=y" as follows.

```
%genreg(modtype=logis,datain=mercury,yvar=merclevel,
        vintrcpt=n,propodds=y,foldcnt=5,expand=y,
        expxvars=weight,contract=y,nocnxint=y);
```

The results of generating a model for an ordinal outcome using the two options of "propodds=y" and "propodds=n" can be used to conduct an assessment of the relative merits of ordinal versus multinomial regression for that outcome. In this case, the simpler ordinal regression model generates the better LCV score 0.61864 (see Sect. 8.9), indicating that it is preferable to the more complex multinomial regression model for these data. If the ordinal regression model generates a smaller LCV score with an insubstantial PD (based on DF = 1), then it is also preferable as a more parsimonious, competitive alternative. Only when the PD is substantial is the complexity of the multinomial regression model justifiable. Of course, if the outcome variable is nominal and not ordinal, then the ordinal regression model should not even be considered.

While all models of Chaps. 8 and 9 are constrained to have intercepts for modeling means, zero intercepts for the means are supported by genreg for models of dichotomous and polytomous outcomes. Zero intercepts for base models for the means are requested using the setting "xintrcpt=n". The option "nocnxint=n" means that the contraction considers removing the intercepts by setting them to zero. For multinomial regression models, all the intercept parameters for the means are set to zero. For ordinal regression models, only the initial intercept parameter for the means is set equal to zero, since intercept parameters for these models must be strictly increasing (see Sect. 8.7.2), otherwise probabilities for one or more of the outcome values will be treated as zero.

Whichever type of polytomous outcome model is used, more general models for the means can be adaptively generated by including multiple primary predictors in the expxvars list, possibly along with "geomcmbn=y" to generate GCs in the expxvars variables. For example, the adaptive ordinal regression model for the means of merclevel in weight, length, river, and GCs in these predictors can be generated as follows.

```
%genreg(modtype=logis,datain=mercury,yvar=merclevel,
        vintrcpt=n,propodds=y,foldcnt=5,expand=y,
        expxvars=weight length river,geomcmbn=y,
        contract=y,nocnxint=y,rprttime=y);
```

The generated model is described in Sect. 8.11. The "rprttime=y" setting requests that the elapsed clock time be reported in the genreg output. This analysis takes about 179.2 s or about 3.0 min of clock time. If the model needs to be regenerated for some reason, it is possible to avoid waiting for it to be adaptively generated. The model can be directly generated in less time as follows.

```
%genreg(modtype=logis,datain=mercury,yvar=merclevel,vintrcpt=n,
        xvars=length,xpowers=1.26,
        xgcs=length 2.5 weight -0.24 : weight 6 length -20 :
             river 1 weight -1.2 length 1 :
             length 2.5 river 1 weight 0.8 :
             length 1.5 weight -0.6,
        xgcpowrs=0.93.11.41 -0.812,propodds=y,foldcnt=5,
        rprttime=y);
```

The xgcs parameter is used to define GCs for modeling the means. Each GC consists of a list of primary predictors with associated powers. For example "length 2.5 weight -0.24" means $length^{2.5} \cdot weight^{-0.24}$. GCs are separated in the list by colons (:). The xgcpowrs parameter is used to power transform the GCs of the xgcs list. Powers are assigned in the same order as GCs are listed in the xgcs list. For example, the first power of 0.9 combined with the first GC generates the transform $(length^{2.5} \cdot weight^{-0.24})^{0.9}$. Due to the "rprttime=y" setting, the elapsed time for generating this model is reported, and it takes only about 2.4 s of clock time. While about 3.0 min as required for the adaptive process in this case is not long to wait, in cases where computation of adaptive models takes substantial amounts of time, regenerating that model in several second provides a distinct reduction in time.

The RA1compare and RA2compare macros (see Sects. 3.8, 3.9 and 9.3) can be used to compare adaptive models for polytomous outcomes to models based on recommended degree 1 and degree 2 sets of powers. The propodds parameter for these macros controls whether the models are ordinal or multinomial as it does for the genreg macro.

9.9   Grouped Residuals for Univariate Polytomous Outcomes

This section provides a formulation (which can be skipped) for conducting residual analyses of grouped data for univariate polytomous outcomes. Both grouped multinomial regression and grouped ordinal regression models are addressed. For polytomous outcomes, scaled residuals, as opposed to standardized residuals as generated for dichotomous outcomes, are generated, which account for correlation between the indicator variables for the outcome variable taking on alternate outcome values.

9.9.1   Multinomial Regression

Using the notation of Sect. 8.7.1, suppose the indexes $s \in S$ for the n observations have been partitioned into G nonempty, disjoint subsets S_g for $1 \leq g \leq G$. For $1 \leq g \leq G$, let $\mathbf{x}_g$ denote the average of the predictor vectors $\mathbf{x}_s$ over $s \in S_g$, n_{gv} the number of observations with indexes $s \in S_g$ satisfying $y_{sv} = 1$ for $0 \leq v \leq K$, and $n_g = n_{g0} + \cdots + n_{gK}$ the number of observations with indexes $s \in S_g$. The grouped data consist of the observations $O_g = (n_{g0}, \cdots, n_{gK}, \mathbf{x}_g)$ for $1 \leq g \leq G$. For $1 \leq g \leq K$, let μ_{gv} denote the common mean for all observations y_{sv} with $s \in S_g$, and model $\mathrm{glogit}(\mu_{gv}) = \mathbf{x}_g^T \cdot \boldsymbol{\beta}_v$ for K $r \times 1$ vectors $\boldsymbol{\beta}_v$ of coefficients, and let $\mu_{g0} = 1 - (\mu_{g1} + \cdots + \mu_{gK})$. The likelihood term L_g for the gth group satisfies

$$\ell_g = \log(L_g) = n_{g0} \cdot \log(\mu_{g0}) + \cdots + n_{gK} \cdot \log(\mu_{gK}).$$

With $\boldsymbol{\theta} = (\boldsymbol{\beta}_1^T, \cdots, \boldsymbol{\beta}_K^T)^T$, the likelihood $L(S; \boldsymbol{\theta})$ is the product of the likelihood terms L_g over $1 \leq g \leq G$ satisfying

$$\ell(S; \boldsymbol{\theta}) = \log(L(S; \boldsymbol{\theta})) = \sum_{1 \leq g \leq G} \ell_g.$$

The maximum likelihood estimate $\boldsymbol{\theta}(S)$ of $\boldsymbol{\theta}$ is computed by solving the estimating equations $\partial\ell(S;\boldsymbol{\theta})/\partial\boldsymbol{\theta} = \mathbf{0}$ obtained by differentiating $\ell(S;\boldsymbol{\theta})$ with respect to $\boldsymbol{\theta}$, where $\mathbf{0}$ denotes the zero vector. For $1 \le g \le G$, the estimated value for the mean μ_{gv} is

$$\mu_{gv}(S) = \frac{\exp(\mathbf{x}_g^T \cdot \boldsymbol{\beta}_v(S))}{1 + \exp(\mathbf{x}_g^T \cdot \boldsymbol{\beta}_1(S)) + \cdots + \exp(\mathbf{x}_g^T \cdot \boldsymbol{\beta}_K(S))}$$

for $1 \le v \le K$ while, for $v = 0$,

$$\mu_{g0}(S) = \frac{1}{\left(1 + \exp\left(\mathbf{x}_g^T \cdot \boldsymbol{\beta}_1(S) + \cdots + \exp\left(\mathbf{x}_g^T \cdot \boldsymbol{\beta}_K(S)\right)\right)\right)}.$$

For $1 \le v \le K$, the random variables n_{gv} equaling the number of $y_{sv} = 1$ with $s \in S_g$ are binomially distributed with estimated means $n_g \cdot \mu_{gv}(S)$ and estimated variances $\sigma_{gv}^2(S) = n_g \cdot \mu_{gv}(S) \cdot (1 - \mu_{gv}(S))$. Associated residuals are defined as $e_{gv}(S) = n_{gv} - n_g \cdot \mu_{gv}(S)$ and are combined into the K-dimensional vectors $\mathbf{e}_g(S)$. The covariance matrix $\boldsymbol{\Sigma}_g(S)$ for $\mathbf{e}_g(S)$ satisfies

$$\boldsymbol{\Sigma}_g(S) = n_g \cdot (\text{diag}(\boldsymbol{\mu}_g(S)) - \boldsymbol{\mu}_g(S) \cdot \boldsymbol{\mu}_g(S)^T)$$

where $\boldsymbol{\mu}_g(S)$ is the K-dimensional vector with entries $\mu_{gv}(S)$ for $1 \le v \le K$ and $\text{diag}(\boldsymbol{\mu}_g(S))$ is the diagonal matrix with diagonal entries $\mu_{gv}(S)$. As in Sect. 8.7.1, scaled residual vectors $\mathbf{sclde}_g(S)$ can then be computed as

$$\mathbf{sclde}_g(S) = (\mathbf{U}_g^T(S))^{-1} \cdot \mathbf{e}_g(S)$$

where $\mathbf{U}_g(S)$ is the square root of the covariance matrix $\boldsymbol{\Sigma}_g(S)$ determined by its Cholesky decomposition. Each y_{sv} with $s \in S_g$ is assigned the residual $e_{sv}(S) = e_{gv}(S)$ and scaled residual $\text{sclde}_{sv}(S) = \text{sclde}_{gv}(S)$. Each observation y_s is thus assigned K different residuals and standardized residuals corresponding to the K non-reference values $1 \le v \le K$. The values of $\text{sclde}_{sv}(S)$ can be combined over all s and all v and analyzed in combination as for independent data. LCV scores can be computed for grouped multinomial regression models using the approach described in Sect. 9.5 for dichotomous outcomes.

Grouped modeling of univariate polytomous outcomes extends readily to include modeling of dispersions as well as means using extended quasi-likelihoods based on multinomial likelihoods. The extension is similar to the extension in Sect. 8.13.2 for ungrouped univariate polytomous outcomes.

9.9.2   Ordinal Regression

Ordinal regression models based on the parameter vectors $\boldsymbol{\theta} = (\alpha_0, \cdots, \alpha_{K-1}, \boldsymbol{\beta}^T)^T$ as defined in Sect. 8.7.2 can be extended to grouped data similarly to the extension for multinomial regression models of Sect. 9.9.1. Grouped residuals and standardized residuals can also be defined in the same way as for multinomial regression but using estimates of μ_{gv} for the K values $0 \le v \le K - 1$ determined by the ordinal regression model generalized to grouped data. LCV scores can be computed for grouped ordinal regression models using the approach described in Sect. 9.5 for dichotomous outcomes. Grouped modeling of univariate ordinal outcomes extends readily to include modeling of dispersions as well as means using extended quasi-likelihoods.

9.10   Grouped Residual Analysis of Merclevel as a Function of Length

Adaptive grouping of lengths for modeling merclevel can be requested as follows.

```
%let wndwval=0.07;
%genreg(modtype=logis,datain=mercury,yvar=merclevel,
        vintrcpt=n,propodds=y,foldcnt=5,regroup=y,
        grpvars=length,window=&wndwval,expand=y,
        expxvars=length,contract=y,nocnxint=y);
```

The choice of 0.07 maximizes the LCV score over multiples of 0.01 from 0.01 to 0.10 for the window parameter generated by varying the value for the wndwval macro variable in the above code. Its LCV score is 0.64683. The PD for the adaptive model based on the ungrouped data with LCV score 0.64103 (as reported in Sect. 8.10) is substantial at 0.90 %, indicating that grouping has distinctly improved the model. The adaptive grouped model is based on the single transform length$^{1.5}$ compared to length$^{2.5}$ for the ungrouped data. The linear model in grouped lengths has LCV score 0.64661 with insubstantial PD of 0.03 %, indicating that the adaptive grouped model is also reasonably close to linear. The resvar and stdrsvar macro parameters determine the names of variables in the dataout data set containing residuals and scaled residuals, respectively. For the above code, these parameters have default settings of res and stdres. Two of each of these types of variables are generated, named res_1 and stdres_1 for predicting a low mercury level and res_2 and stdres_2 for predicting a medium mercury level. Scaled residuals for estimating low and medium levels of mercury are plotted in Fig. 9.4 versus lengths for the grouped data model, distinguishing between low, medium, and high observed values for merclevel. The scaled residuals are all well within ± 3 and even well within ± 2, and so there are no outliers. However, there is asymmetry for large lengths. All fish with lengths greater than about 52 cm have high levels of mercury and generate negative scaled residuals, suggesting consideration of models with the effect of length constant for large lengths, but that issue is not addressed here.

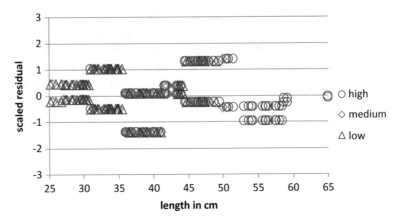

Fig. 9.4 Scaled residuals versus lengths of the fish for predicting low and medium mercury levels using the adaptive ordinal regression model of mercury levels as a function of grouped length values with observed values of low at most 0.72 ppm, medium over 0.72 but at most 1.3 ppm, and high over 1.3 ppm

9.11   Modeling Dispersions as Well as Means for the Dichotomous Outcome Merchigh

Both the dispersions and means for merchigh can be modeled in terms of length as follows.

```
%genreg(modtype=logis,datain=mercury,yvar=merchigh,
        foldcnt=5,expand=y,expxvars=length,
        expvvars=length,contract=y,nocnxint=y,
        cnvzero=y);
```

The expvvars macro parameter provides a list of primary predictors to consider for modeling variances for the normal distribution case and dispersions for other cases like logistic regression. In the above code, the list is the same as for expxvars, but it can be different. The genreg macro supports several other parameters for controlling the variance/dispersion component of the model including vvars, vpowers, vintrcpt, vgcs, and vgcpowrs which work like xvars, xpowers, xintrcpt, xgcs, and xgcpowrs, but address the model for the log of the variances/dispersions (the "v" part of the model) rather than the model for the logits of the means (or the expectations or the "x" part of the model). The default setting "vintrcpt=y" is requested in the above code since it seems better to start the search at the constant dispersions model rather than at the unit dispersions model. However, the default setting "nocnvint=n" is also requested, thereby allowing the intercept term for the dispersions model to be removed during the contraction. Since standard logistic regression models have zero intercepts for the dispersion model, it does not seem

necessary to restrict dispersion models to have non-zero intercepts as it does for the
model for the means. For the same reason, it seems reasonable for the contraction
to generate a model with unit dispersions based on no transforms at all (formally,
zero log dispersions). By default, models for the means and for the dispersions
are not contracted further once they are reduced to a single transform. The setting
"cnvzero=y" means that the contraction should consider the zero log dispersions
model (and hence the unit dispersions model) when the dispersions are based on a
single transform and not stop. The macro parameter cvxzero has the same effect on
the model for the means, but it is unlikely for zero means to be an effective
alternative.

The generated model for the above code has extended quasi-likelihood cross-
validation ($QLCV^+$) score 0.64457 (as also reported in Sect. 8.13.3). This model is
based on one transform for the means: $length^{4.2}$ with an intercept (as for all models
considered in this chapter) and on one transform for the dispersions: $length^{6.6}$ also
with an intercept. In contrast, the unit dispersions model for length (see Sects. 8.5
and 9.4) has $QLCV^+$ score 0.59140 (the same as its LCV score) with substantial
PD of 8.25 % (as also reported in Sect. 8.13.3), indicating that dispersion modeling has substantially improved the model for merchigh as a function of length.
Figure 8.12 displays the estimated dispersions as a function of length. Figure 8.11
displays the estimated probabilities (or means) as a function of length. Whether
there is distinct change to the logit expectation component can be assessed as
follows.

```
%genreg(modtype=logis,datain=mercury,yvar=merchigh,
        foldcnt=15,xvars=length,xpowers=0.5,expand=y,
        expvvars=length,contract=y,contordr=v,
        cnvzero=y,notrxbas=y);
```

The base model for the means depends on $length^{0.5}$ due to the settings of the
xvars and xpowers macro parameters and is not changed in the expansion since
expxvars has its default empty setting. However, by default the contraction considers adjusting the logit expectation component. This is avoided in the above code
by the setting "contordr=v" meaning to contract only the log dispersion component
of the model and not the logit expectation component. If the model is not
contracted, a conditional transformation is executed. This could change the model
for logits of the means, but that is avoided by the "notrxbas=y" setting meaning do
not transform the "x" base model. The generated model has $QLCV^+$ score 0.61097
and substantial PD 5.21 % compared to the nonlinear model for both means and
dispersions (as also reported in Sect. 8.13.3). This indicates that the logit expectation model has distinctly changed when the dispersions are also modeled in terms of
length.

9.12 Modeling Dispersions as Well as Means for the Polytomous Outcome Merclevel

Adaptive models for means and dispersions of polytomous outcomes can be generated similarly to such models for dichotomous outcomes. As described in Sect. 9.8, the type of model is controlled by the propodds macro parameter. Setting "propodds = y" requests a proportional odds or ordinal regression model based on cumulative logits while the default setting "propodds = n" requests a multinomial regression model based on generalized logits. In any case, the estimated dispersion coefficients are the same for all outcome values and do not change with the outcome value as do intercepts for means of ordinal regression models and intercepts and slopes for means of multinomial regression models. For example, an adaptive ordinal regression model for the means and dispersions of merclevel as a function of length, river, and GCs can be generated starting from the constant means and constant dispersions model (using the default settings "xintrcpt=y" and "vintrcpt=y") as follows.

```
%genreg(modtype=logis,datain=mercury,yvar=merclevel,
        propodds=y,foldcnt=5,expand=y,
        expxvars=length river,expvvars=length river,
        geomcmbn=y,contract=y,nocnxint=y,cnvzero=y);
```

The base model for the expansion has constant means and dispersions with $QLCV^+$ score 0.63873 (output not provided). This is expanded (see Table 9.2) to include first the transform $length^{2.5}$ added to the means, then the six transforms $length^{6.62}$, $length^{3.01}$, $VGC\_1 = river \cdot length^{6.8}$, $length^{-6}$, $VGC\_2 = river \cdot length^{5.2}$, and $VGC\_3^{1.1} = (length^3 \cdot river)^{1.1}$ to the dispersions, in that order, and then the expansion stops. The $QLCV^+$ score rounds to 0.72749. It is described in the output as based on a "quasi + likelihood" since extended quasi-likelihoods are used to generate estimates and $QLCV^+$ scores to evaluate models.

The contraction (see Table 9.3) removes the intercept, followed by the transforms $length^{3.01}$ and $VGC\_3^{1.1}$ from the model for the dispersions and then stops. The power of the transform for the means is adjusted to: $length^{6.69}$ while the remaining transforms for the dispersions are adjusted to: $length^{6.658}$, $VGC\_1^{1.005}$, $length^{5.66}$, and $VGC\_2^{1.22}$. The estimated model for the cumulative logits satisfies

$$logit(P(merclevel = 0|length)) = 0.651727 - 2.2 \cdot 10^{-11} \cdot length^{6.69},$$

and

$$logit(P(merclevel \leq 1|length)) = 2.5236445 - 2.2 \cdot 10^{-11} \cdot length^{6.69}.$$

The estimated model for the dispersions satisfies

Table 9.2 Expanded model for mercury levels of low at most 0.72 ppm (merclevel = 0), medium over 0.72 but at most 1.3 ppm (merclevel = 1), and high over 1.3 ppm (merclevel = 2) as a function of length of the fish and the indicator river for being caught in the Waccamaw River

```
          geometric combination log dispersion variables:
                    VGC_1      river*length**(6.8)
                    VGC_2      river*length**(5.2)
                    VGC_3      length**(3)*river
...

                   expanded logit expectation component

       parameter estimates for smaller vs. larger cumulative logits

predictor      power    merclevel=0    merclevel=1      score    order

XINTRCPT           1      4.0762116      6.2188024    0.6387284       0
length           2.5     -0.000565      -0.000565    0.6742635       1

                   expanded log dispersion component

     predictor        power    estimate        score    order

     VINTRCPT             1     -0.65622    0.6387284       0
     length            6.62     -1.83E-11   0.6941912       2
     length            3.01     0.0000366   0.7042338       3
     VGC_1                1     -3.71E-11   0.7145639       4
     length              -6     236854435   0.718714        5
     VGC_2                1     2.7111E-8   0.7228619       6
     VGC_3              1.1     -0.000016   0.7274878       7
...
mth root of quasi+ likelihood using deleted predictions:   0.7274878
```

$$\log(\text{dispersion}) = -9.39 \cdot 10^{-11} \cdot \text{length}^{6.658}$$
$$-2 \cdot 10^{-11} \cdot \left(\text{river} \cdot \text{length}^{6.8}\right)^{1.005} + 4.7049 \cdot 10^{-9} \cdot \text{length}^{5.66}$$
$$+ 1.203 \cdot 10^{-10} \cdot \left(\text{river} \cdot \text{length}^{5.2}\right)^{1.1}.$$

The QLCV$^+$ score rounds to 0.76997. This is a substantial improvement over the unit dispersions model in length, river, and GCs with LCV score 0.64103 (reported in Sect. 8.10) and PD 16.75 %.

An assessment of linearity for the logits in length can be conducted as follows.

```
%genreg(modtype=logis,datain=mercury,yvar=merclevel,
       propodds=y,foldcnt=5,xvars=length,expand=y,
       expvvars=length river,geomcmbn=y,contract=y,
       nocnxbas=y,notrxbas=y,cnvzero=y);
```

The macro parameter xpowers has its default empty value, meaning assign the default power of 1 to the predictor length listed in the xvars setting so that the base

Table 9.3 Contracted model for mercury levels of low at most 0.72 ppm (merclevel = 0), medium over 0.72 but at most 1.3 ppm (merclevel = 1), and high over 1.3 ppm (merclevel = 2) as a function of length of the fish and the indicator river for being caught in the Waccamaw River

```
contracted model adjusted to avoid extreme probability estimates

          contracted logit expectation component

parameter estimates for smaller vs. larger cumulative logits

               predictor old power new power

               XINTRCPT          1           1
               length          2.5        6.69

    predictor      power   merclevel=0   merclevel=1

    XINTRCPT           1     0.651727     2.5236445
    length          6.69    -2.2E-11      -2.2E-11

           old power          score   order

                    .     0.7274878       0

          contracted log dispersion component

    predictor old power new power    estimate

       length          6.62    6.658    -9.39E-11
       VGC_1              1    1.005      -2E-11
       length            -6     5.66   4.7049E-9
       VGC_2              1     1.22   1.203E-10

       discarded    old power        score   order

                            .    0.7274878       0
       VINTRCPT             1    0.7686715       1
       length            3.01    0.7727736       2
       VGC_3             1.1    0.7699678       3
...
mth root of quasi+ likelihood using deleted predictions:   0.7699678
```

model for the logits is linear in length. The logits are not changed by the expansion since expxvars has its default empty setting. It is also not changed by the contraction due to the setting "nocnxbas=y", meaning do not contract the base model for the logit expectation (or x) component of the model and by "notrxbas=y" meaning do not transform that component as well. By default, the contraction removes transforms adjusting powers for the remaining transforms from both the logit expectation and log dispersion components. This is why the "nocnxbas=y" and "notrxbas=y" are needed above. The setting "nocnxbas=y" can be replaced by the setting "contrord=y" meaning contract only the log dispersion component (as demonstrated in Sect. 9.11), but the setting "notrxbas=y" is still needed to avoid transformations in the case a conditional transformation is needed. The generated model has LCV score 0.68728 with substantial PD 10.74 % compared to the model of Table 9.3. Thus, after adjusting for possible non-unit dispersions, the logits for merclevel are distinctly nonlinear in length in contrast to being reasonable close to linear with unit dispersions as reported in Sect. 8.10.

An assessment of non-constant dispersions can be assessed as follows.

```
%genreg(modtype=logis,datain=mercury,yvar=merclevel,
        propodds=y,foldcnt=5,expand=y,
        expxvars=length river,geomcmbn=y,contract=y,
        nocnxint=y);
```

The base model is a constant dispersions model due to using the default setting "vintrcpt=y". This is not changed by the expectation since expvvars has its default empty setting. It is also not changed by the contraction due to using the default setting "nocnxint=y". The generated model has LCV score 0.67426 with substantial PD 12.43 % compared to the model of Table 9.3. Thus, dispersions for merclevel are distinctly non-constant in length.

Figures 9.5 and 9.6 display results for the model for merclevel with non-constant means and dispersions of Table 9.3. The estimated probability of a high mercury level over 1.3 ppm of Fig. 9.5 has an s-shaped pattern with estimated probabilities changing slowly for low lengths ≤ 40 cm and for high lengths ≥ 50 cm, and is the same for both rivers. The estimated dispersions of Fig. 9.6 increase from about 1.2 units for length 25 cm with increased length of the fish for lower values and then decrease to essentially zero by length 55 cm. The dispersions are about the same for the two rivers for lengths up to about 40 cm, after that the dispersions decrease for

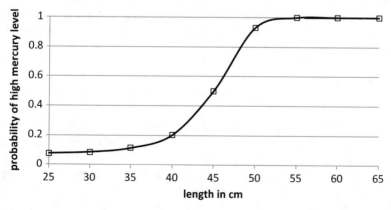

Fig. 9.5 Estimated probability of a high mercury level over 1.3 ppm as a function of length of the fish caught in the Lumber and Waccamaw Rivers

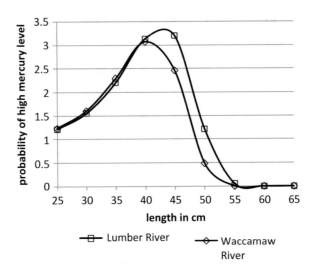

Fig. 9.6 Estimated dispersions for polytomous mercury levels as a function of length of the fish caught in the Lumber and Waccamaw Rivers

fish caught in the Lumber River and continue to increase for fish caught in the Waccamaw River up to about 45 cm. After that, the dispersions decrease for both rivers with increased length, at a higher level for fish caught in the Waccamaw River until the dispersions reach zero for both rivers at about 55 cm.

Logistic regression models can sometimes generate extreme, that is, very low or very high, probability estimates close to 0 or to 1. The minprob macro parameter determines the minimum estimated probability. Its default setting is 0.0001, meaning that probabilities are considered too low when they are < 0.0001. They are considered too high when they are $> (1 - 0.0001 \cdot K)$ where $K + 1$ is the number of unique outcome values. Parameter estimates are adjusted if necessary to these boundary values to avoid generating too low or too high probability estimates. For example, the model of Table 9.3 has been adjusted in this way as indicated in the output. This also occurs for the expanded model but the corresponding output line is not included in Table 9.2.

As pointed out in Sect. 9.8, the cutoff for a substantial PD in the LCV scores for multinomial regression models for outcomes with $K + 1$ unique values is based on $DF = K$ rather than $DF = 1$ as is used for ordinal regression models and for models for continuous outcomes (Chaps. 2–5). This is also the case for $QLCV^+$ scores. The extra DF are needed because the removal or addition of one transform of the model for the means involves the removal or addition of K parameters rather than only one parameter as for other modeling cases. Each transform for the model for the dispersions, though, only involves a single parameter even for multinomial regression models, and so the adaptive modeling process in that case bases the removal or addition of such transforms on $QLCV^+$ ratio tests determined by $DF = 1$.

9.13   Practice Exercises

9.1. The unit dispersions model for the means of merchigh in weight, length, and GCs reported in Sect. 8.6 distinctly outperformed the additive model in weight and length. Consideration of non-unit dispersions may provide improvements as held for the analysis involving only length reported in Sect. 8.13.3. Assess this issue by generating the adaptive model with both means and dispersions depending on weight, length, and GCs. Compare this model to the associated unit-dispersions model of Sect. 8.6. Next generate the adaptive model with both means and dispersions depending additively on weight and length and assess whether there is a benefit to considering GCs or not. For these analyses, start from the constant model for both means and dispersions. Do not allow the contraction to remove the intercept from the model for the means but allow the contraction to consider unit dispersions models. Use 15 folds as justified in Sect. 8.4.

9.2. The unit dispersions model for the means of merchigh in weight, length, river and GCs reported in Sect. 8.6 distinctly outperform the additive model in weight, length, and river. Consideration of non-unit dispersions may provide improvements. Assess this issue by generating the adaptive model with both means and dispersions depending on weight, length, river, and GCs. Start from the constant model for both means and dispersions. Do not allow the contraction to remove the intercept from the model for the means but allow the contraction to consider unit dispersions models. Use 15 folds as justified in Sect. 8.4. Does the generated model substantially improve on the models generated for Practice Exercise 9.1? Is there a distinct effect to river on means and/or dispersions?

9.3. The unit dispersions model for the means of merclevel in weight, length, and GCs is reported in Sect. 8.11. Consideration of non-unit dispersions may provide improvements as held for the analysis involving length and river reported in Sect. 9.12. Assess this issue by generating the adaptive model with both means and dispersions depending on weight, length, and GCs. Compare this model to the associated unit-dispersions model of Sect. 8.11 to see if similar results are produced. Next generate the adaptive model with both means and dispersions depending additively on weight and length and assess whether there is a benefit to considering GCs or not. For these analyses, use adaptive ordinal regression modeling as justified in Sect. 8.9. Start from a constant model for both the means and the dispersions. Do not allow the contraction to remove the intercept from the model for the means but allow the contraction to consider unit dispersions models. Use 5 folds as justified in Sect. 8.9.

9.4. For unit dispersions models in weight, length, and river, there is a distinct effect to river on the means for merclevel (see Sect. 8.11). Consideration of non-unit dispersions models may provide improvements. Assess this issue by generating the adaptive model with both means and dispersions depending on weight, length, river, and GCs. Use adaptive ordinal regression modeling as justified in Sect. 8.9. Start from a constant model for both the means and the dispersions. Do not allow the contraction to remove the intercept from the model for the means but allow the contraction to consider unit dispersions models. Use 5 folds as justified in Sect. 8.9. Does the generated model substantially improve on the model generated for Practice Exercise 9.3? Is there a distinct effect to river on means and/or dispersions?

For Practice Exercises 9.5–9.6, use the Titantic survival data available on the Internet (see Supplementary Materials). Data are available for 756 passengers with no missing data. The outcome variable for this data set is called survived and is the indicator for having survived the sinking of the Titantic. The predictors to be considered are age and the indicator fstclass for the passenger being in first class versus second or third class. The gender of the passenger is also available in the data set but is not used in the practice exercises.

9.5. For the Titantic data, use the adaptive model for having survived as a function of age as the benchmark analysis to set the number of folds for LCV scores. Do not allow the contraction to remove the intercept from the model for the means for all analyses for this practice exercise. Use unit dispersions for all analyses of this practice exercise. Compare the adaptive model in age to the linear polynomial model in age and assess whether the log odds for having survived changes distinctly nonlinearly or not. Generate the adaptive additive model in age and fstclass and the adaptive model in age, fstclass, and GCs. Assess whether being in first class or not distinctly moderates (see Sect. 4.5.3) the effect of age on the chance for surviving. Describe how means for surviving change with the predictors of the most preferable unit dispersions model?

9.6. For the Titantic data, generate adaptive non-unit dispersions models. In these analyses, start from a constant model for both the means and the dispersions, do not allow the contraction to remove the intercept from the model for the means, but allow the contraction to consider unit dispersions models. Use the number of folds determined for Practice Exercise 9.5. First generate the adaptive additive model for means and dispersions depending on age and fstclass. Does the generated model substantially improve on the adaptive additive unit dispersions model generated for Practice Exercise 9.5? Is there a substantial benefit to considering non-unit dispersions? Then generate the adaptive model for means and dispersions depending on age, fstclass, and GCs. Is there a substantial benefit to also considering GCs? For the preferable non-unit dispersions model, how do means and dispersions for having survived change with age for first class passengers compared to second and third class passengers?

References

Allison, P. (2012). *Logistic regression using SAS: Theory and applications* (2nd ed.). Cary, NC: SAS Institute.
SAS Institute. (1995). *Logistic regression examples using the SAS system.* Cary, NC: SAS Institute.
SAS Institute. (2004). *SAS/STAT 9.1 user's guide.* Cary, NC: SAS Institute.
Stokes, M. E., Davis, C. S., & Koch, G. G. (2012). *Categorical data analysis using the SAS system* (3rd ed.). Cary, NC: SAS Institute.
Zelterman, D. (2002). *Advanced log-linear models using SAS.* Cary, NC: SAS Institute.

Chapter 10
Adaptive Logistic Regression Modeling of Multivariate Dichotomous and Polytomous Outcomes

10.1 Chapter Overview

This chapter formulates and demonstrates adaptive fractional polynomial modeling of means and dispersions for repeatedly measured dichotomous and polytomous outcomes with two or more values. A description of how to generate these models in SAS is provided in Chap. 11. Standard models for this context are addressed in several texts (e.g., Fitzmaurice et al. 2011; Molenberghs and Verbeke 2006).

Marginal modeling extends from the multivariate normal outcome context (see Sect. 4.3) to the multivariate dichotomous and polytomous outcome context. However, due to the complexity in general of computing likelihoods and quasi-likelihoods (as needed to account for non-unit dispersions) for general multivariate marginal modeling, generalized estimating equations (GEE) techniques (Liang and Zeger 1986) are often used instead, thereby avoiding computation of likelihoods and quasi-likelihoods. This complicates the extension of adaptive modeling to the GEE context since it is based on cross-validation (CV) scores computed from likelihoods or likelihood-like functions (but see Sects. 10.7 and 10.8). Conditional modeling also extends to the multivariate dichotomous and polytomous outcome context, both transition modeling (see Sect. 4.7) and general conditional modeling (see Sect. 4.9). In contrast to marginal GEE modeling, conditional modeling of means for multivariate dichotomous and polytomous outcomes with unit dispersions is based on pseudolikelihoods that can be used to compute pseudolikelihood CV (PLCV) scores on which to base adaptive modeling of multivariate dichotomous and polytomous outcomes. For this reason, conditional modeling is considered first. PLCV scores are the same as LCV scores for transition models, but not in general. Conditional modeling involving non-unit dispersions is based on extended pseudolikelihoods and extended PLCV ($PLCV^+$) scores. For transition models, $PLCV^+$ scores are the same as their extended quasi-likelihood CV ($QLCV^+$) scores (see Sect. 8.13).

© Springer International Publishing Switzerland 2016
G.J. Knafl, K. Ding, *Adaptive Regression for Modeling Nonlinear Relationships*,
Statistics for Biology and Health, DOI 10.1007/978-3-319-33946-7_10

Section 10.2 describes a dataset with a longitudinal respiratory status outcome that can be analyzed either as dichotomous or polytomous. Section 10.3 formulates conditional modeling, including both transition and general conditional modeling, for multivariate dichotomous outcomes. Section 10.4 then presents analyses of dichotomous respiratory status, but using only transition modeling since that is more appropriate for such longitudinal data than general conditional modeling. Section 10.5 describes the formulation for conditional modeling of multivariate polytomous outcomes. Section 10.6 then presents transition modeling analyses of polytomous respiratory status. Section 10.7 formulates adaptive GEE modeling of multivariate dichotomous and polytomous outcomes. Section 10.8 then presents adaptive GEE analyses, but of only the dichotomous respiratory status outcome for brevity. Sections 10.9 and 10.10 provide overviews of the results of analysis of post-baseline dichotomous and polytomous respiratory status, respectively. Formulation sections are not needed to understand analysis sections.

10.2   The Respiratory Status Data

A data set on respiratory status at baseline and at four post-baseline clinic visits for $n = 111$ patients with respiratory disorder is available on the Internet (see Supplementary Materials). These data were analyzed and are also available in Koch et al. (1989). For the post-baseline data, the variable status0_4 is the original polytomous outcome and contains values for each patient's respiratory status categorized into $0 =$ terrible, $1 =$ poor, $2 =$ fair, $3 =$ good, and $4 =$ excellent. The possible predictor variables are visit (with post-baseline values 1–4), status0_4_0 (the baseline respiratory status), and active (the indicator for the patient being on an active as opposed to a placebo treatment). Miller et al. (1993) analyzed the associated three-level polytomous outcome variable status0_2 with values $0 =$ poor   (original values 0–1), $1 =$ good   (original values 2–3), and $3 =$ excellent   (original value 4) with baseline value status0_2_0 (see their Table 1). Stokes et al. (2012) analyzed the associated dichotomous outcome variable status0_1 with values $0 =$ poor (original values 0–2) and $1 =$ good (original values 3–4) with baseline value status0_1_0. Other predictors are available in the data set including age at baseline, gender, and center (1 or 2) where treated, but these are not considered here. There are a total of 444 post-baseline outcome measurements with four measurements available for each patient, and so none missing. The dichotomous post-baseline outcome variable status0_1 is analyzed in Sect. 10.4 to demonstrate how to conduct logistic regression analyses using transition models accounting for nonlinearity in predictor variables of means and dispersions for repeatedly measured dichotomous outcomes and in Sect. 10.8 to demonstrate adaptive GEE modeling of means and dispersions for such outcomes. The three-level polytomous post-baseline outcome variable status0_2 is analyzed in Sect. 10.7 to demonstrate how to conduct multinomial and ordinal regression analyses using transition models accounting for nonlinearity in predictor variables of means and dispersions for repeatedly measured polytomous outcomes. As for the logistic regression analyses of Chaps. 8–9, in all analyses reported in this chapter, all models for means include an intercept. Also, all models have unit dispersions unless otherwise stated.

10.3   Conditional Modeling of Multivariate Dichotomous Outcomes

This section formulates conditional modeling in the multivariate dichotomous outcome context, first with unit dispersions in Sect. 10.3.1 and then more general dispersions in Sect. 10.3.2. It can be skipped to focus on analyses.

10.3.1   Conditional Modeling of Means Assuming Unit Dispersions

Using the notation of Sects. 4.3.1–4.3.2, 4.7, and 4.9.1, for n matched sets of measurements with indexes $s \in S = \{s : 1 \leq s \leq n\}$, observed data $O_{s,C(s)} = (\mathbf{y}_{s,C(s)}, \mathbf{X}_{s,C(s)})$ are available for possibly different sets $C(s)$ of measurement conditions, subsets of the maximal set of possible conditions $C = \{c : 1 \leq c \leq m\}$, consisting of outcome vectors $\mathbf{y}_{s,C(s)}$ with m(s) entries y_{sc} for $c \in C(s)$ and predictor matrices $\mathbf{X}_{s,C(s)}$ having m(s) rows $\mathbf{x}_{sc}^T$ with entries x_{scj} for $j \in J = \{j : 1 \leq j \leq r\}$ and for $c \in C(s)$. The observed conditional data then consist of $O^{\#}_{sc} = (y^{\#}_{sc}, \mathbf{x}_{sc})$ for the m(SC) measurements $sc \in SC = \{sc : c \in C(s), s \in S\}$ where $y_{sc} = y_{sc}|\mathbf{y}_{s,C(s)\setminus\{c\}}$ is the cth outcome measurement for matched set s conditioned on the other outcome measurements for that matched set. The dependence of $y^{\#}_{sc}$ on the other outcome measurements is modeled using averages PRE(y,i,j) and associated missing indicators PRE(y,i,j,$\varnothing$) (see Sect. 4.7) of prior outcome measurements, averages POST(y,i,j) and associated missing indicators POST(y,i,j,$\varnothing$) (see Sect. 4.9.1) of subsequent outcome measurements, and averages OTHER(y,i,j) and associated missing indicators OTHER(y,i,j,$\varnothing$) (see Sect. 4.9.1) of prior and subsequent outcome measurements, for $1 \leq i \leq j \leq m$. For dichotomous outcomes with values 0 and 1, these averages are also proportions of cases with $y = 1$. To simplify the notation, the predictor matrices $\mathbf{X}_{s,C(s)}$ are assumed to include columns containing observed values for dependence predictors as well as columns for non-dependence predictors. The special case of transition modeling corresponds to cases with dependence based only on prior outcome measurements. Note that dependence predictors can also be computed from prior values of time-varying predictors.

For $sc \in SC$, the mean or expected value $\mu^{\#}_{sc}$ for $y^{\#}_{sc}$ satisfies $\mu^{\#}_{sc} = Ey^{\#}_{sc} = P(y^{\#}_{sc} = 1|\mathbf{x}_{sc})$. With the logit (or log odds) function defined as $\text{logit}(u) = \log(u/(1-u))$ for $0 < u < 1$, model the logit of the mean as

$$\text{logit}\left(\mu^{\#}_{sc}\right) = \mathbf{x}_{sc}^{T} \cdot \boldsymbol{\beta}$$

for a $r \times 1$ vector $\boldsymbol{\beta}$ of coefficients. Solving for $\mu^{\#}_{sc}$ gives $\mu^{\#}_{sc} = \exp(\mathbf{x}_{sc}^{T} \cdot \boldsymbol{\beta})/(1 + \exp(\mathbf{x}_{sc}^{T} \cdot \boldsymbol{\beta}))$. The odds ratio OR for $y^{\#}_{sc} = 1$ under a unit change in a predictor value x_{scj} and adjusted for the other predictor values $x_{scj'}$ for $j' \neq j$ (if any) is computed as $OR = \exp(\beta_{j})$. The conditional variance for $y^{\#}_{sc}$ is $\sigma^{\#}_{sc}{}^{2} = \mu^{\#}_{sc} \cdot (1 - \mu^{\#}_{sc})$.

The pseudolikelihood term PL_{sc} for the scth measurement equals the conditional likelihood $L(O^{\#}_{sc}; \boldsymbol{\beta})$ for the conditional observation $O^{\#}_{sc}$ and satisfies

$$\ell_{sc} = \log(PL_{sc}) = y^{\#}_{sc} \cdot \log\left(\mu^{\#}_{sc}\right) + \left(1 - y^{\#}_{sc}\right) \cdot \log\left(1 - \mu^{\#}_{sc}\right).$$

The pseudolikelihood $PL(SC; \boldsymbol{\beta})$ is the product of the pseudolikelihood terms PL_{sc} over $sc \in SC$ and satisfies

$$\ell(SC; \boldsymbol{\beta}) = \log(PL(SC; \boldsymbol{\beta})) = \sum_{sc \in SC} \ell_{sc}.$$

The maximum pseudolikelihood estimate $\boldsymbol{\beta}(SC)$ of $\boldsymbol{\beta}$ is computed by solving the estimating equations $\partial \ell(SC; \boldsymbol{\beta})/\partial \boldsymbol{\beta} = \mathbf{0}$ obtained by differentiating $\ell(SC; \boldsymbol{\beta})$ with respect to $\boldsymbol{\beta}$, where $\mathbf{0}$ denotes the zero vector. For simplicity of notation, parameter estimates $\boldsymbol{\beta}(SC)$ are denoted as functions of indexes for the data used in their computation without hat (^) symbols. With this notation, the matched-set-wise deletion PLCV formulation of Sect. 4.9.1 and the measurement-wise deletion version of Sect. 4.13 both extend to the multivariate dichotomous outcome logistic regression context. For transition models, the pseudolikelihood is a true likelihood and PLCV scores are also LCV scores.

For $sc \in SC$, the estimated value for the mean $\mu^{\#}_{sc}$ is

$$\mu^{\#}_{sc}(SC) = \frac{\exp(\mathbf{x}_{sc}^{T} \cdot \boldsymbol{\beta}(SC))}{1 + \exp(\mathbf{x}_{sc}^{T} \cdot \boldsymbol{\beta}(SC))}$$

and the corresponding residual is $e^{\#}_{sc}(SC) = y^{\#}_{sc} - \mu^{\#}_{sc}(SC)$. The estimated value for the variance $\sigma^{\#}_{sc}{}^{2}$ is $\sigma^{\#}_{sc}{}^{2}(SC) = \mu^{\#}_{sc}(SC) \cdot (1 - \mu^{\#}_{sc}(SC))$. The standardized or Pearson residual $stde^{\#}_{sc}(SC) = e^{\#}_{sc}(SC)/\sigma^{\#}_{sc}(SC)$ is obtained by standardizing the residual by dividing by the estimated standard deviation.

The predictor vectors $\mathbf{x}_{sc}$ can be based on fractional polynomial transforms of primary predictors of non-dependence type as considered in analyses reported in Chaps. 2, 4, 6, and 8 and of dependence type as considered in analyses of Chaps. 4 and 6. Adaptive fractional polynomial conditional models can be selected using the adaptive modeling process controlled by PLCV scores as in Chap. 4, but with the PLCV scores computed for the logistic regression case. For models based on fractional polynomials, the odds ratio (OR) function for a primary predictor can be generalized as in Sect. 8.3.2 to the exponentiation of the derivative of the logit function with respect to that primary predictor.

10.3.2   Conditional Modeling of Dispersions as Well as Means

Extending the notation of Sect. 8.13.1, dichotomous conditional outcome measurements $y^{\#}_{sc}$ with values 0 and 1 have means $\mu^{\#}_{sc} = P(y^{\#}_{sc} = 1)$, and variances $V(\mu^{\#}_{sc}) = \mu^{\#}_{sc} \cdot (1 - \mu^{\#}_{sc})$. The deviance terms are defined as (McCullagh and Nelder 1999)

$$d(y^{\#}_{sc}; \mu^{\#}_{sc}) = 2 \cdot \left[y^{\#}_{sc} \cdot \log\left(\frac{y^{\#}_{sc}}{\mu^{\#}_{sc}}\right) + (1 - y^{\#}_{sc}) \cdot \log\left(\frac{1 - y^{\#}_{sc}}{1 - \mu^{\#}_{sc}}\right) \right],$$

where $0 \cdot \log(0)$ is set equal to 0. Dispersion parameters $\phi^{\#}_{sc}$ can be incorporated into the conditional logistic model through the extended quasi-pseudolikelihood terms PL_{sc}^{+} satisfying

$$\ell_{sc}^{+} = \log(PL_{sc}^{+}) = -\frac{1}{2} \cdot d(y^{\#}_{sc}; \mu^{\#}_{sc})/\phi^{\#}_{sc} - \frac{1}{2} \cdot \log(\phi^{\#}_{sc}).$$

Let $\boldsymbol{\theta}$ denote the vector of all the parameters determining $\mu^{\#}_{sc}$ and $\phi^{\#}_{sc}$ for $sc \in SC$. Then, the extended quasi-pseudolikelihood $PL^{+}(SC; \boldsymbol{\theta})$ satisfies

$$\begin{aligned}
\ell^{+}(SC; \boldsymbol{\theta}) &= \log\left(PL^{+}(SC; \boldsymbol{\theta})\right) \\
&= \sum_{s \in SC} \ell_{sc}^{+} \\
&= \sum_{sc \in SC} \left((\ell_{sc} - a^{\#}_{sc})/\phi^{\#}_{sc} - \frac{1}{2} \cdot \log(\phi^{\#}_{sc}) \right),
\end{aligned}$$

where $\ell_{sc} = y^{\#}_{sc} \cdot \log(\mu^{\#}_{sc}) + (1 - y^{\#}_{sc}) \cdot \log(1 - \mu^{\#}_{sc})$ are the usual log pseudolikelihood terms and

$$a^{\#}_{sc} = y^{\#}_{sc} \cdot \log\left(y^{\#}_{sc}\right) + \left(1 - y^{\#}_{sc}\right) \cdot \log\left(1 - y^{\#}_{sc}\right) = 0$$

for $sc \in SC$. Extended variances $\sigma^{\#}_{sc}{}^{2}$ can then be defined as $\sigma^{\#}_{sc}{}^{2} = \phi^{\#}_{sc} \cdot V(\mu^{\#}_{sc})$.

Assume as in Sect. 10.3.1 that $\text{logit}(\mu^{\#}_{sc}) = \mathbf{x}_{sc}^{T} \cdot \boldsymbol{\beta}$. When $\phi^{\#}_{sc} = \phi^{\#}$ are constant, $\boldsymbol{\theta} = (\boldsymbol{\beta}^{T}, \phi^{\#})^{T}$, and maximizing $\ell^{+}(SC; \boldsymbol{\theta})$ in $\boldsymbol{\theta}$ generates the same estimates $\boldsymbol{\beta}(SC)$ as maximum pseudolikelihood estimation of $\boldsymbol{\beta}$ under the unit-dispersions conditional model. The maximum extended quasi-pseudolikelihood estimate $\phi^{\#}(SC)$ of $\phi^{\#}$ then satisfies

$$\phi^{\#}(SC) = \frac{1}{m(SC)} \sum_{sc \in SC} d(y^{\#}_{sc}; \mu^{\#}_{sc}(SC)),$$

where $\mu^{\#}_{sc}(SC)$ are the estimates of $\mu^{\#}_{sc}$ determined by $\boldsymbol{\beta}(SC)$. More generally, model the log of the dispersions $\phi^{\#}_{sc}$ as a function of selected dependence and/or non-dependence primary predictors and associated coefficients (similarly to the approach of Sect. 8.13.1). Specifically, let $\log(\phi^{\#}_{sc}) = \mathbf{v}_{sc}^{T} \cdot \boldsymbol{\gamma}$ where, for $sc \in SC$, $\mathbf{v}_{sc}$ is a $q \times 1$ column vector of q predictor values v_{scj} (including unit predictor values if an intercept is to be included) with indexes $j \in Q = \{j : 1 \le j \le q\}$ and $\boldsymbol{\gamma}$ is the associated $q \times 1$ column vector of coefficients. The $(r + q) \times 1$ parameter vector $\boldsymbol{\theta} = (\boldsymbol{\beta}^{T}, \boldsymbol{\gamma}^{T})^{T}$ is estimated through maximum extended quasi-pseudolikelihood estimation. Alternative models can be compared with extended PLCV ($PLCV^{+}$) scores computed as in Sect. 10.3.1 but using extended quasi-pseudolikelihoods rather than pseudolikelihoods and maximum extended quasi-pseudolikelihood estimates of $\boldsymbol{\theta}$ rather than maximum pseudolikelihood estimates. The adaptive modeling process can be extended to search through models for the means and dispersions in combination (see Chap. 20).

As in Sect. 10.3.1, for $sc \in SC$, the estimated value for the mean $\mu^{\#}_{sc}$ is

$$\mu^{\#}_{sc}(SC) = \frac{\exp(\mathbf{x}_{sc}^{T} \cdot \boldsymbol{\beta}(SC))}{1 + \exp(\mathbf{x}_{sc}^{T} \cdot \boldsymbol{\beta}(SC))}$$

and the corresponding residual is $e^{\#}_{sc}(SC) = y^{\#}_{sc} - \mu^{\#}_{sc}(SC)$. The estimated value of the associated dispersion $\phi^{\#}_{sc}$ is $\phi^{\#}_{sc}(SC) = \exp(\mathbf{v}_{sc}^{T} \cdot \boldsymbol{\gamma}(SC))$ and of the extended variance $\sigma^{\#}_{sc}{}^{2}$ is $\sigma^{\#}_{sc}{}^{2}(SC) = \phi^{\#}_{sc}(SC) \cdot V(\mu^{\#}_{sc}(SC))$. The standardized or Pearson residual $stde^{\#}_{sc}(SC) = e^{\#}_{sc}(SC)/\sigma^{\#}_{sc}(SC)$ is obtained by standardizing the residual by dividing by the estimated extended standard deviation.

10.4 Transition Modeling of Post-Baseline Dichotomous Respiratory Status

The cutoff for a substantial percent decrease (PD) in the LCV scores (see Sect. 4.4.2 for the formula) for the 444 post-baseline dichotomous respiratory status measurements is 0.43 %. Reported LCV scores are based on matched-set-wise deletion (Sect. 4.4.1) since there are no missing outcome measurements. See Sect. 4.8 for similar analyses of multivariate continuous outcomes.

10.4.1 Unit Dispersions Models

The adaptive model for post-baseline dichotomous outcome $y = status0\_1$ as a function of PRE(y,1,3) (that is, the average of the up to three prior outcome values) and PRE(y,1,3,∅) (that is, the indicator for there being no prior outcome values with which to compute PRE(y,1,3), in which case PRE(y,1,3) is set to 0) is used as a benchmark analysis for setting the number k of folds (see Sect. 2.8). Geometric combinations (GCs; see Sect. 4.5.4) in these two predictors are not considered because their product PRE(y,1,3) · PRE(y,1,3,∅) = 0. The adaptively generated model for k = 5 is based on the two transforms: PRE(y,1,3)$^{1.1}$ and PRE(y,1,3,∅) with LCV score 0.57507, the same as its pseudolikelihood CV (PLCV) score since it is a transition model. The adaptively generated models for k = 10 and k = 15 are the same and are based on the two untransformed predictors: PRE(y,1,3) and PRE(y,1,3,∅), with LCV scores 0.57359 and 0.57222. Since these scores are smaller than the score for k = 5, k = 5 is used in subsequent analyses of this outcome. In any case, the generated models do not differ much. This is also supported by the 5-fold LCV score 0.57505 for the model linear in PRE(y,1,3) and PRE(y,1,3,∅) with insubstantial PD 0.003 % compared to the adaptive model (that is, smaller than the cutoff 0.43 % for the data). Thus, the logits for post-baseline status0_1 are reasonably close to linear in PRE(y,1,3) and PRE(y,1,3,∅).

The adaptive modeling process, using k = 5, expands the constant base model with LCV score 0.50235 to the model based on the two transforms: PRE(y,1,3)^2 and PRE(y,1,3,∅) in that order, with LCV score 0.57164, and the contraction leaves the model unchanged. However, since the transform PRE(y,1,3)^2 is added to the expanded model first and is not the only transform in the expanded model, it is possible that the LCV score can be improved by adjusting the power of this transform. For this reason, the adaptive modeling process also includes, in cases like this, a conditional model transformation step that considers adjustments to the powers of uncontracted, expanded models. There is no need for such adjustments when terms are removed from the expanded model by the contraction, since remaining terms have their powers adjusted as part of the contraction. In this case, the power for PRE(y,1,3) is adjusted from 2 to 1.1 with improved LCV score 0.57507 as reported earlier. The PD in the LCV scores for the expanded model compared to its adjusted version is substantial at 0.60 %, and so these results justify the inclusion of the conditional model transformation step in the adaptive modeling process.

Basing the transition model on PRE(y,1,3) has the advantage of utilizing all prior outcome values, but transition models based on fewer prior outcome values using PRE(y,1,2) or PRE(y,1) (the same as PRE(y,1,1)) may be more effective. The adaptive model based on PRE(y,1,2) and PRE(y,1,2,∅) includes the two transforms: PRE(y,1,2)$^{0.9}$ and PRE(y,1,2,∅) with smaller LCV score 0.57274 and insubstantial PD 0.41 %. The adaptive model based on PRE(y,1) and PRE(y,1,∅) includes the two untransformed predictors: PRE(y,1) and PRE(y,1,∅) with even smaller LCV score 0.56642 and substantial PD 1.50 %. While the PD for the model based on the prior two outcome values is insubstantial, that model has the same number of terms as the model based on all prior outcome values, and so is not more parsimonious. Consequently, subsequent models are based on PRE(y,1,3) and PRE(y,1,3,∅).

Models for the means have depended so far on only dependence predictors and have been constant in the other available predictors visit, status0_1_0, and active. The effects of the dependence predictors can be kept separate from the effects of the other predictors by starting the adaptive modeling process at the adaptive model generated for PRE(y,1,3) and PRE(y,1,3,∅), that is, with transforms PRE(y,1,3)$^{1.1}$ and PRE(y,1,3,∅), and expanding that base model in only the other predictors. The dependence predictor transforms do not change during the expansion, but can change in the contraction. The advantage of generating models this way is the separate identification of effects on means for the other predictors conditioned on values of the dependence predictors. For example, starting from the adaptive model in PRE(y,1,3) and PRE(y,1,3,∅), the expanded model based on visit includes the extra transform visit^{12} with LCV score 0.57430. The contraction removes this single transform of visit and leaves the dependence predictor transforms unchanged. Consequently, conditioned on the effects of the dependence predictors PRE(y,1,3) and PRE(y,1,3,∅), mean status0_1 is reasonably considered to be constant over the four post-baseline visits.

It is possible that there are effects on mean post-baseline status0_1 to status0_1_0 and active and that there may be an effect to visit once these other effects are addressed. This is addressed by starting from the adaptive model in the dependence predictors PRE(y,1,3) and PRE(y,1,3,∅) and adaptively generating an additive model (that is, without GCs) in visit, status0_1_0, and active. The resulting model is based on the four transforms: PRE(y,1,3)$^{1.1}$, PRE(y,1,3,∅), status0_1_0, and active with improved LCV score 0.59907. Transforms of dependence predictors are unchanged while effects to baseline status0_1 and active treatment are added to the model. The PD for the model based on only dependence predictors is substantial at 4.01 %, and so the effects to status0_1_0 and active are distinct. These results indicate that the dependence predictors still account for all changes in post-baseline status0_1 over clinic visits (since there are no visit transforms in the model) but they do not account for the effects of baseline status0_1 and active. The associated adaptive model adding in additive effects to only visit and status0_1_0, but not active, has lower LCV score 0.59151 with substantial PD of 1.26 %, indicating that the effect of active on status0_1 is substantial. The estimated slope for active in the prior model is positive indicating as expected that post-baseline respiratory status0_1 improves under active treatment compared to placebo treatment. The estimated OR is 2.61 and is constant over time. However, adjustments may be needed if the effect to active treatment interacts with status0_1_0 and/or visit.

When this interaction issue is addressed by repeating the analysis with GCs between visit, status0_1_0, and active also considered in the expansion, the adaptively generated model is based on four transforms: PRE(y,1,3)$^{1.1}$, PRE(y,1,3,∅), (status0_1_0 · visit$^{-0.7}$)$^{0.7}$, and (status0_1_0 · active · visit^{-9})^{2} with improved LCV score 0.60406. The PD in the LCV scores for the model without GCs and with LCV score 0.59907 (as reported above) is substantial at 0.83 %, indicating that, after controlling for possible interactions with visit and status 0_1_0, the active treatment effect does change with visit. The associated adaptive model adding in effects to only visit, status0_1_0, and GCs has lower LCV score 0.59587 with substantial PD of 1.36 %, indicating that these effects of active on post-baseline status0_1 are substantial.

So far, models have kept the effects of dependence predictors PRE(y,1,3) and PRE(y,1,3,∅) separate from the effects of visit, status0_1_0, and active. Consideration of GCs in all of these five predictors might produce distinct improvements. The adaptive model in these five predictors and possible GCs in them is based on $(\text{PRE}(y,1,3)^2 \cdot \text{visit}^{0.5})^{0.7}$, $(\text{status0\_1\_0} \cdot \text{visit}^{-1.4})^{0.8}$, and active $\cdot$ visit^{-1} with LCV score 0.60500. The PD for the model with separate effects to dependence and non-dependence predictors is insubstantial at 0.16 %, indicating that there is not a distinct advantage to modeling dependence and non-dependence predictors jointly rather than separately.

10.4.2   Non-Unit Dispersions Models

Constant dispersions models can be generated by including an intercept term in the model for the log of the dispersions. The adaptive constant dispersions model for the effect of the dependence predictors PRE(y,1,3) and PRE(y,1,3,∅) on mean status0_1 at post-baseline visits 1–4 is based on the two transforms: PRE(y,1,3)$^{1.1}$ and PRE(y,1,3,∅) with extended quasi-likelihood CV (QLCV$^+$) score 0.57631. The corresponding unit dispersions model (see Sect. 10.4.1) has QLCV$^+$ score (the same as its LCV score) 0.57507 with insubstantial PD of 0.22 %. Consequently, in this case, the adaptive unit dispersions model is a parsimonious, competitive alternative to the adaptive constant dispersions model.

Adaptive non-constant dispersions models can be generated by considering models with both means and dispersions depending on transforms of primary predictors. For example, the means and dispersions of post-baseline status0_1 can both be adaptively modeled in terms of PRE(y,1,3) and PRE(y,1,3,∅), starting from a constant model for both the means and dispersions, and allowing the constant dispersions term to be removed in the contraction (thereby allowing for unit dispersions models) but not the constant mean term (as for all other models considered in this chapter). The adaptively generated model for the dispersions is based on only the predictor PRE(y,1,3,∅) without an intercept while the model for the means is based on the two transform: PRE(y,1,3)$^{1.1}$ and PRE(y,1,3,∅) as generated earlier. The QLCV$^+$ score is 0.57887. The associated constant dispersions model has QLCV$^+$ score 0.57631 with substantial PD of 0.44 %. Consequently, accounting for an effect to PRE(y,1,3,∅) provides a distinct improvement over the constant dispersions model (and over the unit dispersions model as well with even smaller QLCV$^+$ score).

The adaptive model for means in terms of PRE(y,1,3), PRE(y,1,3,∅), status0_1_0, visit, active, and GCs and for dispersions in terms of PRE(y,1,3), and PRE$(y,1,3,\varnothing)$, starting from constant means and constant dispersions and allowing for unit dispersions is a unit dispersions model, indicating that unit dispersions are reasonable for predicting mean status0_1 as long as enough predictors are considered. The adaptive model for both means and dispersions in terms of PRE$(y,1,3)$, PRE$(y,1,3,\varnothing)$, status0_1_0, visit, active, and GCs, starting from constant means and constant dispersions and allowing for unit dispersions has means depending on the four transforms: $\left(PRE(y,1,3)^2 \cdot visit^{0.5}\right)^{0.39}$, $\left(status0\_1\_0 \cdot visit^{-1.4}\right)^{0.51}$, $\left(visit^{-1.7} \cdot active \cdot status0\_1\_0\right)^{4.0011}$ and PRE$(y,1,3,\varnothing)$ with an intercept and dispersions depending on active·status0_1_0·PRE$(y,1,3,\varnothing)$, $visit^{0.511}$, and PRE$(y,1,3)^{-2}$, also with an intercept. The QLCV$^+$ score is 0.76753, which is a substantial improvement over the best unit dispersions model with LCV/QLCV$^+$ score 0.60500 and PD 21.18 %. Consequently, the extra predictors: status0_1_0, visit, and active have a distinct effect on the dispersions. The adaptive model with means and dispersions depending on PRE$(y,1,3)$, PRE$(y,1,3,\varnothing)$, status0_1_0, visit, and GCs, but not active, has substantially smaller QLCV$^+$ score 0.65710 with PD 14.39 %, and so active has a distinct effect on both the means and dispersions.

Table 10.1 contains estimated probabilities of a good dichotomous respiratory status based on the best transition model reported above. At any given visit, the probability of good status increases with an increasing average of the prior three dichotomous respiratory status values. There is no effect to being on the active treatment for patients with poor baseline dichotomous respiratory status. Patients on the placebo with good baseline dichotomous respiratory status have an increased chance of having good post-baseline dichotomous respiratory status compared to patients on the placebo or active treatment with poor baseline dichotomous respiratory status. Patients on the active treatment with good baseline dichotomous respiratory status have an increased chance of having good post-baseline dichotomous respiratory status compared to patients with poor baseline dichotomous respiratory status on either the placebo or active treatment at all visits and compared to patients with good respiratory status but only at the first two visits.

Table 10.2 contains estimated dispersions for a good dichotomous respiratory status based on the best transition model reported above for patients either on the placebo treatment or with poor baseline respiratory status. The dispersion at visit 1 is larger than at the other visits except for the largest dispersion value at visit 4. At later visits, the dispersion increases at first with larger averages of prior respiratory status values and then for visits 3 and 4 it decreases. For patients on active treatment and with good baseline respiratory status, the estimated dispersions are the same as reported in Table 10.2 except at visit $= 1$ since then there is not a prior respiratory value to average and PRE$(y,1,3,\varnothing) = 1$. In this case, the estimated dispersion is essentially zero.

Table 10.1 Probability estimates of good dichotomous respiratory status based on the non-unit dispersions transition model

Visit	PRE(y,1,3)	Treatment			
		Placebo		Active	
		Poor baseline status	Good baseline status	Poor baseline status	Good baseline status
1	0	0.37	0.71	0.37	1.00
2	0	0.14	0.29	0.14	0.31
2	1	0.71	0.86	0.71	0.87
3	0	0.14	0.25	0.14	0.25
3	1/2	0.48	0.64	0.48	0.64
3	1	0.76	0.86	0.76	0.86
4	0	0.14	0.23	0.14	0.23
4	1/3	0.39	0.52	0.39	0.52
4	2/3	0.62	0.73	0.62	0.73
4	1	0.79	0.86	0.79	0.86

PRE(y,1,3): average of prior three dichotomous respiratory status values

Table 10.2 Dispersion estimates of good dichotomous respiratory status based on the non-unit dispersions transition model for patients on the placebo treatment or with poor baseline respiratory status

Visit	PRE(y,1,3)	Dispersion
1	0	1.30
2	0	1.01
2	1	1.10
3	0	0.83
3	1/2	1.17
3	1	0.91
4	0	0.70
4	1/3	1.53
4	2/3	0.86
4	1	0.77

PRE(y,1,3): average of prior three dichotomous respiratory status values

10.5 Conditional Modeling of Multivariate Polytomous Outcomes

The formulation of multinomial and ordinal regression of means for univariate polytomous outcomes (see Sect. 8.7) extends to conditional modeling of means for multivariate polytomous outcomes. The extension is straightforward and similar to the extension of standard logistic regression modeling of means for univariate dichotomous outcomes (see Sect. 8.3) to conditional modeling of means for multivariate dichotomous outcomes (see Sect. 10.3.1). The extension of modeling of dispersions along with means for multivariate polytomous outcomes is also straightforward and similar to the extension for multivariate dichotomous outcomes (see Sect. 10.3.2). For this reason, a detailed formulation for multivariate polytomous outcomes is not provided here. The crucial issue is the computation of dependence predictors underlying conditional modeling of polytomous outcomes y with values $v = 0, 1, \cdots, K$. When outcomes y are ordinal, averages PRE(y,i,j), POST(y,i,j), and OTHER(y,i,j) of prior, subsequent, and other outcome measurements and associated missing indicators PRE(y,i,j,$\emptyset$), POST(y,i,j,$\emptyset$), and OTHER(y,i,j,$\emptyset$) are reasonable to use as dependence predictors in either ordinal or multinomial regression models of associated conditional outcomes. However, these dependence predictors seem inappropriate to use to model multivariate nominal outcomes y. The appropriate dependence predictors in that case are the averages PRE(y=v,i,j), POST(y=v,i,j), and OTHER(y=v,i,j) of the indicator variables for prior, subsequent, or other outcome measurements having value v (or, equivalently, proportions of such outcome measurements having value v) and associated missing indicators PRE(y=v,i,j,$\emptyset$), POST(y=v,i,j,$\emptyset$), and OTHER(y=v,i,j,$\emptyset$) for $1 \leq v \leq K$, assuming $v = 0$ is the reference value. These can also be used as dependence predictors for ordinal outcomes.

10.6   Transition Modeling of Post-Baseline Polytomous Respiratory Status

Analyses are reported in this section of the post-baseline three-level polytomous outcome $y = $ status0_2. The cutoff for a substantial percent decrease (PD) in the LCV scores (see Sect. 4.4.2 for the formula) for the $444 \cdot 2 = 888$ effective number (computed similarly to the univariate case of Sect. 8.7.1) of post-baseline polytomous respiratory status measurements is 0.22 %. Reported LCV scores are based on matched-set-wise deletion since there are no missing outcome measurements.

10.6.1   Unit Dispersions Models

Since status0_2 is an ordinal outcome, ordinal regression transition models are considered first. The adaptive model for status0_2 as a function of PRE(y,1,3) and PRE(y,1,3,$\emptyset$) (without GCs since the product of these two variables equals zero for all observations) in these two predictors is used as a benchmark analysis for setting the number k of folds. The adaptively chosen model for $k = 5$ is based on the two transforms: PRE(y,1,3)$^{0.9}$ and PRE(y,1,3,$\emptyset$) with LCV score 0.65933 (the same as its PLCV score). The adaptively generated models for $k = 10$ and $k = 15$ are the same as for $k = 5$ with LCV scores 0.65962 and 0.65874. Thus, $k = 10$ generates the first local maximum in LCV scores and so is used in subsequent analyses of this outcome. The model linear in PRE(y,1,3) and PRE(y,1,3,$\emptyset$) has 10-fold LCV score

0.65940 with insubstantial PD 0.03 % compared to the adaptive model, and so the cumulative logits for post-baseline status0_2 are reasonably close to linear in $PRE(y,1,3)$ and $PRE(y,1,3,\varnothing)$.

Although status0_2 is an ordinal outcome, multinomial regression transition models for status0_2 might provide improvements over ordinal regression transition models. However, the adaptively generated multinomial regression transition model for status0_2 based on the dependence predictors $PRE(y,1,3)$ and $PRE(y,1,3,\varnothing)$ has the smaller LCV score 0.65870. Furthermore, the adaptively generated multinomial regression transition model for status0_2 based on the dependence predictors $PRE(y=1,1,3)$ (that is, the proportions of the up to three prior outcome measurements with value 1), $PRE(y=2,1,3)$ (that is, the proportions of the up to three prior outcome measurements with value 2), and $PRE(y=1,1,3,\varnothing)$ $(PRE(y=2,1,3,\varnothing) = PRE(y=1,1,3,\varnothing)$ since there are no missing outcomes and so is not needed) has a little larger LCV score 0.65898, but not larger than for the ordinal regression model. Thus, ordinal regression transition models for status0_2 are somewhat more effective than multinomial regression transition models and also simpler. For this reason, only ordinal regression transition models are used in subsequent analyses.

It is possible to base transition models on fewer prior outcome values using $PRE(y,1,2)$ or $PRE(y,1,1)$. The adaptive model based on $PRE(y,1,2)$ and $PRE(y,1,2,\varnothing)$ includes the two transforms: $PRE(y,1,2)^{0.9}$ and $PRE(y,1,2,\varnothing)$, with improved LCV score 0.66284. The adaptive model based on $PRE(y,1)$ and $PRE(y,1,\varnothing)$ includes the two untransformed predictors: $PRE(y,1)^{0.91}$ and $PRE(y,1,\varnothing)$, with smaller LCV score 0.65968. Consequently, using dependence predictors based on the prior two outcome measurements produces the best of these three alternative models for post-baseline status0_2, and so subsequent analyses use these dependence predictors. It is also possible to base conditional ordinal regression models on dependence predictors $PRE(y=v,1,j)$ for $v = 1,2$ and $j = 1,2,3$ and associated missing indicators, but that issue is not addressed here.

Starting from the adaptive model in the dependence predictors $PRE(y,1,2)$ and $PRE(y,1,2,\varnothing)$ and adaptively generating an additive model in visit, status0_2_0, and active, the resulting model is based on the four transforms: $PRE(y,1,2)^{0.9}$, $PRE(y,1,2,\varnothing)$, status0_2_0$^{1.2}$, and active with improved LCV score 0.67191. The PD for the prior best model is substantial at 1.35 %, and so the extra effects to status0_2_0 and active in this latter model are distinct. The associated model with active no longer considered has LCV score 0.66902 and substantial PD of 0.43 %, indicating that there is a distinct effect to being on active compared to placebo treatment. Increasing order for the status0_2 values is used to generate the model with the active effect, so the generated proportional OR is based on the odds for lower values compared to higher values, that is, the odds for worse respiratory status compared to better respiratory status. The estimated proportional OR is 0.54. In other words, as expected the odds for worse respiratory status compared to better respiratory status are smaller when on active compared to placebo treatment. However, these results may need adjustment if the effect to active treatment interacts with status0_2_0 and/or visit.

When this interaction issue is addressed by repeating the analysis with GCs between visit, status 0_2_0, and active also considered in the expansion, the adaptive model is based on four transforms: $PRE(y, 1, 2)^{0.83}$, $PRE(y,1,2,\varnothing)$, (active $\cdot$ status0_2_0$^{1.9}$ $\cdot$ visit$^{-0.6}$)$^{0.7}$, and (status0_2_0$^{0.8}$ $\cdot$ visit^{-7})$^{1.6}$ with improved LCV score 0.67609. The PD in LCV scores for the model without GCs is substantial at 0.62 %, indicating that GCs provide a distinct improvement. Moreover, the associated adaptive model without active has LCV score 0.67168 with substantial PD of 0.65 %, indicating that, the effect to active is substantial. This effect changes with status0_2_0 and visit and is limited to patients with good or excellent baseline respiratory status0_2 since (active $\cdot$ status0_2_0$^{1.9}$ $\cdot$ visit$^{-0.6}$)$^{0.7}$ = 0 when status0_2 = 0 whatever the values for active and visit are. For patients with good baseline respiratory status (status0_2_0 = 1), the estimated proportional OR for worse compared to better respiratory status at visit = 1 is 0.49 and increases to 0.62 at visit = 2, 0.69 at visit = 3, and 0.73 at visit = 4. For patients with excellent baseline respiratory status (status0_2_0 = 2), the estimated proportional OR for worse compared to better respiratory status at visit = 1 is 0.07 and increases to 0.17 at visit = 2, 0.25 at visit = 3, and 0.31 at visit = 4. Thus, the effect of active treatment is weaker for later clinic visits.

10.6.2   Non-Unit Dispersions Models

The adaptive model for the means in the dependence predictors $PRE(y,1,2)$ and $PRE(y,1,2,\varnothing)$ with constant dispersions is based on the two transforms: $PRE(y,1,2)^{0.9}$ and $PRE(y,1,2,\varnothing)$ with QLCV$^+$ score 0.68749. The associated unit dispersions model of Sect. 10.6.1 with QLCV$^+$ score 0.66284 (the same as its LCV score) generates a substantial PD of 3.59 %. Consequently, the dispersions for status0_2 are distinctly non-unit. The adaptive model for both means and dispersions in terms of the dependence predictors $PRE(y,1,2)$ and $PRE(y,1,2,\varnothing)$, starting from a constant model for both the means and dispersions but allowing all dispersions terms to be removed in the contraction so that unit dispersions models are considered, has means based on the two transforms: $PRE(y, 1, 2)^{0.9}$ and $PRE(y,1,2,\varnothing)$ with an intercept and the dispersions based on the two transform: $PRE(y,1,2)^{-0.5}$ and $PRE(y,1,2,\varnothing)$ without an intercept, having improved QLCV$^+$ score 0.68906 (the same as its PLCV$^+$ score). The associated adaptive constant dispersions model generates a substantial PD 0.23 %. Consequently, there is a distinct non-constant effect to $PRE(y,1,2)$ on the dispersions. Starting from this revised dependence predictor model for the means and dispersions, the adaptive model with both means and dispersions also depending on visit, status0_1_0, active, and GCs in these three predictors is the model based on four transforms for the means: $PRE(y,1,2,\varnothing)$, $PRE(y,1,2)^{0.9}$, (active $\cdot$ status0_2_0$^{1.9}$ $\cdot$ visit$^{-0.6}$)$^{0.6}$, and visit^{-10} $\cdot$ status0_2_0$^{1.2}$ (with an intercept as always) and the single transform

for the dispersions: $visit^{-0.3}$ without an intercept and improved $QLCV^+$ score
0.69635. The base model with $QLCV^+$ score 0.68906 has substantial PD of 1.05 %,
and so also accounting for non-dependence predictors provides a distinct improvement over only dependence predictors. The associated adaptive model not considering active as a predictor for the means or the dispersions has $QLCV^+$ score
0.69349 and substantial PD of 0.41 %, indicating that the effect of active on the
means is substantial.

Under the model including the effect of active, that effect changes with
status0_2_0 and visit and is limited to patients with good or excellent baseline
respiratory status0_2. For patients with good baseline respiratory status
(status0_2_0 = 1), the estimated proportional OR for worse compared to better
respiratory status at visit = 1 is 0.47 and increases to 0.56 at visit = 2, 0.60 at
visit = 3, and 0.63 at visit = 4. For patients with excellent baseline respiratory
status (status0_2_0 = 2), the estimated proportional OR for worse compared to
better respiratory status at visit = 1 is 0.19 and increases to 0.28 at visit = 2, 0.33 at
visit = 3, and 0.37 at visit = 4. Dispersions decrease from 0.54 at visit 1 to 0.44 at
visit 2, 0.39 at visit 3, and 0.36 at visit 4.

10.7 Adaptive GEE-Based Modeling of Multivariate Dichotomous and Polytomous Outcomes

This section generalizes adaptive modeling of multivariate dichotomous
and polytomous outcomes to allow for GEE parameter estimation. Extended LCV
(LCV^+) scores computed with multivariate normal likelihoods extended to address
dichotomous and polytomous outcomes are used to evaluate and compare models
as part of the adaptive modeling process. Section 10.7.1 provides the formulation
for multivariate dichotomous outcomes and Sect. 10.7.2 for multivariate
polytomous outcomes. LCV^+ scores for GEE-based models are computed with
multivariate normal likelihoods while LCV and $QLCV^+$ scores for transition and
general conditional models are computed with Bernoulli likelihoods for the dichotomous case and categorical likelihoods for the polytomous case, and so these are
not comparable. However, it is possible to compute LCV^+ scores for marginal
models induced by transition models, which can be compared to LCV^+ scores for
GEE-based models. The formulation is provided in Sect. 10.7.3.

10.7.1 Dichotomous Outcomes

Using the notation of Sect. 4.3, for n matched sets of measurements with indexes
$s \in S = \{s : 1 \leq s \leq n\}$, observed data $O_{s,C(s)} = (\mathbf{y}_{s,C(s)}, \mathbf{X}_{s,C(s)})$ are available for
possibly different sets $C(s)$ of measurement conditions, subsets of the maximal set

of possible conditions $C = \{c : 1 \leq c \leq m\}$, consisting of outcome vectors $\mathbf{y}_{s,C(s)}$ with $m(s)$ entries y_{sc} having values 0 and 1 for $c \in C(s)$ and predictor matrices $\mathbf{X}_{s,C(s)}$ having $m(s)$ rows $\mathbf{x}_{sc}^T$ with entries x_{scj} for $j \in J = \{j : 1 \leq j \leq r\}$ and for $c \in C(s)$. The mean or expected value μ_{sc} for y_{sc} satisfies $\mu_{sc} = Ey_{sc} = P(y_{sc} = 1|\mathbf{x}_{sc})$ for $c \in C(s)$ and $s \in S$. With the logit (or log odds) function defined as $\text{logit}(u) = \log(u/(1-u))$ for $0 < u < 1$, model the logit of the mean as $\text{logit}(\mu_{sc}) = \mathbf{x}_{sc}^T \cdot \boldsymbol{\beta}$ for a $r \times 1$ vector $\boldsymbol{\beta}$ of coefficients. Solving for μ_{sc} gives $\mu_{sc} = \exp(\mathbf{x}_{sc}^T \cdot \boldsymbol{\beta})/(1 + \exp(\mathbf{x}_{sc}^T \cdot \boldsymbol{\beta}))$ for $c \in C(s)$, which are combined into the $C(s) \times 1$ vector $\boldsymbol{\mu}_{s,C(s)}$. The odds ratio (OR) for $y_s = 1$ under a unit change in a predictor value x_{scj} and adjusted for the other predictor values $x_{scj'}$ for $j' \neq j$ (if any) is computed as $\text{OR} = \exp(\beta_j)$. The variance for y_{sc} is $V(\mu_{sc}) = \mu_{sc} \cdot (1 - \mu_{sc})$. Assume for now that the dispersions $\phi_{sc} = \phi$ are constant for $c \in C(s)$ and $s \in S$. The errors are $e_{sc} = y_{sc} - \mu_{sc}$ and the standardized errors are $\text{stde}_{sc} = e_{sc}/(\phi \cdot V(\mu_{sc}))^{1/2}$.

For each $s \in S$, define the extended (multivariate normal) likelihood term $L^+(O_{s,C(s)}; \boldsymbol{\theta})$ to satisfy

$$\ell^+(O_{s,C(s)}; \boldsymbol{\theta}) = \log\left(L^+(O_{s,C(s)}; \boldsymbol{\theta})\right)$$
$$= -\frac{1}{2} \cdot \mathbf{e}_{s,C(s)}^T \cdot \boldsymbol{\Sigma}_{s,C(s)}^{-1} \cdot \mathbf{e}_{s,C(s)} - \frac{1}{2} \cdot \log(|\boldsymbol{\Sigma}_{s,C(s)}|) - \frac{1}{2} \cdot m(s) \cdot \log(2 \cdot \pi),$$

where $\mathbf{e}_{s,C(s)} = \mathbf{y}_{s,C(s)} - \boldsymbol{\mu}_{s,C(s)}$ is the $C(s) \times 1$ vector of errors e_{sc} for $c \in C(s)$, $|\boldsymbol{\Sigma}_{s,C(s)}|$ the determinant of the covariance matrix $\boldsymbol{\Sigma}_{s,C(s)} = \phi \cdot \mathbf{A}_{s,C(s)} \cdot \mathbf{R}_{s,C(s)}(\boldsymbol{\rho}) \cdot \mathbf{A}_{s,C(s)}$, $\mathbf{A}_{s,C(s)}$ the diagonal matrix with diagonal entries $V(\mu_{sc})^{1/2}$ for $c \in C(s)$, $\mathbf{R}_{s,C(s)}(\boldsymbol{\rho})$ a $m(s) \times m(s)$ correlation matrix (called the working correlation matrix) determined by a vector $\boldsymbol{\rho}$ of parameters, and π the usual constant. The extended likelihood $L^+(SC; \boldsymbol{\theta})$ is the product of the extended likelihood terms $L^+(O_{s,C(s)}; \boldsymbol{\theta})$ over $s \in S$ where $\boldsymbol{\theta} = (\boldsymbol{\beta}^T, \phi, \boldsymbol{\rho}^T)^T$ is the vector of all model parameters. Differentiating $\ell^+(SC; \boldsymbol{\theta}) = \log(L^+(SC; \boldsymbol{\theta}))$ with respect to $\boldsymbol{\beta}$ gives

$$\partial \ell^+(SC; \boldsymbol{\theta})/\partial \boldsymbol{\beta} = \partial_1 \ell^+(SC; \boldsymbol{\theta})/\partial_1 \boldsymbol{\beta} + \partial_2 \ell^+(SC; \boldsymbol{\theta})/\partial_2 \boldsymbol{\beta},$$

where $\partial_1 \ell^+(SC; \boldsymbol{\theta})/\partial_1 \boldsymbol{\beta}$ is obtained by differentiating the error vectors $\mathbf{e}_{s,C(s)}$ in $\ell^+(SC; \boldsymbol{\theta})$ with respect to $\boldsymbol{\beta}$ holding the other terms of $\ell^+(SC; \boldsymbol{\theta})$ constant in $\boldsymbol{\beta}$ and $\partial_2 \ell^+(SC; \boldsymbol{\theta})/\partial_2 \boldsymbol{\beta}$ is obtained by differentiating the other terms of $\ell^+(SC; \boldsymbol{\theta})$ with respect to $\boldsymbol{\beta}$ holding the error vectors $\mathbf{e}_{s,C(s)}$ in $\ell^+(SC; \boldsymbol{\theta})$ constant in $\boldsymbol{\beta}$. The first of these derivative terms satisfies

$$\partial_1 \ell^+(SC; \boldsymbol{\theta})/\partial_1 \boldsymbol{\beta} = \sum_{s \in S} \mathbf{D}_{s,C(s)}^T \cdot \boldsymbol{\Sigma}_{s,C(s)}^{-1} \cdot \mathbf{e}_{s,C(s)}$$

with $\mathbf{D}_{s,C(s)} = \partial \boldsymbol{\mu}_{s,C(s)}/\partial \boldsymbol{\beta}$. GEE estimates $\boldsymbol{\beta}_{\text{GEE}}(SC)$ of $\boldsymbol{\beta}$ are obtained by solving the generalized estimating equations $\partial_1 \ell^+(SC; \boldsymbol{\theta})/\partial_1 \boldsymbol{\beta} = \mathbf{0}$, that is, generalized from the estimating equations for the independence case to incorporate covariance (without considering the extended likelihood). Chaganty (1997) appears to be the first to have recognized this justification of GEE estimates in terms of multivariate normality (specifically, he uses $e_{s,C(s)}^T \cdot \Sigma_{s,C(s)}^{-1} \cdot e_{s,C(s)}$ to define what he calls quasi-least squares estimates). For simplicity of notation, parameter estimates are denoted as functions of the index set SC for the observed data used in their computation without hat (^) symbols.

In GEE modeling, the dispersion parameter ϕ and the working correlation matrices $\mathbf{R}_{s,C(s)}(\boldsymbol{\rho})$ are estimated using the standardized errors $stde_{sc}$ with estimates determined by the structure for the matrices $\mathbf{R}_{s,C(s)}(\boldsymbol{\rho})$. For example, under exchangeable correlations (EC), all the off-diagonal entries of $\mathbf{R}_{s,C(s)}(\boldsymbol{\rho})$ are the same with common value ρ (and so $\boldsymbol{\rho} = (\rho)$). Given a value $\boldsymbol{\beta}$ for the expectation parameter vector, ρ is estimated as

$$\rho_{GEE}(\boldsymbol{\beta}) = \frac{1}{m(CC) - r} \sum_{c'c \in CC} stde_{sc'}(\boldsymbol{\beta}) \cdot stde_{sc}(\boldsymbol{\beta}),$$

where $CC = \{c'c : c' < c, \ c',c \in C(S), \ s \in S\}$ and $m(CC)$ is the number of pairs $c'c$ of indexes in CC and the standardized errors $stde_{sc'}(\boldsymbol{\beta})$ and $stde_{sc}(\boldsymbol{\beta})$ are computed using the estimate $\phi_{GEE}(\boldsymbol{\beta})$ of ϕ given by

$$\phi_{GEE}(\boldsymbol{\beta}) = \sum_{sc \in SC} e_{sc}(\boldsymbol{\beta})^2 / (V(\mu_{sc}) \cdot (m(SC) - r)).$$

These are bias-corrected estimates since the denominators are adjusted for bias by subtracting the number r of expectation parameters. Unadjusted estimates are also possible by not subtracting r in the denominators. The unadjusted estimate of the dispersion ϕ is also the maximum extended likelihood estimate of ϕ given the value of $\boldsymbol{\beta}$ for the expectation parameter vector and assuming independence. Similar estimates of the correlation matrices can be obtained under other structures like autoregressive (AR) and unstructured (UN) correlations (for details see SAS Institute 2004). The estimating equations are solved to obtain the estimate $\boldsymbol{\beta}_{GEE}(SC)$ using a Gauss-Newton-like iterative algorithm. The Hessian matrix for the usual Gauss-Newton algorithm is replaced in this algorithm by

$$\partial_1^2 \ell^+(SC; \theta)/(\partial_1\boldsymbol{\beta}\partial_1\boldsymbol{\beta}^T) = \sum_{s \in S} \mathbf{D}_{s,C(s)}^T \cdot \Sigma_{s,C(s)}^{-1} \cdot \mathbf{D}_{s,C(s)},$$

where $\partial_1^2 \ell^+(SC; \boldsymbol{\theta})/(\partial_1\boldsymbol{\beta}\partial_1\boldsymbol{\beta}^T)$ denotes the derivative with respect to $\boldsymbol{\beta}$ of the error vectors $e_{s,C(s)}$ in $\partial_1\ell^+ SC; \boldsymbol{\theta})/\partial_1\boldsymbol{\beta}$ holding the other terms constant in $\boldsymbol{\beta}$. Using the notation of SAS Institute (2004, p. 1676), the model-based estimator, assuming the structure of the working correlation matrix is the true correlation structure, of the covariance matrix of the estimate $\boldsymbol{\beta}_{GEE}(SC)$ of $\boldsymbol{\beta}$ is $\Sigma_m(\boldsymbol{\beta}_{GEE}(SC)) = \mathbf{I}_0^{-1}$ where

$$\mathbf{I}_0 = \partial_1{}^2 \ell^+(SC; \boldsymbol{\theta}_{GEE}(SC))/(\partial_1 \boldsymbol{\beta} \partial_1 \boldsymbol{\beta}^T)$$

and

$$\boldsymbol{\theta}_{GEE}(SC) = \left(\boldsymbol{\beta}_{GEE}(SC)^T, \boldsymbol{\phi}_{GEE}(\boldsymbol{\beta}_{GEE}(SC)), \boldsymbol{\rho}_{GEE}(\boldsymbol{\beta}_{GEE}(SC))^T \right)^T$$

is the GEE estimate of the complete set of model parameters. The robust empirical estimator of that covariance matrix is $\boldsymbol{\Sigma}_e(\boldsymbol{\beta}_{GEE}(SC)) = \mathbf{I}_0{}^{-1} \cdot \mathbf{I}_1 \cdot \mathbf{I}_0{}^{-1}$ where

$$\mathbf{I}_1 = \sum_{s \in S} \partial_1 \ell^+\left(O_{s,C(s)}; \boldsymbol{\theta}_{GEE}(SC) \right)/\partial_1 \boldsymbol{\beta} \cdot \left(\partial_1 \ell^+\left(O_{s,C(s)}; \boldsymbol{\theta}_{GEE}(SC) \right)/\partial_1 \boldsymbol{\beta} \right)^T.$$

While GEE was initially formulated to avoid computing likelihoods or quasi-likelihoods, the above formulation indicates that it can be considered a kind of "semi-likelihood" estimation method, using a part $\partial_1 \ell^+(SC; \boldsymbol{\theta})/\partial_1 \boldsymbol{\beta}$ of the derivative $\partial \ell^+(SC; \boldsymbol{\theta})/\partial \boldsymbol{\beta}$ of the extended likelihood underlying the data, based on the multivariate normal distribution extended to handle dichotomous data. Alternate GEE-related estimates are also possible by maximizing the extended likelihood. For example, the usual GEE estimates of the correlation matrices $\mathbf{R}_{s,C(s)}(\boldsymbol{\rho})$ and of the dispersion ϕ can be combined with the maximum extended likelihood estimate $\boldsymbol{\beta}(SC)$ of $\boldsymbol{\beta}$ obtained by maximizing the log-likelihood $\ell(SC; \boldsymbol{\theta}) = \log(L(SC; \boldsymbol{\theta}))$ in $\boldsymbol{\beta}$. This is achieved by solving the estimating equations $\partial \ell^+(SC; \boldsymbol{\theta})/\partial \boldsymbol{\beta} = \mathbf{0}$, thereby incorporating $\partial_2 \ell^+(SC; \boldsymbol{\theta})/\partial_2 \boldsymbol{\beta}$ in the estimates along with $\partial_1 \ell^+(SC; \boldsymbol{\theta})/\partial_1 \boldsymbol{\beta}$. Another alternative is to use the full maximum extended likelihood estimate $\boldsymbol{\theta}(SC)$ of $\boldsymbol{\theta}$ obtained by maximizing the log-extended-likelihood

$$\ell^+(SC; \boldsymbol{\theta}) = \log(L^+(SC; \boldsymbol{\theta}))$$

over all possible parameter vectors $\boldsymbol{\theta}$, solving the estimating equations $\partial \ell^+(SC; \boldsymbol{\theta})/\partial \boldsymbol{\theta} = \mathbf{0}$. However, these alternative estimates are not addressed any further here.

An advantage of the formulation of the extended likelihood underlying GEE estimation is that the extended likelihood can be used to compute extended LCV (LCV^+) scores for evaluating and comparing GEE models, using either matched-set-wise deletion as in Sect. 4.4.1 or measurement-wise deletion as in Sect. 4.13. The adaptive modeling process then also extends to GEE modeling by basing it on such LCV^+ scores. It is also possible to compute extended penalized likelihood criteria (see Sect. 2.10.1) adding the usual penalty factors to extended likelihoods giving the extended AIC (AIC^+), extended BIC (BIC^+), and extended TIC (TIC^+), which are assumed to be adjusted to larger is better form for use in adaptive model selection (see Sect. 2.10.1). These are alternatives to the quasi-likelihood information criterion (QIC) of Pan (2001), which extends to the dichotomous and polytomous outcome context from the continuous outcome context of Sect. 4.11.1. AIC^+, BIC^+, and TIC^+ are not based in part on results for independent correlations as is QIC but are wholly based on the working correlation structure.

The above formulation extends to modeling of dispersions as well as means similarly to the extension of Sect. 4.15.1 for marginal models of continuous outcomes. The covariance matrices $\Sigma_{s,C(s)}$ are assumed to satisfy

$$\Sigma_{s,C(s)} = B_{s,C(s)} \cdot R_{s,C(s)}(\rho) \cdot B_{s,C(s)},$$

where $B_{s,C(s)}$ are the diagonal matrices with diagonal entries $\sigma_{sc} = (\phi_{sc} \cdot V(\mu_{sc}))^{1/2}$ representing extended standard deviations for the outcome measurements y_{sc} with associated dispersions ϕ_{sc} for $c \in C(s)$ and $s \in S$. The logs of the dispersions ϕ_{sc} are then modeled as functions of selected predictor variables and associated coefficients. Specifically, let $\log(\phi_{sc}) = v_{sc}^T \cdot \gamma$ where, for $s \in S$ and $c \in C(s)$, v_{sc} is a $q \times 1$ column vector of q predictor values v_{scj} (including unit predictor values if an intercept is to be included) with indexes $j \in Q = \{j : 1 \leq j \leq q\}$ and γ is the associated $q \times 1$ column vector of coefficients. The parameter vector $\theta = (\beta^T, \gamma^T, \rho^T)^T$ is estimated by jointly solving the GEE equations $\partial_1 \ell^+(SC; \theta)/\partial_1 \beta = 0$ for β and the maximum extended likelihood equations $\partial \ell(SC; \theta)/\partial \gamma = 0$ for γ using the GEE estimate $\rho_{GEE}(\beta_{GEE}(SC))$ of the correlation parameter vector. These latter estimates are computed from estimates of the standardized errors $\text{stde}_{sc} = e_{sc}/(\phi_{sc} \cdot V(\mu_{sc}))^{1/2}$. Define $V_{s,C(s)}$ to be the $m(s) \times q$ matrix with rows v_{sc}^T for, $c \in C(s)$ and $s \in S$, and let $O_{s,C(s)} = (y_{s,C(s)}, X_{s,C(s)}, V_{s,C(s)})$ denote the observed data for each $s \in S$. With this notation, the above formulation extends to combined adaptive GEE-based modeling of means and dispersions for multivariate dichotomous outcomes. As in Sect. 4.3.3, scaled residual vectors $\text{sclde}_s(SC)$ can be computed as $\text{sclde}_s(SC) = U_s^T(SC)^{-1} \cdot e_s(SC)$ where $U_s(SC)$ is the square root of the covariance matrix $\Sigma_s(SC)$ determined by its Cholesky decomposition, for either constant or non-constant dispersions models. The entries of $\text{sclde}_s(SC)$ can be combined over all s and analyzed in combination as for independent data.

10.7.2 Polytomous Outcomes

Using notation like that of Sect. 8.7.1 for univariate multinomial regression, the formulation of Sect. 10.7.1 for multivariate dichotomous logistic regression can be extended to multivariate multinomial regression as follows (see also Lipsitz et al. 1994; Miller et al. 1993). For $0 \leq v \leq K$, let y_{scv} be the indicator for $y_{sc} = v$. Conditioned on the observed predictor vector value x_{sc}, the mean or expected value μ_{scv} for y_{scv} is $\mu_{scv} = Ey_{scv} = P(y_{sc} = v|x_{sc})$ for $c \in C(s)$ and $s \in S$. Using generalized logits, model

$$\text{glogit}(\mu_{scv}) = \log\left(\frac{\mu_{scv}}{\mu_{sc0}}\right) = x_{sc}^T \cdot \beta_v$$

for $1 \leq v \leq K$ (and so with $v = 0$ as the reference value) and $K r \times 1$ vectors β_v of coefficients. Solving for μ_{scv} gives

$$\mu_{scv} = \frac{\exp(\mathbf{x}_{sc}^T \cdot \boldsymbol{\beta}_v)}{1 + \exp(\mathbf{x}_{sc}^T \cdot \boldsymbol{\beta}_1) + \cdots + \exp(\mathbf{x}_{sc}^T \cdot \boldsymbol{\beta}_K)}$$

for $1 \le v \le K$ and $\mu_{sc0} = 1/(1 + \exp(\mathbf{x}_{sc}^T \cdot \boldsymbol{\beta}_1) + \cdots + \exp(\mathbf{x}_{sc}^T \cdot \boldsymbol{\beta}_K))$ for $v = 0$. The variance for y_{scv} is $V(\mu_{scv}) = \mu_{scv} \cdot (1 - \mu_{scv})$.

Let $\mathbf{y}_{sc}$ be the $K \times 1$ vector with entries y_{scv} for $1 \le v \le K$ and $\mathbf{y}_{s,C(s)}$ the $(m(s) \cdot K) \times 1$ vector combining the vectors $\mathbf{y}_{sc}$ over $c \in C(s)$ and $s \in S$. Similarly define the mean vectors $\boldsymbol{\mu}_{sc}$ and $\boldsymbol{\mu}_{s,C(s)}$ from the means μ_{scv}, the error vectors $\mathbf{e}_{sc}$ and $\mathbf{e}_{s,C(s)}$ from the errors $e_{scv} = y_{scv} - \mu_{scv}$, and the standardized error vectors $\mathbf{stde}_{sc}$ and $\mathbf{stde}_{s,C(s)}$ from the standardized errors $stde_{scv} = e_{scv}/(\phi \cdot V(\mu_{scv}))^{1/2}$. With the observed data $O_{s,C(s)} = (\mathbf{y}_{s,C(s)}, \mathbf{X}_{s,C(s)})$, the constant dispersions formulation of Sect. 10.7.1 extends to the multivariate multinomial case. The diagonal matrices $\mathbf{A}_{s,C(s)}$ have diagonal entries $V(\mu_{scv})^{1/2}$ over $1 \le v \le K$ and $c \in C(s)$ for $s \in S$. For each $s \in S$, the $(m(s) \cdot K) \times (m(s) \cdot K)$ working correlation matrix $\mathbf{R}_{s,C(s)}(\boldsymbol{\rho})$ is composed of blocks $\mathbf{R}_{scc'}$ representing correlation submatrices for $\mathbf{y}_{sc}$ and $\mathbf{y}_{sc'}$ over c, $c' \in C(s)$. Since $\mathbf{y}_{sc}$ is multinomially distributed, the main diagonal submatrices $\mathbf{R}_{scc} = \mathbf{A}_{s,c}^{-1/2} \cdot (\mathrm{diag}(\boldsymbol{\mu}_s(S)) - \boldsymbol{\mu}_s(S) \cdot \boldsymbol{\mu}_s(S)^T) \cdot \mathbf{A}_{s,c}^{-1/2}$ (see Lipsitz et al. 1994, p. 1154). The off-diagonal submatrices $\mathbf{R}_{scc'}$ for $c' < c$ need to be estimated. For $c' > c$, the submatrices $\mathbf{R}_{sc'c} = \mathbf{R}_{scc'}^T$.

For example, under exchangeability all $\mathbf{R}_{scc'}$ for $c' < c$ are the same with $K \times K$ common value $\mathbf{R}_0$. For a given parameter vector $\boldsymbol{\beta}$, $\mathbf{R}_0$ can be estimated as

$$\mathbf{R}_0(\boldsymbol{\beta}) = \frac{1}{m(CC) - r} \sum_{c'c \in CC} \mathbf{stde}_{sc'}(\boldsymbol{\beta}) \cdot \mathbf{stde}_{sc}(\boldsymbol{\beta})^T,$$

where $CC = \{c'c : c' < c, \; c', c \in C(S), \; s \in S\}$, $m(CC)$ is the number of pairs $c'c$ of indexes in CC, and the standardized error vectors $\mathbf{stde}_{sc'}(\boldsymbol{\beta})$ and $\mathbf{stde}_{sc}(\boldsymbol{\beta})$ are computed using the estimate $\phi_{GEE}(\boldsymbol{\beta})$ of ϕ given by

$$\phi_{GEE}(\boldsymbol{\beta}) = \frac{1}{m(SC) - r} \sum_{scv \in SCV} \frac{e_{scv}(\boldsymbol{\beta})^2}{V(\mu_{scv})},$$

where $SCV = \{scv : 1 \le v \le K, \; c \in C(S), \; s \in S\}$. These are bias-corrected estimates since the denominators are adjusted for bias by subtracting the number r of expectation parameters. Unadjusted estimates are also possible by not subtracting r in the denominators. These are also dispersion-adjusted, that is, the estimate of the dispersion is included in the estimate of the correlation submatrix $\mathbf{R}_0$, as for GEE correlation estimates in the multivariate dichotomous case. Lipsitz et al. (1994), on the other hand, use non-dispersion-adjusted correlation estimates (see, for example, their Example 1 covering exchangeability). They define the standardized errors as $stde'_{scv} = e_{scv}/(V(\mu_{scv}))^{1/2}$ without including the dispersion ϕ and define the estimate $\mathbf{R}_0(\boldsymbol{\beta})$ for exchangeability as above using associated estimates $stde'_{scv}(\boldsymbol{\beta})$ of these standard errors without including an estimate for the dispersion. An estimate

$\beta_{GEE}(SC)$ of β can be obtained by solving the GEE equations and model-based and robust empirical estimators of the covariance matrix of the estimate $\beta_{GEE}(SC)$ can be obtained as in Sect. 10.7.1.

As in Sect. 10.7.1, extended LCV (LCV^+) scores can be computed for GEE models of polytomous outcomes, using either matched-set-wise deletion or measurement-wise deletion. The adaptive modeling process then also extends to GEE modeling of polytomous outcomes by basing it on such LCV^+ scores. It is also possible to compute extended penalized likelihood criteria adding the usual penalty factors to extended likelihoods giving the extended AIC (AIC^+), the extended BIC (BIC^+), and the extended TIC (TIC^+). Modeling of dispersions along with means is formulated similarly to the extension of Sect. 10.7.1 for multivariate dichotomous outcomes. As for univariate polytomous outcomes (see Sect. 8.13.2), dispersions are treated as the same for all values of the outcome rather than changing with those values, as do the means. Scaled residual vectors $\mathbf{sclde}_s(SC)$ can also be computed as $\mathbf{sclde}_s(SC) = (\mathbf{U}_s^T(SC))^{-1} \cdot \mathbf{e}_s(SC)$ where $\mathbf{U}_s(SC)$ is the square root of the covariance matrix $\Sigma_s(SC)$ determined by its Cholesky decomposition. The entries of $\mathbf{sclde}_s(SC)$ can be combined over all s (and $1 \leq v \leq K$ since $\mathbf{sclde}_s(SC)$ has m(s)·K entries) and analyzed in combination as for independent data.

The formulation for multivariate ordinal regression is similar to that of multivariate multinomial regression. The extensions to non-constant dispersions for both of these cases are similar to the extension for multivariate dichotomous outcomes, and so detailed formulations are not presented here.

10.7.3   Comparing Transition Models to Marginal GEE-Based Models

Using the notation of Sects. 10.3.1 and 10.7.1, assume that a transition model for a conditional dichotomous outcome with values $y^{\#}_{sc}$ has parameter vector θ, means $\mu^{\#}_{sc}$, dispersions $\phi^{\#}_{sc}$, and extended variances $\sigma^{\#}_{sc}{}^2 = \phi^{\#}_{sc} \cdot V(\mu^{\#}_{sc})$ for $c \in C(s)$ and $s \in S$. The error vectors $\mathbf{e}^{\#}_{s,C(s)}$ have entries $e^{\#}_{sc} = y^{\#}_{sc} - \mu^{\#}_{sc}$ while the standardized error vectors $\mathbf{stde}^{\#}_{s,C(s)}$ have entries $stde^{\#}_{sc} = e^{\#}_{sc}/\sigma^{\#}_{sc}$. Using the independence correlation structure $\mathbf{R}_{s,C(s)}(\rho) = \mathbf{I}_{C(s)}$ for $s \in S$, the associated extended likelihood terms $L^+(O^{\#}_{s,C(s)}; \theta)$ induced by the conditional model satisfy

$$\ell^+(O^{\#}_{s,C(s)}; \theta) = \log\left(L^+(O^{\#}_{s,C(s)}; \theta)\right)$$
$$= -\frac{1}{2} \cdot \mathbf{stde}^{\#}_{s,C(s)}{}^T \cdot \mathbf{stde}^{\#}_{s,C(s)} - \frac{1}{2} \cdot \sum_{c \in C(s)} \log(\sigma^{\#}_{sc}{}^2) - \frac{1}{2} \cdot m(s) \cdot \log(2 \cdot \pi)$$

for $s \in S$. The associated extended likelihood $L^+(SC; \theta)$ is the product of these extended likelihood terms $L^+(O^{\#}_{s,C(s)}; \theta)$ over $s \in S$. The formulation for polytomous outcomes is similar except that the working correlation $\mathbf{R}_{s,C(s)}(\rho)$ has

diagonal   blocks $\mathbf{R}_{scc} = \mathbf{A}_{s,c}^{-1/2} \cdot (\mathrm{diag}(\boldsymbol{\mu}^{\#}_{s}(S)) - \boldsymbol{\mu}^{\#}_{s}(S) \cdot \boldsymbol{\mu}^{\#}_{s}(S)^{T}) \cdot \mathbf{A}_{s,c}^{-1/2}$
where $\boldsymbol{\mu}^{\#}_{s}(S)$ is the vector with entries $\mu^{\#}_{sc}(S)$ for $c \in C(s)$ as in Sect. 10.7.2 and
zero off-diagonal blocks $\mathbf{R}_{sc'c} = \mathbf{0}$ for $c' \neq c$.

These conditional-model-induced extended likelihoods can be used in comput-
ing conditional-model-induced LCV^{+} scores using parameter vectors $\boldsymbol{\theta}(S\backslash F(h))$
estimated with the conditional model over complements $S\backslash F(h)$ of folds $F(h)$ for
$h \in H$, either with matched-set-wise deletion (Sect. 4.4.1) or measurement-wise
deletion (Sect. 4.13). These LCV^{+} scores can be compared to LCV^{+} scores for
GEE-based models to assess the effectiveness of conditional modeling compared to
GEE-based modeling.

10.8   Adaptive GEE-Based Modeling of Post-Baseline Respiratory Status

For brevity, only dichotomous respiratory status is analyzed and all models have
constant dispersions. Also all extended LCV (LCV^{+}) scores are based on $k = 5$
folds as for transition modeling of these data. The adaptive GEE-based model for
status0_1 in visit with EC correlation structure is the constant model with LCV^{+}
score 0.57059. The corresponding adaptive GEE-based model with AR1 correlation
structure is also the constant model with smaller LCV^{+} score 0.55526. Consequently, EC is the more appropriate correlation structure for these data and is used
in subsequent analyses.

The adaptive GEE-based model in status0_1_0, visit, and GCs is based on the
single predictor: status0_1_0 · visit$^{-0.14}$ with improved LCV^{+} score 0.58989. This is
a distinct improvement over the constant model generating a substantial PD of 3.27 %.
The associated adaptive constant dispersions transition model, starting from the
model based on $\mathrm{PRE}(y,1,3)^{1.1}$ and $\mathrm{PRE}(y,1,3,\varnothing)$ and allowing for the extra
primary predictors status0_1_0, visit, and GCs, is based on the three transforms:
$\mathrm{PRE}(y,1,3)^{1.1}$, $\mathrm{PRE}(y,1,3,\varnothing)$, and status0_1_0 · visit^{-1}. It induces a marginal model
with LCV^{+} score 0.58992, which is an improvement over the associated GEE-based
model, but the PD in the LCV^{+} scores of 0.01 % is insubstantial. The adaptive
constant dispersions transition model in $\mathrm{PRE}(y,1,3)$, $\mathrm{PRE}(y,1,3,\varnothing)$, status0_1_0,
visit, and GCs in these four primary predictors is based on the three transforms:
$(\mathrm{PRE}(y,1,3)^{2} \cdot \mathrm{visit}^{0.5})^{0.6}$, $(\mathrm{status0\_1\_0} \cdot \mathrm{visit}^{-1.4})^{0.7}$, and visit$^{-4.5}$. It induces a
marginal model with LCV^{+} score 0.59825, which is a distinct improvement over
the GEE-based model with the best LCV^{+} score 0.58989 and substantial PD of
1.40 %. Moreover, it requires only about 1.7 min of clock time to compute
compared to about 18.4 min for the associated GEE-based model. These results
indicate that transition models for multivariate dichotomous outcomes can induce
marginal models that distinctly outperform associated GEE-based marginal models
while requiring substantially less computation time.

10.9 Overview of Analyses of Post-Baseline Dichotomous Respiratory Status

1. For post-baseline dichotomous respiratory status (Sect. 10.2), analyses use $k = 5$ folds (Sect. 10.4.1).

2. Using unit dispersions, post-baseline dichotomous respiratory status is best modeled in terms of the average of the prior three outcome measurements compared to averages of the prior one or two outcome measurements and so this is used in subsequent analyses (this and the following results reported in Sect. 10.4.1). Modeling post-baseline dichotomous respiratory status in the average of the prior three outcome measurements and the associated indicator of no prior outcome measurements separately from visit, baseline dichotomous respiratory status, and being on active compared to placebo treatment generates a competitive model compared to modeling post-baseline dichotomous respiratory status in both sets of these predictors in combination. Under the generated model for the separate effects case, there is a distinct effect to being on active compared to placebo treatment. Section 11.3 provides a residual analysis for the separate effects model.

3. Using constant dispersions does not distinctly improve on using unit dispersions (this and the following results reported in Sect. 10.4.2). However, using non-constant dispersions does distinctly improve on using constant dispersions, and so also on unit dispersions. For the best non-constant dispersions model, being on active compared to placebo treatment has a distinct effect on the log odds for post-baseline dichotomous respiratory status but only for patients with good baseline respiratory status and only better than patients on placebo treatment with good baseline respiratory status at early visits (see Table 10.1). The dispersions for patients on the placebo treatment or with poor baseline respiratory status (see Table 10.2) change with visit and the average of the prior three outcome measurements, but the only difference for patients on active treatment is at the first visit when they also have good baseline respiratory status, in which case the dispersion is almost zero.

4. Using constant dispersions and GEE parameter estimation, exchangeable correlations are more appropriate to use than order 1 autoregressive correlations (this and the following results reported in Sect. 10.8). The model for the log odds is distinctly improved by consideration of visit, baseline respiratory status, and GCs in these two predictors. However, this GEE-based model is distinctly outperformed by the marginal model induced by the constant dispersions transition model in the average of the prior three outcome measurements, the associated indicator of no prior outcome measurements, visit, baseline respiratory status, and GCs in these predictors.

10.10   Overview of Analyses of Post-Baseline Polytomous Respiratory Status

1. For post-baseline polytomous respiratory status (Sect. 10.2), analyses use k = 10 folds (Sect. 10.6.1).
2. Ordinal regression is more appropriate for analyzing post-baseline polytomous respiratory status than multinomial regression, and so is used in subsequent analyses (this and the following results reported in Sect. 10.6.1). Using unit dispersions, post-baseline polytomous respiratory status is best modeled in terms of the average of the prior two outcome measurements compared to averages of the prior one or three outcome measurements and so this is used in subsequent analyses. Modeling post-baseline polytomous respiratory status in the average of the prior two outcome measurements and the associated indicator of no prior outcome measurements separately from visit, baseline polytomous respiratory status, and being on active compared to placebo treatment, there is a distinct effect to being on active compared to placebo treatment. The proportional odds for worse versus better polytomous respiratory status are lower for patients on active compared to placebo treatment, but with less of an improvement at later visits. There is no effect to being on active compared to placebo treatment for patients with poor baseline polytomous respiratory status, but there is otherwise with more of an improvement for patients with excellent baseline polytomous respiratory status compared to patients with good baseline polytomous respiratory status.
3. Using constant dispersions distinctly improves on using unit dispersions (this and the following results reported in Sect. 10.6.2). Using non-constant dispersions distinctly improve on using constant dispersions. Modeling means and dispersions for post-baseline polytomous respiratory status in the average of the prior two outcome measurements and the associated indicator of no prior outcome measurements separately from visit, baseline polytomous respiratory status, and being on active compared to placebo treatment, there is a distinct effect to being on active compared to placebo treatment. The proportional odds for worse versus better polytomous respiratory status are lower for patients on active compared to placebo treatment, but with less of an improvement at later visits. There is no effect to being on active compared to placebo treatment for patients with poor baseline polytomous respiratory status, but there is otherwise with more of an improvement for patients with excellent baseline polytomous respiratory status compared to patients with good baseline polytomous respiratory status. Dispersions decrease with visit.

10.11 Chapter Summary

This chapter presents a series of analyses of the respiratory status data, addressing how respiratory status over four post-baseline clinic visits categorized as poor or good and as poor, good, or excellent depends on visit, baseline respiratory status, and active versus placebo treatment for n = 111 patients with respiratory distress using both adaptive transition models and adaptive marginal models with generalized estimating equations (GEE) parameter estimation. These analyses demonstrate adaptive logistic regression modeling of multivariate outcomes using fractional polynomials, including modeling of dichotomous outcomes, extensions to adaptive multinomial and ordinal regression for polytomous outcomes, and how to model dispersions as well as means. The chapter has also provided formulations for these alternative regression models; for associated k-fold likelihood cross-validation (LCV) scores for unit dispersions transition models, extended quasi-likelihood cross-validation (QLCV$^+$) scores for non-unit dispersions transition models, pseudolikelihood cross-validation (PLCV) and extended PLCV (PLCV$^+$) scores for general conditional models of means and/or dispersions, and extended LCV (LCV$^+$) scores for GEE models of means and/or dispersions; for odds ratio (OR) functions generalizing the OR of standard logistic regression; and for standardized or Pearson residuals and scaled residuals.

The example analyses demonstrate assessing whether the log odds of a dichotomous and polytomous outcome are nonlinear in individual predictors, whether those relationships are better addressed with multiple predictors in combination compared to using singleton predictors, whether those relationships interact using geometric combinations (GCs), whether ordinal polytomous outcomes are better modeled with ordinal or multinomial regression, and whether there is a benefit to considering constant or non-constant dispersions over unit dispersions. The example analyses also demonstrate how to compare GEE-based marginal models to marginal models induced by transition models. The result of this comparison indicate that transition models for multivariate dichotomous outcomes can induce marginal models that distinctly outperform associated GEE-based marginal models while requiring substantially less computation time. Thus, it seems reasonable not to consider GEE-based marginal models when analyzing multivariate dichotomous outcomes and most likely multivariate polytomous outcomes as well. Example residual analyses are not reported in this chapter. See Chap. 11 for a description of how to conduct analyses of multivariate dichotomous and polytomous outcomes in SAS including an example residual analysis.

References

Chaganty, N. R. (1997). An alternative approach to the analysis of longitudinal data via generalized estimating equations. *Journal of Statistical Planning and Inference, 63*, 39–54.

Fitzmaurice, G. M., Laird, N. M., & Ware, J. H. (2011). *Applied longitudinal analysis* (2nd ed.). Hoboken, NJ: Wiley.

Koch, G. G., Carr, C. F., Amara, I. A., Stokes, M. E., & Uryniak, T. J. (1989). Categorical data analysis. In D. A. Berry (Ed.), *Statistical methodology in the pharmaceutical sciences* (pp. 391–475). New York: Marcel Dekker.

Liang, K.-Y., & Zeger, S. L. (1986). Longitudinal data analysis using generalized linear models. *Biometrika, 73*, 13–22.

Lipsitz, S. R., Kim, K., & Zhao, L. (1994). Analysis of repeated categorical data using generalized estimating equations. *Statistics in Medicine, 13*, 1149–1163.

McCullagh, P., & Nelder, J. A. (1999). *Generalized linear models* (2nd ed.). Boca Raton, FL: Chapman & Hall/CRC.

Miller, M. E., Davis, C. S., & Landis, J. R. (1993). The analysis of longitudinal polytomous generalized estimating equations and connections with weighted least squares. *Biometrics, 49*, 1033–1044.

Molenberghs, G., & Verbeke, G. (2006). *Models for discrete longitudinal data*. New York: Springer.

Pan, W. (2001). Akaike's information criterion in generalized estimating equations. *Biometrics, 57*, 120–125.

SAS Institute. (2004). *SAS/STAT 9.1 user's guide*. Cary, NC: SAS Institute.

Stokes, M. E., Davis, C. S., & Koch, G. G. (2012). *Categorical data analysis using the SAS system* (3rd ed.). Cary, NC: SAS Institute.

Chapter 11
Adaptive Logistic Regression Modeling of Multivariate Dichotomous and Polytomous Outcomes in SAS

11.1 Chapter Overview

This chapter describes how to use the genreg macro for adaptive logistic regression modeling of multivariate dichotomous and polytomous outcomes, as described in Chap. 10, and its generated output. See Supplementary Materials for a more complete description of the macro. See Allison (2012), SAS Institute (1995), Stokes et al. (2012) for details on standard generalized estimating equations (GEE) modeling of multivariate dichotomous and polytomous outcomes in SAS. Familiarity with adaptive modeling in SAS of univariate logistic outcomes as described in Chap. 9 and of transition modeling in SAS as described in Chap. 5 is assumed in this chapter.

Section 11.2 describes the respiratory status data (see Sect. 10.2) used in the analyses of Chap. 10. Section 11.3 provides examples of transition modeling of dichotomous respiratory status while Sect. 11.4 provides examples of GEE-based marginal modeling of dichotomous respiratory status. Section 11.5 provides examples of both transition modeling and GEE-based marginal modeling of polytomous respiratory status.

11.2 Loading in the Respiratory Status Data

Analyses are conducted in Chap. 10 of respiratory status for $n = 111$ patients with respiratory disorder (see Sect. 10.2). Assume that these respiratory status data have been loaded into the default library (for example, by importing them from a spreadsheet file) in wide format (see Sect. 5.2) under the name wideresp. An output title line, selected system options, labels for the variables, and formats for values of selected variables can be assigned using the code that follows. Patients were cared for in one of two centers with 56 patients at Center 1 and 55 at Center 2.

© Springer International Publishing Switzerland 2016
G.J. Knafl, K. Ding, *Adaptive Regression for Modeling Nonlinear Relationships*,
Statistics for Biology and Health, DOI 10.1007/978-3-319-33946-7_11

Patient identifiers in the variable id start at 1 for both centers and so identifiers for Center 2 are increased by 56 to make them unique. The respiratory status outcome measurements at visits 0–4 are in the variables status0–status4. Formats are created with PROC FORMAT for the values of the group, gender, and status0–status4 variables and assigned with the format statement in the data step. The five possible values for status0–status4 are described in the stat0_4fmt format. Indicator variables active and male are created from the group and gender variables, respectively, and assigned the nyfmt format. Formats are also created for the alternative simplified respiratory status outcome variables yet to be computed.

```
options nodate pageno=1 pagesize=53 linesize=76;
title1 "Respiratory Status Data";
proc format;
  value $grpfmt "P"="Placebo" "A"="Active";
  value $gndrfmt "F"="Female" "M"="Male";
  value stat0_4fmt 0="0:Terrible" 1="1:Poor" 2="2:Fair"
                   3="3:Good" 4="4:Excellent";
  value stat0_2fmt 0="0:Poor" 1="1:Good" 2="2:Excellent";
  value stat0_1fmt 0="0:Poor" 1="1:Good"; value nyfmt 0="no" 1="yes";
run;
data wideresp;
  set wideresp;
  if center=2 then id=id+56; * so patient identifiers are unique;
  active=(group="A"); male=(gender="M");
  label id="Patient Identifier" center="Center" group="Treatment Group"
        gender="Gender" age="Age in Years"
        status0="Respiratory Status at Visit 0"
        status1="Respiratory Status at Visit 1"
        status2="Respiratory Status at Visit 2"
        status3="Respiratory Status at Visit 3"
        status4="Respiratory Status at Visit 4"
        active="Active or Not" male="Male or Not";
  format group $grpfmt. gender $gndrfmt. status0-status4 stat0_4fmt.
         active male nyfmt.;
run;
```

The following code converts the data to long format and stores it in the longresp data set.

```
data longresp;
 set wideresp;
 array status{5} status0-status4;
 do i=1 to 5;
  visit=i-1; status0_4=status{i}; status0_4_0=status0; output;
 end;
 label visit="Visit" status0_4="Respiratory Status 0-4"
       status0_4_0="Baseline Respiratory Status 0-4";
 format status0_4 status0_4_0 stat0_4fmt.; drop i status0-status4;
run;
data longresp;
 set longresp;
 if status0_4<=1 then status0_2=0;
 else if status0_4<=3 then status0_2=1; else status0_2=2;
 if status0_4_0<=1 then status0_2_0=0;
 else if status0_4_0<=3 then status0_2_0=1; else status0_2_0=2;
 status0_1=(status0_4>2); status0_1_0=(status0_4_0>2);
 label status0_2="Respiratory Status 0-2"
       status0_1="Respiratory Status 0-1"
       status0_2_0="Baseline Respiratory Status 0-2"
       status0_1_0="Baseline Respiratory Status 0-1";
 format status0_1 status0_1_0 stat0_1fmt. status0_2 status0_2_0
        stat0_2fmt.;
run;
```

The five-valued respiratory status variable status0_4 is created from status0–status4 and used to compute the reduced three valued variable status0_2 with values described in stat0_2fmt and the further reduced two valued variable status0_1 with values described in stat0_1fmt. The variables status0_4_0, status0_2_0, and status0_1_0 are loaded with baseline values for the three alternative respiratory status outcome variables. These are baseline values for modeling post-baseline respiratory status using the postresp data set created as follows.

```
data postresp;
 set longresp;
 if visit=0 then delete;
run;
```

The cutoff for a substantial percent decrease (PD) in the likelihood cross-validation (LCV) scores for analyses of post-baseline status0_1 with $4 \cdot 111 = 444$ measurements is 0.43 % (as reported in Sect. 10.4) while it is 0.22 % for analyses of post-baseline status0_2 with $2 \cdot 444 = 888$ effective measurements (as reported in Sect. 10.6). Post-baseline status0_4 is not analyzed in Chap. 10, and so the associated cutoff is not reported. Since there are no missing measurements, LCV scores are computed with matched-set-wise deletion.

11.3 Transition Modeling of Dichotomous Respiratory Status

Assume that copies y and w of status0_1 and visit, respectively, have been loaded in the longresp and postresp data sets. Assume also that genreg has been loaded into SAS (see Supplementary Materials). An adaptive transition model for post-baseline status0_1 can be generated as follows.

```
%genreg(modtype=logis,datain=postresp,yvar=status0_1,
        matchvar=id,withinvr=visit,conditnl=y,
        corrtype=IND,vintrcpt=n,foldcnt=5,expand=y,
        expxvars=pre_y_w_1_3 pre_y_w_1_3_m,contract=y,
        nocnxint=y);
```

The parameter setting "modtype=logis" requests a logistic regression model. The datain parameter specifies the input data set, in this case the postresp data set. The yvar parameter specifies the dichotomous or polytomous outcome variable, in this case the dichotomous outcome variable status0_1. A conditional model is requested since "conditnl=y". This requires an independent correlation structure as requested with "corrtype=IND". It also requires that the matchvar and withinvr parameters have nonempty settings specifying, respectively, the variable whose unique values determine the matched sets, the variable id in this case, and the variable whose values indicate the different conditions under which the outcome variable has been measured, the variable visit in this case. The option "vintrcpt=n" requests a unit dispersions model (formally, a zero log dispersions model). The parameter setting "foldcnt=5" (as justified in Sect. 10.4.1) requests that 5-fold LCV scores be computed for models and is used in all further analyses of status0_1. The parameter setting "expand=y" requests that the base model be expanded. The model for the means is expanded by adding in transforms of primary predictor variables listed in the setting for the expxvars parameter. The model for the dispersions is not changed since the expvvars macro parameter has its default empty setting. The parameter setting "contract=y" requests that the expanded model be contracted. The option "nocnxint=y" requests that the contraction not remove the intercept from the model for the means (as for all analyses of Chaps. 10–11). In this case, the two dependence predictors pre_y_w_1_3 and pre_y_w_1_3_m (called PRE(y,1,3) and PRE(y,1,3,$\emptyset$), respectively, in Chap. 10) are considered in the expansion (see Sect. 5.4 for more on how dependence predictors are specified). Using the copies y and w shortens the names of these predictors. Using the shorter name w for visit is optional but not the shorter name y for status0_1. The variable names used in specifying dependence predictors must not contain underscores (_). Underscores are used by genreg to decompose a dependence predictor name into its components. Using pre_status0_1_visit_1_3 would generate an error since genreg would treat the outcome variable as being status0 and not status0_1 and the within variable as 1 and not visit. The yvar variable can be character valued, but then it needs to be recoded as numeric for use in dependence predictors since these currently can only be based on numeric variables. Alternate transition models can be generated by changing the expxvars list to depend on pre_y_w_1_2 or pre_y_w_1_1 (called PRE(y,1,2) and PRE(y,1,1) in Chap. 10, respectively).

The default setting "measdlte=n" is requested so that generated LCV scores are based on matched-set-wise deletion with all measurements of a matched set assigned to the same fold (see Sect. 4.4.1). Measurement-wise deletion (see Sect. 4.13) with individual measurements assigned to folds instead can be requested with the setting "measdlte=y". For transition and general conditional models, partial measurement-wise deletion (Sect. 4.13) can be requested with the setting "measdlte=p".

The base model is generated first, in this case the model with constant means (since the default settings of "xintrcpt=y" and "xvars=" are used), unit dispersions, and LCV score 0.50235. This is expanded by adding in the two transforms for the means: pre_y_w_1_3^2 and pre_y_w_1_3_m, in that order, with associated LCV score 0.57164, and the contraction leaves this expanded model unchanged. However, the expanded model might be improved by adjusting the power of its first transform, and so a conditional transformation step occurs (due to the default setting "condtrns = y"; see Sect. 3.3). Table 11.1 contains part of the output describing the conditionally transformed expanded model. The component of the

Table 11.1 Conditionally transformed expanded transition model for dichotomous respiratory status

```
              transformed logit expectation component

     parameter estimates for logits relative to smallest status0_1=0

          predictor            power          status0_1=1

          XINTRCPT                 1              -1.48671
          pre_y_w_1_3            1.1              3.059236
          pre_y_w_1_3_m           1              1.8324555
```

adjusted	old power	new power	score	order
	.	.	0.5716416	0
pre_y_w_1_3	2	1.1	0.5750678	1

```
          transformed log dispersion component

          predictor            power            estimate

          VZERO                    1                   0

          log dispersion component unchanged
```

```
...
   mth root of likelihood using deleted predictions:        0.5750678
     same as deleted mth root of quasi+ likelihood with dispersion=1
```

model for the logits of the expectations or means (called the logit expectation component in the output) is described first. It is based on an intercept parameter (denoted as XINTRCPT), the transform of the primary predictor pre_y_w_1_3 raised to the power 1.1, and the untransformed primary predictor pre_y_w_1_3_m. The order that terms have their powers adjusted is indicated in the output. The base model for the transformation with order 0 has LCV score rounding to 0.57164. The transform of pre_y_w_1_3 has its power changed from 2 to 1.1 first since that change has order 1, and then the transformation stops. Estimates of coefficients are interpreted in the same way as for univariate dichotomous outcomes and can also be used to calculate odds ratio (OR) functions in the same way (see Sects. 8.3.2 and 10.3.1). The component of the model for the log of the dispersions is described next. It is based on a zero intercept parameter (denoted as VZERO) as requested by the "vintrcpt=n" option. Several values describing the model are generated last. Of these, only the LCV score is included in Table 11.1, rounded to seven digits. The number of chararacter positions and hence digits for LCV scores can be changed with the screchrs macro parameter with default value 9. The LCV score for the transformed model rounds to 0.57507 (and provides a distinct improvement as justified in Sect. 10.4.1). This is the same as its extended quasi-LCV (QLCV$^+$) score as indicated in the output (by describing that score as based on a "quasi+ likelihood"), and so can be compared to QLCV$^+$ scores for non-unit dispersions models.

An adaptive model in the baseline value status0_1_0, the within-patient variable visit, the indicator variable active, and geometric combinations (GCs) in these three predictors, starting from the model of Table 11.1 as the base model, can be generated as follows.

```
%genreg(modtype=logis,datain=postresp,yvar=status0_1,
        matchvar=id,withinvr=visit,conditnl=y,
        corrtype=IND,vintrcpt=n,foldcnt=5,
        xvars=pre_y_w_1_3 pre_y_w_1_3_m,xpowers=1.1 1,
        expand=y,expxvars=status0_1_0 visit active,
        geomcmbn=y,contract=y,nocnxint=y);
```

The base model is set using the xvars and xpowers settings. The primary predictors for the expansion are set through the expxvars parameter. GCs are requested as part of this expansion with the "geomcmbn=y" setting. The default setting "geomcmbn=n" generates the associated additive model. The expansion adds four transforms to the base model: $active \cdot status0\_1\_0 \cdot visit^{-1.8}$, $status0\_1\_0 \cdot visit^{-0.7}$, $active \cdot visit^{-0.4}$, and $(status0\_1\_0 \cdot active \cdot visit^{-9})^2$ with LCV score 0.60591. This is contracted to the model based on the four transforms: $pre\_y\_w\_1\_3^{1.1}$, $pre\_y\_w\_1\_3\_m$, $(status0\_1\_0 \cdot visit^{-0.7})^{0.7}$, and $(status0\_1\_0 \cdot active \cdot visit^{-9})^2$ with LCV score 0.60406. Odds ratios (ORs) associated with terms like $(status0\_1\_0 \cdot active \cdot visit^{-9})^2$ are not generated by genreg but can be simply computed (for example, in a spreadsheet tool) from the estimated slope of 7.3846659 (as reported in the genreg output). Just multiply this estimate by

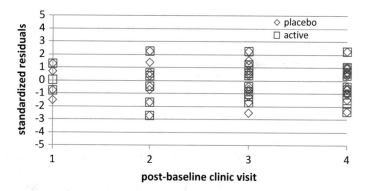

Fig. 11.1 Standardized residuals versus post-baseline clinic visit by group (on placebo or active treatment) for the adaptive model of dichotomous respiratory status

status0_1_0 · visit^{-18} with status0_1_0 set to each of its two possible values 0–1 and visit set to each of its four possible post-baseline values 1–4 and then exponentiate. Confidence intervals would not be reported for these ORs since the significance of this active effect is addressed instead with a LCV ratio test.

Residual analyses can be conducted for transition models for multivariate dichotomous outcomes similarly to those for univariate dichotomous outcomes (see Sects. 9.4 and 9.6). Since values for the predictors of the above model have limited ranges, there is little benefit to grouping the data (as in Sect. 9.6). A residual analysis for the above ungrouped model can be conducted using the stdres variable in the dataout data set. Figure 11.1 displays these standardized residuals. They are reasonably close to being symmetric. Furthermore, they are all within ±3, and so there are no outlying observations. This is a reasonable model for these data.

Effects for dependence and the other predictors do not have to be separate. An adaptive model in all these predictors and GCs is generated using the following code.

```
%genreg(modtype=logis,datain=postresp,yvar=status0_1,
        matchvar=id,withinvr=visit,conditnl=y,
        corrtype=IND,vintrcpt=n,foldcnt=5,expand=y,
        geomcmbn=y,expxvars=pre_y_w_1_3 pre_y_w_1_3_m
        status0_1_0 visit active,
        contract=y,nocnxint=y);
```

The generated model has three transforms: $(pre\_y\_w\_1\_3^2 \cdot visit^{0.5})^{0.7}$, $(status0\_1\_0 \cdot visit^{-1.4})^{0.8}$, and active · visit^{-1} with improved LCV score 0.60500, but the PD for the prior best model is insubstantial at 0.16 %, as also reported in Sect. 10.4.1.

Adaptive models for both the means and dispersions can also be generated. For example, the following code generates a model with both means and dispersions a function of the dependence predictors pre_y_w_1_3 and pre_y_w_1_3_m.

```
%genreg(modtype=logis,datain=postresp,yvar=status0_1,
        matchvar=id,withinvr=visit,conditnl=y,
        corrtype=IND,foldcnt=5,expand=y,geomcmbn=y,
        expxvars=pre_y_w_1_3 pre_y_w_1_3_m,
        expvvars=pre_y_w_1_3 pre_y_w_1_3_m,contract=y,
        nocnxint=y,cnvzero=y);
```

The setting "cnvzero=y" means consider zero log dispersions models (or, equivalently, unit dispersions models) in the contraction. The default setting "vintrcpt=y" is requested, so the base model is a constant dispersions model. The default setting "nocnvint=n" is also requested, so the intercept for the log dispersions model is considered for removal in the contraction. The generated model for the means has two transforms: $pre\_y\_w\_1\_3^{1.1}$ and $pre\_y\_w\_1\_3\_m$ with an intercept and for the dispersions the single transform: $pre\_y\_w\_1\_3\_m$ without an intercept. The $QLCV^+$ score is 0.57887, which substantially improves on the associated unit dispersions model (see Sect. 10.4.2).

11.4 Marginal GEE-Based Modeling of Dichotomous Respiratory Status

An adaptive GEE-based model can be generated for post-baseline status0_1 in terms of visit as follows.

```
%genreg(modtype=logis,datain=postresp,yvar=status0_1,
        matchvar=id,withinvr=visit,GEE=y,corrtype=EC,
        biasadj=y,foldcnt=5,expand=y,expxvars=visit,
        contract=y,nocnxint=y,rprttime=y);
```

Only constant dispersions models are considered since the default settings "vintrcpt=y", "expvvars=" (that is, the empty setting), and "cnvzero=n" are requested. The setting "GEE=y" requests a GEE-based model (see Sect. 10.7.1). The default setting is "GEE=n", but that is only supported for marginal models with "modtype=norml". The corrtype parameter has the same meaning as for marginal models of continuous outcomes (see Sect. 5.3.1). Exchangeable correlations (EC) are requested in this case. The setting "biasadj=y" requests that correlation and dispersions estimates be bias-corrected (see Sect. 10.7.1) adjusting the number of measurements by subtracting the number of terms in the model for the means as is standard for GEE-based modeling. The default setting "biasadj=n" means compute those estimates without adjusting for bias, dividing instead by the unadjusted number of measurements.

The search starts at the constant means and dispersions model with extended LCV (LCV^+) score 0.57059. The expansion adds in the single transform $visit^{1.5}$

with somewhat improved LCV^+ score 0.57099 and then the contraction removes this transform leaving the constant model as the selected model. The "rprttime=y" setting requests that clock time be generated. It takes about 200.0 s or about 3.3 min of clock time to generate this model. In comparison, the adaptive transition model in pre_y_w_1_3, pre_y_w_1_3_m, and visit with constant dispersions requires about 18.5 s. The adaptive GEE-based model takes about 10.8 times as much clock time as the comparable transition model. While the total time of 3.3 min does not seem too long, the extra time to conduct a complete analysis with several steps and considering multiple predictors and GCs can be considerable. For example, as reported in Sect. 10.8 the adaptive GEE-based marginal model with EC correlations and with means depending on status0_1_0, visit, and GCs requires about 18.4 min of clock time. Moreover, as demonstrated in Sect. 10.8, adaptively generated transition models can induce marginal models that distinctly outperform GEE-based marginal models, and so consideration of just transition models can be a reasonable strategy and this can substantially reduce computation times.

LCV^+ scores for GEE-based models of dichotomous and polytomous outcomes are computed with extended multivariate normal likelihoods while LCV and $QLCV^+$ scores for transition and general conditional models of dichotomous and polytomous outcomes are computed with Bernoulli and categorical likelihoods, respectively, and so these two types of scores are not comparable. However, transition and general conditional models for dichotomous and polytomous outcomes induce marginal models (see Sect. 10.7.3), whose LCV^+ scores can be compared to those for GEE-based marginal models. The induced score for a model is reported when requested with the setting "GEEscore=y".

The use of penalized likelihood criteria (PLCs) has the potential to speed up adaptive GEE computations. For example, an adaptive model in status0_1_0, visit, and GCs with constant dispersions based on the extended Akaike information criterion (AIC^+) is generated as follows.

```
%genreg(modtype=logis,datain=postresp,yvar=status0_1,
        matchvar=id,withinvr=visit,GEE=y,corrtype=EC,
        biasadj=y,scretype=AIC,expand=y,
        expxvars=status0_1_0 visit,geomcmbn=y,contract=y,
        nocnxint=y,rprttime=y);
```

The scretype macro parameter controls the type of scores used by the adaptive modeling process to evaluate and compare models. The default "scretype=LCV" requests the use of CV scores based on likelihoods or likelihood-like functions, in particular LCV^+ scores for GEE-based models. The setting "scretype=AIC" for GEE-based models requests the use of AIC^+ scores (assumed to be in larger is better form; see Sect. 10.7.1). However, the expanded model is based on five transforms with four removed in the contraction, and so the total clock time is still fairly long at about 15.2 min compared to 18.4 min required using LCV^+ scores (as also reported in Sect. 10.8). Consequently, model selection based on PLCs can sometimes require relatively long amounts of clock time. Furthermore, as demonstrated in Sect. 4.8.4, the use of PLCs can sometimes generate distinctly inferior models to those generated by LCV scores. Also, as demonstrated in Sect. 2.10.2, when they generate competitive LCV scores, they can be more highly influenced by outlying observations, and these results are likely to hold for models based on extended PLC scores like AIC^+, BIC^+, and TIC^+ as well.

SAS PROC GENMOD generates quasi-likelihood information criterion (QIC) scores for GEE-based model selection (see Sect. 10.7.1), but these are not supported by the genreg macro for adaptive model selection. So consider the fixed GEE-based model for status0_1 with means depending on regression effects to active, visit, and their interaction, with unit dispersions, and EC correlation structure. The estimated correlation for this model is 0.50, the QIC score is 595.2554, and the LCV^+ score is 0.57150. When the correlation structure is changed to the independence structure setting the correlation to zero, the QIC score improves (i.e., decreases) a little to 595.2542, suggesting that the apparently substantial correlation estimate of 0.50 is actually insubstantial. However, the LCV^+ score decreases to 0.49633 with very substantial PD of 13.15 %. In this case, the QIC score provides a misleading assessment of the correlation structure, most likely due to being computed in part using the independence correlation structure and not completely based on the current working correlation structure as is LCV^+. Similar results also hold for extended PLCs. The EC-based model has AIC^+ score 0.57503, BIC^+ score using the number of measurements 0.56452, BIC^+ score using the number of matched sets 0.56805, TIC^+ score 0.57483, and these decrease for the model with independent correlations to 0.49825, 0.48914, 0.49221, and 0.49594, respectively, all with substantial PDs at least 13.35 %. While extended PLCs may be problematic for generating adaptive models, these results indicate that they can be effective in simpler model selection settings, like choosing an appropriate correlation structure for a given fixed effects model.

11.5 Modeling of Polytomous Outcomes

Transition models for multivariate polytomous outcomes like status0_2 can be generated similarly to transition models for multivariate dichotomous outcomes like status0_1 as presented in Sect. 11.3. As for univariate polytomous outcomes (see Sects. 9.8 and 9.12), the propodds macro parameter controls whether the model is ordinal or multinomial. If the outcome values are loaded in the variable yy and the values of the withinvr variable in w, prior dependence predictors like pre_yy_w_1_3 (denoted as PRE(y,1,3) in Sect. 10.6) are based on averages of prior outcome values. When the outcome values are nominal, such averages are not meaningful. It is then better to create indicator variables yy1, yy2, $\cdots$ for yy taking on its first, second, $\cdots$ value and using the prior dependence predictors pre_yy1_w_1_3, pre_yy2_w_1_3, $\cdots$ (denoted as PRE(y=1,1,3), PRE(y=2,1,3), $\cdots$ in Sect. 10.6). These could also be considered for ordinal polytomous outcomes, but dependence predictors like pre_yy_w_1_3 should be considered in any case for ordinal polytomous outcomes. Marginal GEE-based models for polytomous outcomes like status0_2 can also be generated similarly to marginal GEE-based models for dichotomous outcomes like status0_1 as presented in Sect. 11.4. However, processing times for generating adaptive models can be prohibitive.

11.6   Practice Exercises

11.1. A model is generated in Sect. 10.4.2 for status0_1 with both means and dispersions depending on the two prior dependence predictors pre_y_w_1_3 and pre_y_w_1_3_m (but called there PRE(y,1,3) and PRE(y,1,3,∅)). However, the baseline status variable status0_1_0 also represents an aspect of the prior measurements. Conduct an adaptive analysis of both the means and dispersions of status0_1 in terms of status0_1_0, pre_y_w_1_3, pre_y_w_1_3_m, and GCs. Start from a constant model for both the means and the dispersions. Do not allow the contraction to remove the intercept from the model for the means but allow the contraction to consider the unit dispersions model. Use 5 folds as justified in Sect. 10.4.1. Does this provide a distinct improvement over the model of Sect. 10.4.2?

11.2. Starting from the better of the two models considered in Practice Exercise 11.1, generate the adaptive model that adds in transforms of active, visit, and GCs to both the means and dispersions for status0_1. Do not allow the contraction to remove the intercept from the model for the means but allow the contraction to consider the unit dispersions model. Use 5 folds as justified in Sect. 10.4.1. Does the generated model improve on the base model for this analysis? What is the effect of active and visit on the means and dispersions of merchigh?

11.3. The gender of patients is also available in the data set and might have an effect on status0_1. Starting from the better of the two models considered in Practice Exercise 11.1, generate the adaptive model that adds in transforms of male, active, visit, and GCs to both the means and dispersions for status0_1. Do not allow the contraction to remove the intercept from the model for the means but allow the contraction to consider the unit dispersions model. Use 5 folds as justified in Sect. 10.4.1. Does the generated model improve on the model generated for Practice Exercise 11.2? What is the effect of gender on the conclusions for Practice Exercise 11.2?

11.4. The baseline age of patients is also available in the data set and might have an effect on status0_1. Age varies for patients from 11 to 68 years. To reduce the complexity of assessing the effect of age, create a data set called extended with a copy of the postresp data set with the following two indicator variables added: "agelo = (age < =25);" and "agelomid = (age < =37);". There are 32.4 % of the patients with age < =25 and 65.8 % with age < =37, and so this is close to a tertile split of the data. Using the extended data and starting from the better of the two models considered in Practice Exercise 11.1, generate the adaptive model that adds in transforms of agelo, agelomid, active, visit, and GCs to both the means and dispersions for status0_1. Do not allow the contraction to remove the intercept from the model for the means but allow the contraction to consider the unit dispersions model. Use 5 folds as justified in Sect. 10.4.1. Does the generated model improve on the model generated for Practice Exercise 11.2? What is the effect of agelo and agelomid on the conclusions for Practice Exercise 11.3?

11.5. A model is generated in Sect. 10.6.2 for status0_2 with the dependence of means and dispersions on the prior dependence predictors pre_yy_w_1_2 and pre_yy_w_1_2_m (but called there PRE(y,1,2) and PRE(y,1,2,∅)) separate from the predictors status0_2_0, visit, and active. Generate the adaptive ordinal regression model with both means and dispersions depending on pre_yy_w_1_2, pre_yy_w_1_2_m, status0_1_0, visit, active, and GCs. Start from a constant model for both the means and the dispersions. Do not allow the contraction to remove the intercept from the model for the means but allow the contraction to consider the unit dispersions model. Use 10 folds as justified in Sect. 10.6.1. Does this provide a distinct improvement over the model of Sect. 10.6.2 with the best $QLCV^+$ score? If so, generate the adaptive model under the same conditions except without active in the primary predictors for the means and dispersions. Is there a distinct effect to active in this context? Under the final selected model, which primary predictors have effects on the means and which on the dispersions?

For Practice Exercises 11.6–11.7, use the toxicity data available on the Internet (see Supplementary Materials) and initially analyzed in Price et al. (1985). Data are available for 1,028 pups from 94 mice litters. The outcome variable malform for this data set is the indicator for pups being malformed or not. The predictors to be considered are dose (0, 750, 1,500, and 3,000 mg/kg/day) of the toxin ethylene glycol and fetalwgt (the weight of the pup). The matched sets are determined by the variable litterid while the variable pup is the index for pups within these matched sets. Since these data are clustered, use general conditional modeling to analyze them based on the dependence predictor other_y_pup_1_end (that is, the average of malform measurements for the other pups in the same litter or the proportion of those pups that are malformed). There are 1–16 pups per litter. There is only one litter with one pup, so there is no need for the missing indicator other_y_pup_1_end_miss, which equals zero for all but this one pup. The analyses for these practice exercises can be time-consuming (requiring up to about 1 h) so non-constant dispersions modeling and GEE-based modeling have not been addressed.

11.6. For the toxicity data, use the adaptive model for malform as a function of other_y_pup_1_end as the benchmark analysis to set the number of folds for $QLCV^+$ scores. Do not allow the contraction to remove the intercept from the model for the means, use constant dispersions, and measurement-wise dele-tion (since the matched sets have varying sizes) for all analyses of this practice exercise. Starting from the selected model for other_y_pup_1_end, generate the adaptive model in dose (treating it as a continuous predictor), fetalwgt, and geometric combinations (GCs). Does this model distinctly improve on the model in only other_y_pup_1_end? Next, rerun the prior analysis but restricting to additive models. Assess whether fetal weight distinctly moderates (see Sect. 4.5.3) the effect of dose of ethylene glycol on the chance for malformation.

11.7. For the toxicity data, dose can be considered an analysis of variance factor rather than as a continuous predictor. This can be addressed by using the indicator variables over0, over750, and over1500 for dose >0, dose >750, and dose >1,500 mg/kg/day, respectively. These variables are created by the load code for the toxicity data available on the Internet. Do not allow the contraction to remove the intercept from the model for the means, use constant dispersions, and measurement-wise deletion (since the matched sets have varying sizes) for all analyses of this practice exercise. Use the number of folds determined in Practice Exercise 11.6. Starting from the model for other_y_pup_1_end selected in Practice Exercise 11.6, generate the adaptive model in over0, over750, over1500, fetalwgt, and geometric combinations (GCs). Compare this model to the associated model of Practice Exercise 11.6. Next, rerun the prior analysis but restricting to additive models. Assess moderation of the effect of dose as an analysis factor by fetalwgt. Is the conclusion about moderation of the effect of dose on malform different when dose is treated as an analysis of variance factor or as a continuous predictor?

References

Allison, P. (2012). *Logistic regression using SAS: Theory and applications* (2nd ed.). Cary, NC: SAS Institute.

Price, C. J., Kimmel, C. A., Tyl, R. W., & Marr, M. C. (1985). The developmental toxicity of ethylene glycol in rats and mice. *Toxicological Applications in Pharmacology, 81*, 113–127.

SAS Institute. (1995). *Logistic regression examples using the SAS system*. Cary, NC: SAS Institute.

Stokes, M. E., Davis, C. S., & Koch, G. G. (2012). *Categorical data analysis using the SAS system* (3rd ed.). Cary, NC: SAS Institute.

Part III
Adaptive Poisson Regression Modeling

Chapter 12
Adaptive Poisson Regression Modeling of Univariate Count Outcomes

12.1 Chapter Overview

This chapter formulates and demonstrates adaptive fractional polynomial modeling of univariate count outcomes with either unit, constant, or non-constant dispersions, possibly adjusted to rate outcomes through offsets. A description of how to generate these models in SAS is provided in Chap. 13. A familiarity with Poisson regression modeling is assumed, for example, as treated in Stokes et al. (2012) or Zelterman (2002). A data set with a univariate rate outcome is described in Sect. 12.2. The formulation for Poisson regression modeling of count/rate outcomes is provided in Sect. 12.3, both modeling of means alone and modeling of dispersions along with means. Section 12.4 conducts analyses of the count/rate outcome of Sect. 12.2. Section 12.5 provides an overview of the results of analysis of skin cancer rates. Formulations can be skipped to focus on analyses.

12.2 The Skin Cancer Data

A data set on skin cancer incidence for women living in either St. Paul, Minnesota or Fort Worth, Texas is available on the Internet (see Supplementary Materials). These data are analyzed here to demonstrate how to conduct Poisson regression analyses that account for nonlinearity in predictor variables. The variable cases, containing numbers of women with skin cancer, is the outcome variable for this data set. There are 15 observations corresponding to eight age groups (with minimum ages of 15, 25, $\cdots$, 85 years) for the two different cities (with no data for the 75-year minimum age category for St. Paul). The predictors are agemin, containing the minimum age corresponding to each count in the cases variable and the indicator variable city for residing in Fort Worth. The variable population contains the population size corresponding to each count in the cases variable

© Springer International Publishing Switzerland 2016
G.J. Knafl, K. Ding, *Adaptive Regression for Modeling Nonlinear Relationships*,
Statistics for Biology and Health, DOI 10.1007/978-3-319-33946-7_12

with values ranging from 7,583 to 181,343. It is used as the offset variable, thereby converting counts of skin cancer occurrences into skin cancer rates. The cutoff for a substantial percent decrease (PD) in the LCV and QLCV$^+$ scores for these data with 15 measurements is 12.0 % (using the formula of Sect. 4.4.2).

12.3   Multiple Poisson Regression Modeling of Count Outcomes

This section contains formulations (which can be skipped) for Poisson regression modeling of univariate count outcomes, possibly adjusted to rate outcomes using offsets. Section 12.3.1 addresses the unit dispersions case while Sect. 12.3.2 the non-unit dispersions case.

12.3.1   Unit Dispersions Formulation

The data for Poisson regression models, as considered in the analyses of Sect. 12.4.1, consist of observations $O_s = (y_s, x_s, o_{Es})$ for subjects $s \in S = \{s : 1 \leq s \leq n\}$ where each outcome measurement y_s is a count with values $0, 1, \cdots$; x_s is a $r \times 1$ column vector of r predictor values x_{sj} (including unit predictor values if an intercept is included in the model) with indexes $j \in J = \{j : 1 \leq j \leq r\}$; and o_{Es} is an offset value for modeling the expectations (hence the subscript "E") or means. The expected value or mean μ_s for y_s satisfies $\mu_s = E(y_s | x_s, o_{Es})$ for $s \in S$. Model the log of the mean as $\log(\mu_s) = x_s^T \cdot \beta + o_{Es}$ for a $r \times 1$ vector β of coefficients. The conditional variance for y_s is $\sigma_s^2 = \mu_s$.

The likelihood term L_s for the sth subject is based on the Poisson distribution and satisfies

$$\ell_s = \log(L_s) = y_s \cdot \log(\mu_s) - \mu_s - \log(y_s!),$$

where $y_s!$ is the usual factorial notation. The likelihood $L(S;\beta)$ is the product of the individual likelihood terms L_s over $s \in S$ and satisfies

$$\ell(S; \beta) = \log(L(S; \beta)) = \sum_{s \in S} \ell_s.$$

The maximum likelihood estimate $\beta(S)$ of β is computed by solving the estimating equations $\partial \ell(S;\beta)/\partial \beta = 0$ obtained by differentiating $\ell(S;\beta)$ with respect to β, where 0 denotes the zero vector. For simplicity of notation, parameter estimates $\beta(S)$ are denoted as functions of indexes for the data used in their computation without hat ($\wedge$) symbols. With this notation, the LCV formulation of Sect. 2.5.3 extends to the Poisson regression case. For $s \in S$, the estimated value for the mean μ_s of the counts y_s are $\mu_s(S) = \exp(x_s^T \cdot \beta(S) + o_{Es})$. The associated estimated rates are

$\mu_s(S)/\exp(o_{Es}) = \exp(\mathbf{x}_s^T \cdot \boldsymbol{\beta}(S))$. For incidence data like the skin cancer data, these can be converted to rates per 100,000 by multiplying them by 100,000. The corresponding residuals are $e_s(S) = y_s - \mu_s(S)$. The estimated values for the variances σ_s^2 are $\sigma_s^2(S) = \mu_s(S)$. The standardized or Pearson residuals $\text{stde}_s(S) = e_s(S)/\sigma_s(S)$ are obtained by standardizing residuals by dividing by estimated standard deviations.

The predictor vectors $\mathbf{x}_s$ can be based on fractional polynomial transforms of primary predictors as considered in analyses reported in Chaps. 2, 4, 6, 8, and 10. Adaptive fractional polynomial models can also be selected using the adaptive modeling process controlled by LCV scores as in those chapters, but with the LCV scores computed for the Poisson regression case.

12.3.2 Non-Unit Dispersions Formulation

For standard Poisson regression models, outcome measurements y_s have means μ_s and variances $V(\mu_s) = \mu_s$ equal to those means. Consequently, variances are functions of the means and not separate parameters as for the normal distribution. The deviance terms are defined as (McCullagh and Nelder 1999)

$$d(y_s; \mu_s) = 2 \cdot \left[y_s \cdot \log\left(\frac{y_s}{\mu_s}\right) - (y_s - \mu_s) \right],$$

where $0 \cdot \log(0)$ is set equal to 0. Dispersion parameters ϕ_s can be incorporated into the Poisson model through the extended quasi-likelihood terms QL_s^+ (McCullagh and Nelder 1999) satisfying

$$\ell_s^+ = \log(QL_s^+) = -\frac{1}{2} \cdot \frac{d(y_s; \mu_s)}{\phi_s} - \frac{1}{2} \cdot \log(\phi_s).$$

Let $\boldsymbol{\theta}$ denote the vector of all the parameters determining μ_s and ϕ_s for $s \in S$. Then, the extended quasi-likelihood $QL^+(S; \boldsymbol{\theta})$ satisfies

$$\ell^+(S; \boldsymbol{\theta}) = \log\left(QL^+(S; \boldsymbol{\theta})\right) = \sum_{s \in S} \ell_s^+ = \sum_{s \in S} \left(\frac{\ell_s + a_s}{\phi_s} - \frac{1}{2} \cdot \log(\phi_s) \right),$$

where ℓ_s are the log-likelihood terms defined in Sect. 12.3.1 and

$$a_s = \log(y_s!) + y_s - y_s \cdot \log(y_s)$$

for $s \in S$. Extended variances σ_s^2 incorporating the dispersions can then be defined as $\sigma_s^2 = \phi_s \cdot V(\mu_s)$.

The data are now assumed to consist of observations $O_s = (y_s, \mathbf{x}_s, o_{Es}, o_{Ds})$ for subjects $s \in S$ where o_{Ds} is an offset value for modeling the dispersions (hence the subscript "D"). While the offset for the dispersions is allowed to differ from the one for the expectations in this formulation, they will usually be the same. Assume as in Sect. 12.3.1 that $\log(\mu_s) = \mathbf{x}_s^T \cdot \boldsymbol{\beta} + o_{Es}$. Model the log of the dispersions ϕ_s as a function of selected predictor variables and associated coefficients (similarly to the way variances are modeled in Sect. 2.19.1 and dispersions are modeled in Sect. 8.13.1). Specifically, let $\log(\phi_s) = \mathbf{v}_s^T \cdot \boldsymbol{\gamma} + o_{Ds}$ where, for $s \in S$, $\mathbf{v}_s$ is a $q \times 1$ column vector of q predictor values v_{sj} (including unit predictor values if an intercept is to be included) with indexes $j \in Q = \{j : 1 \leq j \leq q\}$ and $\boldsymbol{\gamma}$ is the associated $q \times 1$ column vector of coefficients. When $\phi_s = \phi$ are constant, $\boldsymbol{\theta} = (\boldsymbol{\beta}^T, \phi)^T$, and maximizing $\ell^+(S; \boldsymbol{\theta})$ in $\boldsymbol{\theta}$ generates the same estimates $\boldsymbol{\beta}(S)$ as maximum likelihood estimation of $\boldsymbol{\beta}$ under the unit-dispersions Poisson regression model. The maximum extended quasi-likelihood estimate $\phi(S)$ of ϕ then satisfies $\phi(S) = \sum_{s \in S} d(y_s; \mu_s(S))/n$ where $\mu_s(S)$ are the estimates of μ_s determined by $\boldsymbol{\beta}(S)$. The general $(r + q) \times 1$ parameter vector $\boldsymbol{\theta} = (\boldsymbol{\beta}^T, \boldsymbol{\gamma}^T)^T$ is estimated through maximum extended quasi-likelihood estimation.

As in Sect. 12.3.1, for $s \in S$, the estimated value for the mean μ_s is $\mu_s(S) = \exp(\mathbf{x}_s^T \cdot \boldsymbol{\beta}(S) + o_{Es})$ with corresponding residual $e_s(S) = y_s - \mu_s(S)$ while the estimated value of the associated dispersions ϕ_s is $\phi_s(S) = \exp(\mathbf{v}_s^T \cdot \boldsymbol{\gamma}(S) + o_{Ds})$. These can be converted to means and dispersions for rates in the same way as means are converted to rates in Sect. 12.3.1. For incidence data like the skin cancer data these means and dispersions for rates can be converted to means and dispersions for rates per 100,000 by multiplying by 100,000. The estimated value for the extended variance σ_s^2 is $\sigma_s^2(S) = \phi_s(S) \cdot V(\mu_s(S))$. The standardized or Pearson residual $\text{stde}_s(S) = e_s(S)/\sigma_s(S)$ is obtained by standardizing the residual by dividing by the estimated extended standard deviation.

Alternative models can be compared with extended quasi-likelihood cross-validation (QLCV$^+$) scores computed as LCV scores are computed in Sect. 12.3.1, but using extended quasi-likelihoods rather than likelihoods and maximum extended quasi-likelihood estimates $\boldsymbol{\theta}(S)$ of $\boldsymbol{\theta}$ rather than maximum likelihood estimates. The adaptive modeling process can be extended to search through models for the means and dispersions in combination (see Chap. 20).

12.4   Skin Cancer Rates as a Function of the Minimum Age and City of Residence

12.4.1   Modeling Means for Skin Cancer Rates with Constant Dispersions Models

Unless otherwise stated, models considered in this section have constant dispersions, in the sense that logs of dispersions are modeled as a constant, and use the log of the population size (in the variable population) as the offsets for both the models of the means and the dispersions (so while the dispersions are based on a constant model, they are actually not constant due to including offsets). Since the sample size 15 is small, fold sizes can be relatively large. For example, for $k = 5$, fold sizes range from 1 to 5 so that the fold complement sizes can be as small as 10 or only 67 % of the sample. Estimates generated by such small subsamples may not be reliable. For that reason, leave-one-out (LOO) cross-validation is used in this chapter for model evaluation and comparison. The adaptively chosen model for cases as a function of agemin is based on the single power transform agemin$^{-0.43}$ without an intercept with LOO extended quasi-likelihood cross-validation (QLCV$^+$) score 0.11679. The model linear in agemin has QLCV$^+$ score 0.08161 with PD of 30.1 % compared to the adaptive model and so is substantial (that is, larger than the cutoff 12.0 % for the data). Consequently, the log of mean cases is distinctly nonlinear in agemin.

The adaptive constant dispersions model without offsets has the component for the means constant in agemin (that is, based on only an intercept) and with essentially zero QLCV$^+$ score. Consequently, including offsets based on population sizes in the dispersions model provides a very substantial improvement in this case. The adaptive unit-dispersions model (and also without offsets) has component for the means based on agemin$^{-0.42}$ without an intercept and LCV score (the same as its QLCV$^+$ score) only 0.00004 with extremely substantial PD rounding to 100 % compared to the constant dispersions model with offsets for the dispersions. Consequently, dispersions are more appropriately treated as constant than as unit in this case, suggesting that unit dispersions models should usually not be considered for count/rate outcomes.

How skin cancer rates depend on agemin might change with the city in which the women live (an issue called moderation or modification; see Sect. 4.5.3). This can be addressed with the adaptive model based on agemin, city, and geometric combinations (GCs) in these two predictors (see Sect. 4.6 for the definition of GCs). The generated model is based on the two transforms: agemin$^{-0.49}$ and (city·agemin$^{-0.98}$)$^{0.85}$ without an intercept and has QLCV$^+$ score 0.37479. This is a substantial improvement over the model based on only agemin, whose QLCV$^+$ score generates a substantial PD of 68.8 %. Furthermore, the additive model based on agemin and city without GCs is based on agemin$^{-0.399}$ and city without an intercept and with QLCV$^+$ score 0.28586 and substantial PD 23.7 %. Thus, the dependence of skin cancer rates on agemin is distinctly moderated by city, that is, it changes differently with the minimum age for the two cities. Estimated skin cancer rates per 100,000 women generated by the GC-based model are plotted in Fig. 12.1. The estimated skin cancer rates increase with increasing minimum age as would be expected and at a faster rate of change and to higher levels for women living in Fort Worth with more chance for exposure to the sun than for women living in St. Paul.

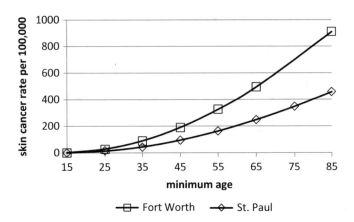

Fig. 12.1 Estimated skin cancer rates per 100,000 women as a function of minimum age in years moderated by the city in which the women reside based on adaptive Poisson regression modeling with constant dispersions

12.4.2   Modeling Dispersions as Well as Means for Skin Cancer Rates

The adaptive modeling process can be applied to model both the means and the dispersions of the outcome variable cases in combination. When this process is applied using the singleton predictor agemin for both means and dispersions, the generated model has QLCV$^+$ score 0.16946. The adaptive model with only means depending on agemin has QLCV$^+$ score 0.11679 and so with substantial PD of 31.1 %. Consequently, the dispersions change distinctly with agemin. The means in this model depend on agemin$^{-0.46}$ without an intercept while the dispersions depend on agemin$^{-0.33}$ without an intercept.

The adaptive model with means and dispersions depending on agemin, city, and GCs is a constant dispersions model and has the same model for the means as generated with constant dispersions, suggesting that the dispersions do not depend on agemin or city. The adaptive additive model with means and dispersions depending on agemin and city, but not GCs, has means based on the two transforms: agemin$^{-0.4201}$ and city without an intercept and dispersions based on the single transform: agemin$^{-0.2}$ without an intercept. Its QLCV$^+$ score is 0.49011 so that the best constant dispersions model with QLCV$^+$ score 0.37479 generates a substantial PD of 23.5 %. Consequently, dispersions for skin cancer rates are distinctly non-constant, depending on agemin but not city, and this can only be identified by consideration of additive models. Furthermore, under this model the dependence of the log of the means on agemin is not moderated by city, as suggested by constant-dispersions modeling, but does change additively with city by the same amount for all minimum ages.

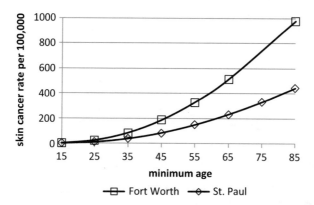

Fig. 12.2 Estimated skin cancer rates per 100,000 women as an additive function of minimum age in years and the city in which the women live based on adaptive Poisson regression modeling with non-constant dispersions

Estimated cancer rates per 100,000 women generated by the additive non-constant dispersions model are plotted in Fig. 12.2. As before the estimated cancer rates increase with increasing minimum age and at a faster rate of change and to higher levels for women living in Fort Worth than for women living in St. Paul. Compared to the estimates in Fig. 12.1, the estimated cancer rates increase to a higher rate at the oldest minimum age of 85 years for women in Fort Worth but to a similar rate for women in St. Paul. Estimated dispersions for skin cancer rates per 100,000 are plotted in Fig. 12.3. They change in the same way for both cities and increase nonlinearly with the minimum age but at faster rates of change for older minimum ages.

12.5   Overview of Analyses of Skin Cancer Rates

1. For the skin cancer rates (Sect. 12.2), analyses use LOO QLCV^{+} (Sect. 12.4.1).
2. Models for skin cancer rates based on constant dispersions with offsets are distinctly better than models based on constant dispersions without offsets and on unit dispersions without offsets (this and the following results reported in Sect. 12.4.1). Using constant dispersions with offsets, the effect of minimum age on skin cancer rates is distinctly moderated by city. Results are displayed in Fig. 12.1.
3. Using non-constant dispersions with offsets, the effect of minimum age on skin cancer rates is not distinctly moderated by city but city has a main effect. Dispersions change with minimum age in the same way for both cities. Results are displayed in Figs. 12.2 and 12.3. See Sect. 13.4 for a residual analysis for this model .

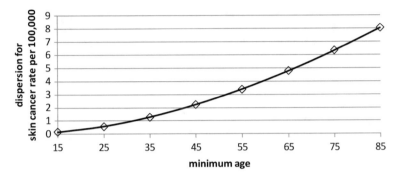

Fig. 12.3 Estimated dispersions for skin cancer rates per 100,000 as a function of minimum age in years based on adaptive Poisson regression modeling

12.6   Chapter Summary

This chapter presents a series of analyses of the skin cancer incidence data. These analyses address how skin cancer rates for women in St. Paul, Minnesota and Fort Worth, Texas depend on the their age and city of residence. Using constant dispersions with offsets, the logs of the mean skin cancer rates depend distinctly nonlinearly on the age of the women, and this relationship changes with the city in which they reside (a moderation effect). Moreover, non-constant dispersions with offsets are more appropriate for these data. The logs of the mean cancer rates still change with the age of the women, but following the same pattern with age and shifted up for Fort Worth compared to St. Paul, rather than following different patterns for the two cities as suggested by constant dispersions modeling.

These analyses demonstrate adaptive Poisson regression modeling of univariate count outcomes, possibly adjusted to rates using offsets, with fractional polyno-mials, including modeling of only the means as well as modeling of dispersions as well as means. The chapter also provides formulations for Poisson regression models; for k-fold likelihood cross-validation (LCV) scores for unit dispersions models; for extended quasi-likelihood cross-validation (QLCV$^+$) scores for non-unit dispersions models based on extended quasi-likelihoods; and for residuals and standardized (or Pearson) residuals. The example analyses demonstrate assessing whether the logs of the means of an outcome are nonlinear in individual predictors, whether the relationships are better addressed with multiple predictors in combination compared to using singleton predictors, whether the relationships are additive in predictors, whether the predictors interact using geometric combi-nations, and whether there is a benefit to considering constant dispersions compared to unit dispersions and non-constant dispersions compared to constant dispersions. Example residual analyses are not reported in this chapter. See Chap. 13 for a description of how to conduct analyses of univariate count/rate outcomes in SAS including an example residual analysis.

References

McCullagh, P., & Nelder, J. A. (1999). *Generalized linear models* (2nd ed.). Boca Raton, FL: Chapman & Hall/CRC.

Stokes, M. E., Davis, C. S., & Koch, G. G. (2012). *Categorical data analysis using the SAS system* (3rd ed.). Cary, NC: SAS Institute.

Zelterman, D. (2002). *Advanced log-linear models using SAS*. Cary, NC: SAS Institute.

Chapter 13
Adaptive Poisson Regression Modeling of Univariate Count Outcomes in SAS

13.1   Chapter Overview

This chapter describes how to use the genreg macro for adaptive Poisson regression modeling as described in Chap. 12 and its generated output in the special case of univariate count/rate outcomes. Familiarity with the use of the genreg macro as presented in Chap. 3 is assumed. See Supplementary Materials for a more complete description of this macro. See Stokes et al. (2012) and Zelterman (2002) for details on standard approaches for Poisson regression modeling in SAS. Section 13.2 provides a description of the skin cancer data analyzed in Chap. 12. Section 13.3 provides code for modeling means for skin cancer rates in terms of age and city of residence of the women in the study while Sect. 13.4 provides code for modeling both means and dispersions of these skin cancer rates.

13.2   Loading in the Skin Cancer Data

Analyses are conducted in Chap. 12 of skin cancer rates for $n = 15$ counts in the variable cases of skin cancer occurrences for population groups of women of sizes in the variable population categorized by the minimum age in the variable minage and city of residence in the variable city (see Sect. 12.2). Assume that these skin cancer data have been loaded into the default library (for example, by importing them from a spreadsheet file) under the name skin. An output title line, selected system options, labels for the variables, and formats for values of selected variables can be assigned as follows.

```
options nodate pageno=1 pagesize=53 linesize=76;
title1 "Skin Cancer Data";
```

© Springer International Publishing Switzerland 2016   265
G.J. Knafl, K. Ding, *Adaptive Regression for Modeling Nonlinear Relationships*,
Statistics for Biology and Health, DOI 10.1007/978-3-319-33946-7_13

```
proc format;
 value cityfmt 0="St Paul" 1="Forth Worth";
run;
data skin;
 set skin;
 xoffset=log(population);
 voffset=log(population);
 label
    cases="Number of Skin Cancer Cases" city="City"
    agemin="Minimum Age in Population" population="Population Size"
    xoffset="Expectation Offset Variable"
    voffset="Dispersion Offset Variable"
 ;
 format city cityfmt.;
run;
```

A format is created with PROC FORMAT for the two values of the variable city and assigned with the format statement in the data step. The offset variables xoffset and voffset for the means ("x") and dispersions ("v"), respectively, are both computed as logs of population sizes in the variable population. This converts Poisson regression models for skin cancer counts into models for the associated skin cancer rates. The cutoff for a substantial percent decrease (PD) for analyses of cases with 15 observations is 12.0 % (as reported in Sect. 12.2).

13.3   Modeling Means for Skin Cancer Rates

Assuming that the genreg macro has been loaded into SAS (see Supplementary Materials), an adaptive model for cases as a function of agemin with a constant dispersions model using a leave-one-out (LOO) extended quasi-likelihood cross-validation (QLCV$^+$) can be generated as follows.

```
%genreg(modtype=poiss,datain=skin,yvar=cases,
        xoffstvr=xoffset,voffstvr=voffset,foldcnt=,
        LOO=y,expand=y,expxvars=agemin,contract=y);
```

The parameter setting "modtype=poiss" requests a Poisson regression model. The datain parameter specifies the input data set, in this case the skin data set. The yvar parameter specifies the count outcome variable, in this case the variable cases. The xoffset and voffset parameters specify the offset variables for the expectation and dispersion models, respectively. The base models for both the means and dispersions by default are both constant, intercept-only models plus associated offsets. The parameter setting "LOO=y" requests a LOO QLCV$^+$ (because the default setting "vintrcpt=y" requests a constant dispersions model). It requires the empty setting "foldcnt=" for the foldcnt parameter (or the setting "foldcnt=."). This is used to maximize the sizes of the fold complements at 14 each to avoid deleted parameter estimates based on even smaller subsets of the data. The parameter setting "expand=y" requests that the base model be expanded. The model for the means is expanded by adding in transforms of primary predictor variables listed in the setting for the expxvars parameter. In this case, only agemin is considered for expansion. The model for the dispersions is not changed since the expvvars macro parameter has its default empty setting. The parameter setting "contract=y" requests that the expanded model be contracted. Parameters like xintrcpt, xvars, xoffset, and expxvars are used to control settings for the mean, expectation or "x" component of the model while corresponding parameters like vintrcpt, vvars, voffset, and expvvars are used to control the variance/dispersion or "v" component of the model (see Sect. 13.4).

The expanded model generated by the above code has means based on the single transform $agemin^{-0.5}$ with LOO QLCV$^+$ score 0.10124. The contraction removes the intercept for the means, adjusts the remaining transform to $agemin^{-0.43}$ with QLCV$^+$ score 0.11679 (as also reported in Sect. 12.4.1), which is a substantial improvement on the expanded model with PD 13.3 % (that is, larger than the cutoff of 12.0 % for the data). This latter model is also the adaptive monotonic model for these data since it is based on a single transform of agemin. Note that this is an example of a zero-intercept adaptive model distinctly improving on a nonzero-intercept adaptive model.

The RA1compare macro (see Sect. 3.8) can be used to compare adaptive models for count/rate outcomes to models based on the recommended degree 1 set of powers (Sect. 2.12) as follows.

```
%RA1compare(modtype=poiss,datain=skin,yvar=cases,xvar=agemin,
            xoffstvr=xoffset,voffstvr=voffset,foldcnt=,LOO=y,
            scorefmt=9.7);
```

The modtype, datain, yvar, xoffset, voffset, foldcnt, and LOO macro parameters have the same meaning as for the genreg macro. The xvar macro parameter is like the xvars macro parameter of genreg, but it can only specify a single predictor variable for the means. The scorefmt macro parameter requests that QLCV$^+$ scores generated by RA1compare be formatted with the SAS w.d format (where w is the width and d is the number of decimal digits) with value 9.7, that is, with scores printed out in 9 character positions and rounded to 7 decimal digits. The power generating the best QLCV$^+$ score among recommended degree 1 powers is -0.5, and so the same as the adaptive expanded model based on $agemin^{-0.5}$ with an intercept. Consequently, the adaptive monotonic model provides a distinct improvement over this best recommended degree 1 power.

The RA2compare macros (see Sect. 3.9) can be used to compare adaptive models for count/rate outcomes to models based on the recommended degree 2 set of powers (Sect. 2.13). Just change "RA1" to "RA2" in the above code, leaving everything else the same. The powers generating the best QLCV$^+$ score among recommended degree 2 powers are -2 and -1 with QLCV$^+$ score 0.09385 and even larger PD of 19.6 % over the adaptive monotonic model. Consequently, the adaptive monotonic model also provides a distinct improvement over this best pair of recommended degree 2 powers. Since the recommended degree 2 models include products of power transforms of agemin and its log, the adaptive model generated by RA2compare is based on agemin, log(agemin), and geometric combinations (GCs; see Sect. 4.5.4) between these two primary predictors. Since the recommended degree 2 powers are based on products of at most 2 transforms, RA2compare restricts the search to GCs based on products of only 2 transforms. This is achieved by including the setting "maxterms=2" in the RA2compare call to genreg. By default, the maxterms parameter has an empty setting, meaning any number of transforms can be included in GCs. The maxterms parameter can be used in general to reduce the complexity of generated GCs and so improve the interpretability of associated models. The generated model in this case has means based on the single transform $(\log(agemin))^{-1.7}$ with QLCV$^+$ score 0.11683. The adaptive model in agemin, not considering its log transform, has competitive QLCV$^+$ score 0.11679 with insubstantial PD 0.03 %.

The linear polynomial model in agemin can be generated as follows using the xvars parameter.

```
%genreg(modtype=poiss,datain=skin,yvar=cases,xoffstvr=xoffset,
        voffstvr=voffset,foldcnt=,LOO=y,xvars=agemin);
```

An adaptive model with constant dispersions but no offset variable for the dispersions can be generated as follows by removing the setting "voffstvr=voffset" so that the voffstvr parameter has its default empty setting.

```
%genreg(modtype=poiss,datain=skin,yvar=cases,xoffstvr=xoffset,
        foldcnt=,LOO=y,expand=y,expxvars=agemin,contract=y);
```

An adaptive model for the means in agemin with unit dispersions can be generated as follows by adding the setting "vintrcpt=n".

```
%genreg(modtype=poiss,datain=skin,yvar=cases,
        xoffstvr=xoffset,vintrcpt=n,foldcnt=,LOO=y,
        expand=y,expxvars=agemin,contract=y);
```

An adaptive model in agemin, city, and GCs in these two predictors with constant dispersions plus offsets can be generated as follows.

```
%genreg(modtype=poiss,datain=skin,yvar=cases,
        xoffstvr=xoffset,voffstvr=voffset,foldcnt=,
        LOO=y,expand=y,expxvars=agemin city,geomcmbn=y,
        contract=y);
```

GCs are requested with the "geomcmbn=y" setting. The default setting "geomcmbn=n" is used to generate an additive model in agemin and city. The base constant plus offsets model has LOO QLCV$^+$ score 0.04052 (output not reported). The expansion adds in the transforms: $\text{agemin}^{-0.5}$, $(\text{city} \cdot \text{agemin}^{-0.98})^{0.89}$, and $\text{city} \cdot \text{agemin}^{-2.9}$ in that order with final QLCV$^+$ score 0.30490. The contraction first removes $\text{city} \cdot \text{agemin}^{-2.9}$, then the intercept, and stops adjusting the powers for the remaining transforms to $\text{agemin}^{-0.49}$ and $(\text{city} \cdot \text{agemin}^{-0.98})^{0.85}$. This final model has QLCV$^+$ score 0.37479 as also reported in Sect. 12.4.1.

13.4 Modeling Dispersions as Well as Means for Skin Cancer Rates

Both the dispersions and means for skin cancer rates can be modeled in terms of agemin, city, and GCs as follows.

```
%genreg(modtype=poiss,datain=skin,yvar=cases,
        xoffstvr=xoffset,voffstvr=voffset,foldcnt=,
        LOO=y,expand=y,expxvars=agemin city,
        expvvars=agemin city,geomcmbn=y,contract=y);
```

The expvvars macro parameter provides a list of primary predictors to consider for modeling variances for the normal distribution case and dispersions for other cases like Poisson regression. In the above code, the list is the same as for expxvars, but it can be different. The genreg macro supports several other parameters for controlling the variances/dispersions including vvars, vpowers, vintrcpt, vgcs, and vgcpowrs which work like xvars, xpowers, xintrcpt, xgcs, and xgcpowrs, but address the model for the log of the variances/dispersions (the "v" part of the model) rather than the model for the log of the means (or the expectations or the "x" part of the model). The default settings of "xintrcpt=y" and "vintrcpt=y" are requested in the above code to start the search at the model with constant means and dispersions, both with offsets.

The base model is generated first with constant means and dispersions plus offsets and QLCV$^+$ score 0.04052. Table 13.1 contains part of the output describing the expanded model. The component of the model for the log of the expectations or means is described first. It is based on an intercept parameter (denoted as XINTRCPT) together with the transforms $\text{agemin}^{-0.5}$, $(\text{city} \cdot \text{agemin}^{-0.98})^{0.89}$, and $\text{city} \cdot \text{agemin}^{-2.9}$. The component of the model for the log of the dispersions is described next. It is based on only an intercept parameter (denoted as VINTRCPT). The order that terms are added into the model is indicated in the output. The two intercept terms have order 0 indicating they were in the base model. The three transforms for the log expectation component are the terms added to the model in the order they are listed in the output and then the expansion stops. The QLCV$^+$ score for the expanded model rounds to 0.30490.

Table 13.1 Expanded model for skin cancer rates as a function of the minimum age, city of residence, and geometric combinations

```
                               expanded model

                geometric combination log expectation variables:
                        XGC_1    city*agemin**(-0.98)
                        XGC_2    city*agemin**(-2.9)
...

                       expanded log expectation component

  predictor      power              estimate           score       order

  XINTRCPT         1              -0.382589          0.0405185        0
  agemin          -0.5           -45.23658           0.1012383        1
  XGC_1            0.89           27.307113           0.3249203        2
  XGC_2            1            -4135.521             0.3048965        3

                       expanded log dispersion component

  predictor      power              estimate           score       order

  VINTRCPT         1              -11.22219           0.0405185        0
...
mth root of quasi+ likelihood using deleted predictions:   0.3048965
```

The contraction (see Table 13.2) removes the transform $city \cdot agemin^{-2.9}$ from the log expectation component, followed by the intercept (XINTRCPT), and then stops. The log expectation component is based on the two transforms: $agemin^{-0.49}$ and $(city \cdot agemin^{-0.98})^{0.85}$ with somewhat adjusted powers. The log dispersion component remains unchanged. The $QLCV^+$ score rounds to 0.37479. This is the same model generated with constant dispersions modeling.

An adaptive additive model in agemin and city, that is, without GCs, can be generated as follows using the default setting "geomcmbn=n".

```
%genreg(modtype=poiss,datain=skin,yvar=cases,
        xoffstvr=xoffset,voffstvr=voffset,foldcnt=,
        LOO=y,expand=y,expxvars=agemin city,
        expvvars=agemin city,contract=y);
```

The expanded model includes the two transforms for the means: $agemin^{-0.5}$ and city along with the one transform for the dispersions: $agemin^{0.5}$. The $QLCV^+$ score is 0.36254. The contraction removes the intercept for the means, followed by the intercept for the dispersions, and then stops. The contracted model is based on two transforms for the means: $agemin^{-0.4201}$ and city without an intercept and one transform for the dispersions: $agemin^{-0.2}$ also without an intercept The $QLCV^+$ score is 0.49011 so that the best constant dispersions model (the same as the one in Table 13.2) generates a substantial PD 23.5 % as also reported in Sect. 12.4.2.

Table 13.2 Contracted model for skin cancer rates as a function of the minimum age, city of residence, and geometric combinations

	contracted log expectation component		
predictor	old power	new power	estimate
agemin	-0.5	-0.49	-46.38243
XGC_1	0.89	0.85	22.259312
discarded	old power	score	order
	.	0.3048965	0
XGC_2	1	0.3923262	1
XINTRCPT	1	0.3747876	2
	contracted log dispersion component		
predictor	old power	new power	estimate
VINTRCPT	1	1	-10.9753
	log dispersion component unchanged		

...

mth root of quasi+ likelihood using deleted predictions: 0.3747876

Residual analyses can be conducted for adaptive Poisson regression models. The genreg macro generates standardized or Pearson residuals for these models as defined for unit dispersions models in Sect. 12.3.1 and for non-unit dispersions models in Sect. 12.3.2. These are loaded into a variable named stdres in a data set called dataout (along with a variety of other generated variables; see Supplementary Materials). The name of the variable can be changed with the stdrsvar parameter and the name of the data set with the dataout parameter.

A residual analysis can be requested for the adaptive additive model in agemin city with the best overall QLCV$^+$ score as follows.

```
%genreg(modtype=poiss,datain=skin,yvar=cases,
        xoffstvr=xoffset,voffstvr=voffset,foldcnt=,LOO=y,
        xintrcpt=n,xvars=agemin city,xpowers=-0.4301 1,
        vintrcpt=n,vvars=agemin,vpowers=-0.2,ranlysis=y);
```

The plot for this model of the standardized residuals versus agemin is displayed in Fig. 13.1, distinguishing between observations from the two cities. The standardized residuals are all with ± 2 except for a value of -3.08 for minimum age 15 years in St. Paul. A sensitivity analysis (see Sects. 5.3.3 and 5.4.2 for examples) could be conducted to see if the inclusion of this observation has highly influenced the results, but that is not addressed here for brevity.

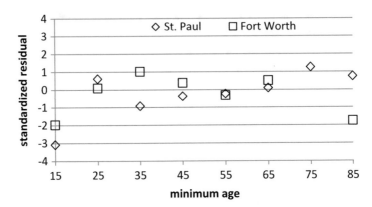

Fig. 13.1 Standardized residuals versus minimum age by city of residence for the adaptive additive model of means and dispersions for skin cancer rates as a function of minimum age in years and city of residence

The dataout data set also contains a variable named yhat (whose name is determined by the yhatvar macro parameter) containing, in the Poisson regression context, estimated mean counts and a variable named vhat (whose name is determined by the vhatvar macro parameter) containing, in the Poisson regression context, estimated dispersions for counts. When there are nonzero offsets, these variables need adjustment to generate estimated means (as in Figs. 12.1 and 12.2) and estimated dispersions (as in Fig. 12.3) for associated rates. For the skin cancer data, this can be accomplished as follows.

```
data adjusted;
  set dataout;
  adjyhat=yhat/population;
  adjvhat=vhat/population;
run;
proc plot data=adjusted;
  plot adjyhat*agemin=city;
  plot adjvhat*agemin=city;
  format city;
run;
```

The y-axes of the two plots generated in the above code are based on estimated means and dispersions for skin cancer rates, respectively, while the x-axes are based on minimum age values. The plotted points will be either 0 for observations from St. Paul or 1 for observations from Fort Worth because the variable city is listed on the right hand side of the equal sign (=) in the two plot statements. Values of 0 and 1 are used because the format command turned off the format for the variable city temporarily for the execution of the PROC PLOT step, meaning use actual values of the city variable in the plots. If the format statement is removed, the first letters "S" and "F" of the formatted values are used instead. The data used in these plots can be exported to a spreadsheet (like Excel if working in Windows) and used to generate a more sophisticated plot (as were the plots of Figs. 12.1, 12.2, and 12.3). The plots generated above are for rates per person while the plots of Figs. 12.1, 12.2, and 12.3 are for rates per 100,000. These latter rates can be obtained by multiplying the above rates by 100,000.

13.5 Practice Exercises

13.1. Models for skin cancer rates considered in Chaps. 12 and 13 treat the minimum age as a continuous predictor and so are regression models. It is possible that minimum age might be more appropriately modeled as an analysis of variance (ANOVA) factor. Assume that indicator variables amin15, amin25, $\cdots$, amin85 for agemin having respective values 15, 25, $\cdots$, 85 years exist in the skin cancer data set (for example, amin15 is created with the command "amin15=(agemin=15);"). In all analyses, use LOO QLCV$^+$ starting from the model with constant means with offset variable xoffset and constant dispersions with offset variable voffset. First, generate the adaptive ANOVA model in minimum age for both means and dispersions. Do this using as expansion variables the indicator variables amin15, amin25, $\cdots$, amin65, and amin85 thereby treating the reference category as a minimum age of 75 years since it has a missing value for St. Paul. Next, generate the adaptive additive ANOVA model for both means and dispersions using as expansion variables the indicator variables amin15, amin25, $\cdots$, amin65, amin85, and city. Finally, generate the adaptive ANOVA model for both means and dispersions using as expansion variables the indicator variables amin15, amin25, $\cdots$, amin65, amin85, city, and GCs. Which of these three alternative adaptive ANOVA models generates the best QLCV$^+$ score? Do any of the other adaptive ANOVA models generate competitive QLCV$^+$ scores? Compare the adaptive ANOVA model with the best QLCV$^+$ score to the adaptive regression model in agemin with the best QLCV$^+$ score of Sect. 13.4. Does adaptive ANOVA modeling or adaptive regression modeling generate distinctly more effective models for the skin cancer data or are they equally effective (in the sense that the smaller of the best QLCV$^+$ scores for the two cases generates a competitive PD compared to the larger QLCV$^+$ score)?

For Practice Exercises 13.2–13.3, use the lung cancer data available on the Internet (see Supplementary Materials). There are 36 observations. The outcome variable for this data set is called dead and contains counts of deaths within population groups of sizes in the variable population. The predictors to be considered are the minimum age for the groups with values 40, 45, $\cdots$, 80 years in the variable agemin and the indicator smoker for individuals in the groups being smokers or not. For all models use offsets for means and dispersions set equal to the logs of population sizes so that the Poisson regression models for lung cancer death counts are converted into models for lung cancer death rates. The data set created with the code available on the Internet contains the variables xoffset and voffset loaded with these offset values.

13.2. For the lung cancer data, use as the benchmark analysis to set the number of folds for QLCV$^+$ scores the adaptive model for the means of the lung cancer death rates as a function of minimum age in the variable agemin. Use constant dispersions with offsets for all analyses of this practice exercise. Use the number of folds determined in this first analysis for all other analyses of this practice exercise. Compare the adaptive model in minimum age to the linear polynomial model for the means in age and assess whether logs of mean lung cancer death rates change distinctly nonlinearly or not. Generate the adaptive additive model for the means in agemin and smoker and the adaptive moderation model for the means in agemin, smoker, and GCs. Assess whether or not smoker distinctly moderates (see Sect. 4.5.3) the effect of agemin on mean lung cancer death rates. Describe how means for lung cancer death rates change with the predictors of the most preferable constant dispersions with offsets model generated in this practice analysis.

13.3. For all analyses of this practice exercise, use the number of folds for QLCV$^+$ scores determined in Practice Exercise 13.2. Start all adaptive analyses using the base model with constant means and constant dispersions, both with offsets. Generate the adaptive model for the means and the dispersions in agemin by itself, the adaptive additive model for the means and the dispersions in agemin and smoker, and the adaptive moderation model for the means and the dispersions in agemin, smoker, and GCs. Compare these three models for the means and dispersions to assess whether or not consideration of smoker along with agemin provides a substantial improvement over just using agemin and whether or not smoker distinctly moderates (see Sect. 4.5.3) the effect of age on the lung cancer death rates. Compare the model for this practice exercise having the largest QLCV$^+$ score to the model for the means with constant dispersions plus offsets having the largest QLCV$^+$ score of the models considered in Practice Exercise 13.2 to assess whether dispersions for the lung cancer death rates have a distinct impact on lung cancer rates.

References

Stokes, M. E., Davis, C. S., & Koch, G. G. (2012). *Categorical data analysis using the SAS system* (3rd ed.). Cary, NC: SAS Institute.
Zelterman, D. (2002). *Advanced log-linear models using SAS*. Cary, NC: SAS Institute.

Chapter 14
Adaptive Poisson Regression Modeling of Multivariate Count Outcomes

14.1 Chapter Overview

This chapter formulates and demonstrates adaptive fractional polynomial modeling of means and dispersions for repeatedly measured count outcomes, possibly converted to rates using offsets. A description of how to generate these models in SAS is provided in Chap. 15. Standard models for this context are addressed in several texts (e.g., Fitzmaurice et al. 2011; Molenberghs and Verbeke 2006).

Marginal modeling extends from the multivariate normal outcome context (see Sect. 4.3) to the multivariate count/rate outcome context. However, due to the complexity in general of computing likelihoods and quasi-likelihoods (as needed to account for non-unit dispersions) for general multivariate marginal modeling, generalized estimating equations (GEE) techniques (Liang and Zeger 1986) are often used instead, thereby avoiding computation of likelihoods and quasi-likelihoods. This complicates the extension of adaptive modeling to the GEE context since it is based on cross-validation (CV) scores computed from likelihoods or likelihood-like functions (but see Sect. 14.5). Conditional modeling also extends to the multivariate count/rate outcome context, both transition modeling (see Sect. 4.7) and general conditional modeling (see Sect. 4.9). In contrast to marginal GEE-based modeling, conditional modeling of means for multivariate count/rate outcomes with unit dispersions is based on pseudolikelihoods that can be used to compute pseudolikelihood CV (PLCV) scores on which to base adaptive modeling of multivariate count/rate outcomes. For this reason, conditional modeling is considered first. PLCV scores are the same as LCV scores for transition models, but not in general. Conditional modeling involving non-unit dispersions is based on extended pseudolikelihoods and extended PLCV (PLCV$^+$) scores. For transition models, PLCV$^+$ scores are the same as their extended quasi-likelihood CV (QLCV$^+$) scores (see Sect. 12.3.2).

Section 14.2 describes a dataset with longitudinal count outcome containing seizure counts/rates for 59 epileptics over time. Section 14.3 formulates conditional modeling, including both transition and general conditional modeling, for

© Springer International Publishing Switzerland 2016
G.J. Knafl, K. Ding, *Adaptive Regression for Modeling Nonlinear Relationships*,
Statistics for Biology and Health, DOI 10.1007/978-3-319-33946-7_14

multivariate count/rate outcomes. Section 14.4 then presents analyses of the seizure rates per week, but using only transition modeling since that is more appropriate for such longitudinal data than general conditional modeling. Section 14.5 formulates adaptive GEE-based modeling of multivariate count/rate outcomes. Section 14.6 then presents adaptive GEE analyses of seizure rates per week. Section 14.7 provides an overview of the results of analysis of post-baseline seizure rates. Formulation sections are not needed to understand analysis sections.

14.2   The Epileptic Seizures Data

A data set on seizure counts at baseline and at four post-baseline clinic visits for 59 patients with epilepsy is available on the Internet (see Supplementary Materials). These data were analyzed and first published by Thall and Vail (1990). The outcome variable count contains numbers of seizures. The possible predictor variables for the post-baseline counts are visit (with values 1–4), rate0 (the baseline seizure rate per week, based on a period of 8 weeks), and int (the indicator for the patient being in the intervention group given the antiepileptic drug progabide as opposed to the control group given a placebo). The associated numbers of weeks for the seizure counts are loaded into the variable dltatime, but all post-baseline periods are 2 weeks long. The offsets log(dltatime) are used to convert Poisson regression models for seizure counts into models for seizure rates per week, but these are equivalent since all post-baseline measurement periods have the same length. Age at baseline is also available in the data set, but is not considered here. There are a total of 236 post-baseline outcome measurements with four measurements available for each patient, and so none missing. The outcome variable post-baseline seizure rate is analyzed in this chapter to demonstrate how to conduct Poisson regression analyses using transition as well as adaptive GEE-based models accounting for nonlinearity in predictor variables for log-transformed means and dispersions.

The cutoff for a substantial percent decrease (PD) in the LCV scores (see Sect. 4.4.2 for the formula) for the 236 post-baseline seizure rates per week is 0.81 %. Reported CV scores are based on matched-set-wise deletion (Sect. 4.4.1) since there are no missing outcome measurements.

14.3   Conditional Modeling of Multivariate Count Outcomes

This section formulates conditional modeling in the multivariate count/rate outcome context, first with unit dispersions in Sect. 14.3.1 and then more general dispersions in Sect. 14.3.2. It can be skipped to focus on analyses.

14.3.1 Conditional Modeling of Means Assuming Unit Dispersions

Using the notation of Sects. 4.3, 4.7, and 4.9.1, for n matched sets of measurements with indexes $s \in S = \{s : 1 \leq s \leq n\}$, observed data $O_{s,C(s)} = (\mathbf{y}_{s,C(s)}, \mathbf{X}_{s,C(s)}, \mathbf{o}_{Es,C(s)})$ are available for possibly different sets C(s) of measurement conditions, subsets of the maximal set of possible conditions $C = \{c : 1 \leq c \leq m\}$, consisting of outcome vectors $\mathbf{y}_{s,C(s)}$ with m(s) count entries y_{sc} for $c \in C(s)$, predictor matrices $\mathbf{X}_{s,C(s)}$ having m(s) rows $\mathbf{x}_{sc}^T$ with entries x_{scj} for $j \in J = \{j : 1 \leq j \leq r\}$ and for $c \in C(s)$, and expectation offset vectors $\mathbf{o}_{Es,C(s)}$ with m(s) entries o_{Esc} for $c \in C(s)$. The observed conditional data then consist of $O_{sc}^\# = (y_{sc}^\#, \mathbf{x}_{sc}, o_{Esc})$ for the m(SC) measurements $sc \in SC = \{sc : c \in C(s), s \in S\}$ where $y_{sc}^\# = y_{sc} | \mathbf{y}_{s,C(s) \setminus \{c\}}$ is the cth outcome measurement for matched set s conditioned on the other outcome measurements for that matched set. The dependence of the rates $y_{sc}^\# / \exp(o_{Esc})$ (or counts $y_{sc}^\#$ when o_{Esc} always equals 0) on the other outcome measurements is modeled using averages PRE(y,i,j) and associated missing indicators PRE(y,i,j,$\varnothing$) (see Sect. 4.7) of prior outcome rate measurements, averages POST(y,i,j) and associated missing indicators POST(y,i,j,$\varnothing$) (see Sect. 4.9.1) of subsequent outcome rate measurements, and averages OTHER(y,i,j) and associated missing indicators OTHER(y,i,j,$\varnothing$) (see Sect. 4.9.1) of prior and subsequent outcome rate measurements, for $1 \leq i \leq j \leq m$. Note that outcome rates are used to compute these dependence predictors to account for offset values and not the counts unless the offset values are all zero. To simplify the notation, the predictor matrices $\mathbf{X}_{s,C(s)}$ are assumed to include columns containing observed values for dependence predictors as well as columns for non-dependence predictors. The special case of transition modeling corresponds to cases with dependence based only on prior outcome measurements. Note that dependence predictors can also be computed from prior values of time-varying predictors.

For $sc \in SC$, the mean or expected value $Ey_{sc}^\# = \mu_{sc}^\#$ for $y_{sc}^\#$ is modeled as $\log(\mu_{sc}^\#) = \mathbf{x}_{sc}^T \cdot \boldsymbol{\beta} + o_{Esc}$ for a $r \times 1$ vector $\boldsymbol{\beta}$ of coefficients. Solving for $\mu_{sc}^\#$ gives $\mu_{sc}^\# = \exp(\mathbf{x}_{sc}^T \cdot \boldsymbol{\beta} + o_{Esc})$. The conditional variance for $y_{sc}^\#$ is $\sigma_{sc}^{\#2} = \mu_{sc}^\#$.

The pseudolikelihood term PL_{sc} for the scth measurement equals the conditional likelihood $L(O_{sc}^\#; \boldsymbol{\beta})$ for the conditional observation $O_{sc}^\#$ and satisfies

$$\ell_{sc} = \log(PL_{sc}) = y_{sc}^\# \cdot \log(\mu_{sc}^\#) - \mu_{sc}^\# - \log(y_{sc}^\#!),$$

where $y_{sc}^\#!$ is the usual factorial notation. The pseudolikelihood PL(SC; $\boldsymbol{\beta}$) is the product of the pseudolikelihood terms PL_{sc} over $sc \in SC$ and satisfies

$$\ell(SC; \boldsymbol{\beta}) = \log(PL(SC; \boldsymbol{\beta})) = \sum_{sc \in SC} \ell_{sc}.$$

The maximum pseudolikelihood estimate $\boldsymbol{\beta}(SC)$ of $\boldsymbol{\beta}$ is computed by solving the estimating equations $\partial \ell(SC; \boldsymbol{\beta})/\partial \boldsymbol{\beta} = \mathbf{0}$ obtained by differentiating $\ell(SC; \boldsymbol{\beta})$ with respect to $\boldsymbol{\beta}$, where $\mathbf{0}$ denotes the zero vector. For simplicity of notation, parameter estimates $\boldsymbol{\beta}(SC)$ are denoted as functions of indexes for the data used in their computation without hat ($\wedge$) symbols. With this notation, the matched-set-wise deletion PLCV formulation of Sect. 4.9.1 and the measurement-wise deletion version of Sect. 4.13 both extend to the multivariate count/rate outcome Poisson regression context. For transition models, the pseudolikelihood is a true likelihood and PLCV scores are also LCV scores.

For $sc \in SC$,   the   estimated   value   for   the   mean $\mu^{\#}_{sc}$ is $\mu^{\#}_{sc}(SC) = \exp(\mathbf{x}_{sc}^{T} \cdot \boldsymbol{\beta}(SC) + o_{Esc})$ and the corresponding residual is $e^{\#}_{sc}(SC) = y^{\#}_{sc} - \mu^{\#}_{sc}(SC)$. The estimated value for the variance $\sigma^{\#}_{sc}{}^{2}$ is $\sigma^{\#}_{sc}{}^{2}(SC) = \mu^{\#}_{sc}(SC)$. The standardized or Pearson residual $stde^{\#}_{sc}(SC) = e^{\#}_{sc}(SC)/\sigma^{\#}_{sc}(SC)$ is obtained by standardizing the residual by dividing by the estimated standard deviation.

The predictor vectors $\mathbf{x}_{sc}$ can be based on fractional polynomial transforms of primary predictors of non-dependence type as considered in analyses reported in Chaps. 2, 4, 6, 8, 10, and 12 and of dependence type as considered in analyses of Chaps. 4, 6, 10, and 12. Adaptive fractional polynomial conditional models can be selected using the adaptive modeling process controlled by PLCV scores as in Chap. 12, but with the PLCV scores computed for the Poisson regression case.

14.3.2 Conditional Modeling of Dispersions as Well as Means

Extending the notation of Sect. 12.3.2, conditional count outcome measurements $y^{\#}_{sc}$ with nonnegative integer values have means $\mu^{\#}_{sc}$ and variances $V(\mu^{\#}_{sc}) = \mu^{\#}_{sc}$. The deviance terms are defined as (McCullagh and Nelder 1999)

$$d(y^{\#}_{sc}; \mu^{\#}_{sc}) = 2 \cdot \left[y^{\#}_{sc} \cdot \log\left(\frac{y^{\#}_{sc}}{\mu^{\#}_{sc}}\right) - (y^{\#}_{sc} - \mu^{\#}_{sc}) \right],$$

where $0 \cdot \log(0)$ is set equal to 0. Dispersion parameters $\phi^{\#}_{sc}$ can be incorporated into the conditional Poisson model through the extended quasi-pseudolikelihood terms $PL_{sc}{}^{+}$ satisfying

$$\ell_{sc}{}^{+} = \log(PL_{sc}{}^{+}) = -\frac{1}{2} \cdot \frac{d(y^{\#}_{sc}; \mu^{\#}_{sc})}{\phi^{\#}_{sc}} - \frac{1}{2} \cdot \log(\phi^{\#}_{sc}).$$

Let $\boldsymbol{\theta}$ denote the vector of all the parameters determining $\mu^{\#}_{sc}$ and $\phi^{\#}_{sc}$ for $sc \in SC$. Then, the extended quasi-pseudolikelihood $PL^{+}(SC; \boldsymbol{\theta})$ satisfies

$$\ell^+(SC; \boldsymbol{\theta}) = \log(PL^+(SC; \boldsymbol{\theta}))$$

$$= \sum_{s \in SC} \ell_{sc}^+ = \sum_{sc \in SC} \left(\frac{\ell_{sc} + a_{sc}^\#}{\phi_{sc}^\#} - \frac{1}{2} \cdot \log(\phi_{sc}^\#) \right),$$

where $\ell_{sc} = y_{sc}^\# \cdot \log(\mu_{sc}^\#) - \mu_{sc}^\# - \log(y_{sc}^\#!)$ are the usual log pseudolikelihood terms and

$$a_{sc}^\# = \log(y_{sc}^\#!) + y_{sc}^\# - y_{sc}^\# \cdot \log(y_{sc}^\#)$$

for $sc \in SC$. Extended variances $\sigma_{sc}^{\#2}$ can then be defined as $\sigma_{sc}^{\#2} = \phi_{sc}^\# \cdot V(\mu_{sc}^\#)$.

Assume as in Sect. 14.3.1 that $\log(\mu_{sc}^\#) = \mathbf{x}_{sc}^T \cdot \boldsymbol{\beta} + o_{Esc}$. When $\phi_{sc}^\# = \phi^\#$ are constant $\boldsymbol{\theta} = (\boldsymbol{\beta}^T, \phi^\#)^T$, and maximizing $\ell^+(SC; \boldsymbol{\theta})$ in $\boldsymbol{\theta}$ generates the same estimates $\boldsymbol{\beta}(SC)$ as maximum pseudolikelihood estimation of $\boldsymbol{\beta}$ under the unit-dispersions conditional model. The maximum pseudolikelihood estimate $\phi^\#(SC)$ of $\phi^\#$ then satisfies

$$\phi^\#(SC) = \frac{1}{m(SC)} \sum_{sc \in SC} d\left(y_{sc}^\#; \mu_{sc}^\#(SC)\right),$$

where $\mu_{sc}^\#(SC)$ are the estimates of $\mu_{sc}^\#$ determined by $\boldsymbol{\beta}(SC)$. More generally, model the log of the dispersions $\phi_{sc}^\#$ as a function of selected dependence and/or non-dependence primary predictors and associated coefficients (similarly to the approach of Sect. 12.13.2) and offsets. Specifically, let $\log(\phi_{sc}^\#) = \mathbf{v}_{sc}^T \cdot \boldsymbol{\gamma} + o_{Dsc}$ where, for $sc \in SC$, $\mathbf{v}_{sc}$ is a $q \times 1$ column vector of q predictor values v_{scj} (including unit predictor values if an intercept is to be included) with indexes $j \in Q = \{j : 1 \le j \le q\}$, $\boldsymbol{\gamma}$ is the associated $q \times 1$ column vector of coefficients, and o_{Dsc} is the associated offset value for dispersion modeling. The $(r + q) \times 1$ parameter vector $\boldsymbol{\theta} = (\boldsymbol{\beta}^T, \boldsymbol{\gamma}^T)^T$ is estimated through maximum extended quasi-pseudolikelihood estimation. Alternative models can be compared with extended PLCV (PLCV$^+$) scores computed as in Sect. 14.3.1 but using extended quasi-pseudolikelihoods rather than pseudolikelihoods and maximum extended quasi-pseudolikelihood estimates of $\boldsymbol{\theta}$ rather than maximum pseudolikelihood estimates. The adaptive modeling process can be extended to search through models for the means and dispersions in combination (see Chap. 20).

As in Sect. 14.3.1, for $sc \in SC$, the estimated value for the mean $\mu_{sc}^\#$ is $\mu_{sc}^\#(SC) = \exp(\mathbf{x}_{sc}^T \cdot \boldsymbol{\beta}(SC) + o_{Esc})$ and the corresponding residual is $e_{sc}^\#(SC) = y_{sc}^\# - \mu_{sc}^\#(SC)$. The estimated value of the associated dispersion $\phi_{sc}^\#$ is $\phi_{sc}^\#(SC) = \exp(\mathbf{v}_{sc}^T \cdot \boldsymbol{\gamma}(SC) + o_{Dsc})$ and of the extended variance $\sigma_{sc}^{\#2}$ is $\sigma_{sc}^{\#2}(SC) = \phi_s^\#(SC) \cdot V(\mu_{sc}^\#(SC))$. The standardized or Pearson residual $stde_{sc}^\#(SC) = e_{sc}^\#(SC)/\sigma_{sc}^\#(SC)$ is obtained by standardizing the residual by dividing by the estimated extended standard deviation.

14.4   Transition Modeling of Post-Baseline Seizure Rates

This section describes transition modeling of seizure rates, first using constant dispersions models (with offsets) in Sect. 14.4.1 and then using non-constant dispersions models in Sect. 14.4.2. See Sects. 4.8, 10.4, and 10.6 for similar analyses of multivariate continuous, dichotomous, and polytomous outcomes, respectively.

14.4.1   Constant Dispersions Models

All models for means have offsets log(dltatime). Unless otherwise stated, all models for dispersions are constant with offsets log(dltatime). The adaptive model for the post-baseline seizure rates corresponding to the count outcome variable $y =$ count as a function of PRE$(y,1,4)$ is used as a benchmark analysis for setting the number k of folds (see Sect. 2.8). Note that even though only the post-baseline rates are modeled, the values of PRE$(y,1,4)$ are computed as averages of the up to four prior outcome values including the baseline value. Moreover, since an offset variable is included, the values of PRE$(y,1,4)$ are computed from prior rates rather than prior counts. This would have no effect if the baseline values were not included since dltatime is constant (2 weeks each) for post-baseline measurements, but there is a difference since the baseline dltatime is different (8 weeks). The variable PRE$(y,1,4,\varnothing)$ (that is, the indicator for there being no prior outcome values with which to compute PRE$(y,1,4)$, in which case PRE$(y,1,4)$ is set to 0) is not needed since there is always at least one prior outcome measurement, the baseline measurement, so that PRE$(y,1,4,\varnothing)$ has all zero values. The adaptively generated model for $k = 5$ is based on the transform PRE$(y,1,4)^{0.05}$ with an intercept and extended quasi-likelihood CV (QLCV$^+$) score 0.31873, the same as its extended pseudolikelihood CV (PLCV$^+$) score since it is a transition model. The adaptively generated model for $k = 10$ is based on the two transform PRE$(y,1,4)^{-0.406}$ and PRE$(y,1,4)^{0.27}$ without an intercept and with QLCV$^+$ score 0.31518 while the model for $k = 15$ is based on the transform PRE$(y,1,4)^{0.089}$ with an intercept and with QLCV$^+$ score 0.31565. Since these latter two scores are smaller than the score for $k = 5$, $k = 5$ is used in subsequent analyses of this outcome. The linear polynomial model in PRE$(y,1,4)$ has QLCV$^+$ score 0.04233 with very substantial PD 86.72 % (that is, larger than the cutoff of 0.81 % for the data) compared to the adaptive model. Thus, the log of mean post-baseline seizure rate is distinctly nonlinear in PRE$(y,1,4)$.

Using unit dispersions without offsets, the adaptive model considering the single predictor PRE$(y,1,4)$ is also based on a single transform: PRE$(y,1,4)^{0.05}$ with an intercept but with LCV score (the same as its QLCV$^+$ score) 0.20400 and substantial PD of 36.00 %. Using unit dispersions with offsets, the adaptive model is based on the single transform PRE$(y,1,4)^{0.05}$ with an intercept and the QLCV$^+$ score improves to 0.29256 but the PD is a substantial 8.21 %. Using constant dispersions without offsets, the adaptive model is based on the same transform $PRE(y,1,4)^{0.05}$ with an intercept, $QLCV^+$ score 0.23178, and substantial PD of 27.28 %. Note that $PRE(y,1,4)$ is computed as the average of the prior seizure counts in y without offsets and as the average of the prior seizure rates with offsets. If the baseline values were not included as prior outcome variables, there would have not been any difference since the post-baseline offset values are constant (at 2 weeks), but there is difference when baseline values are included since they have a different offset value (8 weeks). These results indicate the importance of using constant dispersions with offsets when modeling multivariate rate outcomes. While the same model is generated in all cases, the $QLCV^+$ score is substantially worse with unit dispersions and/or no offsets.

Basing the transition model on $PRE(y,1,4)$ has the advantage of utilizing all prior outcome values, but transition models based on fewer prior outcome values using $PRE(y,1,3)$, $PRE(y,1,2)$, or $PRE(y,1)$ (the same as $PRE(y,1,1)$) may be more effective. The adaptive model based on $PRE(y,1,3)$ includes the transform: $PRE(y,1,3)^{0.06}$ with an intercept and smaller $QLCV^+$ score 0.31546. For $PRE(y,1,2)$ and $PRE(y,1,1)$ even smaller $QLCV^+$ scores of 0.31190 and 0.28324 are generated. Consequently, subsequent models are based on $PRE(y,1,4)$.

Models for the means have depended so far on only dependence predictors and not on other available predictors. The adaptive additive model in $PRE(y,1,4)$, rate0, and visit is the same model as generated for $PRE(y,1,4)$ alone, indicating that mean seizure rates do not change distinctly with the baseline seizure rate or over post-baseline clinic visit, when considered additively. The adaptive additive model in $PRE(y,1,4)$, rate0, visit, and int is the same model as generated not considering int, indicating that treatment group does not have a constant effect over all clinic visits. However, it may have an effect that changes with clinic visit (or with the other predictors). This can be addressed with geometric combinations (GCs; see Sect. 4.5.4). The adaptive model in $PRE(y,1,4)$, visit, rate0, int, and GCs in these four predictors is based on the four transforms: $PRE(y,1,4)^{0.073}$, $(PRE(y,1,4)^{-0.8} \cdot rate0^{1.5} \cdot visit^{-1})^{3.27}$, $int \cdot PRE(y,1,4)^{-0.7} \cdot visit^{-0.7} \cdot rate0^{-0.1}$, and $(rate0^{-5} \cdot PRE(y,1,4)^{2.1} \cdot visit^{1.2})^{2.92}$ with an intercept and $QLCV^+$ score 0.33995. In comparison, the adaptive model in $PRE(y,1,4)$, rate0, visit, and GCs, not considering int, is based on the four transforms: $PRE(y,1,4)^{0.055}$, $(PRE(y,1,4)^{-0.8} \cdot rate0^{1.5} \cdot visit^{-1})^{3.4}$, $rate0^{-9.5} \cdot visit^{11} \cdot PRE(y,1,4)^{-1}$, and $(PRE(y,1,4)^{-1} \cdot rate0^2)^{1.97}$ with an intercept and $QLCV^+$ score 0.33706. The PD compared to the model also considering int is an insubstantial 0.59 %, indicating that mean seizure rates are reasonably considered not to differ for the two treatments. However, this might change with consideration of non-constant dispersions.

14.4.2   Non-Constant Dispersions Models

Adaptive non-constant dispersions models can be generated by considering models with both means and dispersions depending on transforms of primary predictors. For example, the means and dispersions of post-baseline seizure rates can both be adaptively modeled in terms of $PRE(y,1,4)$, visit, rate0, int, and GCs, starting from constant means and dispersions models. In this case, the adaptively generated model for the means is based on the one transform: $PRE(y,1,4)^{0.056}$ with an intercept. The adaptively generated model for the dispersions is based on the four transforms: $PRE(y,1,4)^{0.3}$, $(visit^9 \cdot PRE(y,1,4))^{1.001}$, and $(visit^3 \cdot int \cdot PRE(y,1,4))^{1.1}$ without an intercept. The $QLCV^+$ score is 0.36552, which is a distinct improvement over the best constant dispersions model of Sect. 14.4.1 with $QLCV^+$ score 0.33995 and substantial PD of 7.00 %, indicating that the seizure rates have distinctly non-constant dispersions. For the adaptive model for means and dispersions in terms of $PRE(y,1,4)$, visit, rate0, and GCs, not considering int, the means are based on the three transform: $PRE(y,1,4)^{0.05}$, $(rate0^{-10} \cdot visit^2 \cdot PRE(y,1,4)^{-1.2})^{1.2}$, and $(PRE(y,1,4)^{-1.111} \cdot visit^{-2} \cdot rate0^2)^{-3.489}$ with an intercept while the dispersions are based on the two transforms: $PRE(y,1,4)^{0.75}$ and $(visit^9 \cdot PRE(y,1,4))^{2.04}$ without an intercept. The $QLCV^+$ score is 0.35606 with substantial PD of 3.24 % compared to the model also considering int. Consequently, non-constant dispersions modeling supports the conclusion that the dispersions change with taking probagide compared to a placebo but not the means (since none of those transforms depend on int). The estimated slope for the transform $(visit^3 \cdot int \cdot PRE(y,1,4))^{1.1}$ is negative so that taking the drug progabide decreases the dispersions for seizure rates. However, only transition models have been considered so far. The conclusions might change with consideration of GEE-based marginal models.

14.5   Adaptive GEE-Based Modeling of Multivariate Count Outcomes

The formulation for adaptive modeling of multivariate count/rate outcomes using GEE parameter estimation is similar to the formulation for the multivariate dichotomous logistic regression case given in Sect. 10.7.1. The outcome variable y has count values rather than 0–1 values, its variance equals its mean μ so that $V(\mu) = \mu$, offsets are included in models for means and dispersions, and means are log-transformed rather than logit-transformed, but otherwise the formulation is the same and so is not provided. This formulation includes scaled residuals as also used in the continuous case of Sect. 4.3.3 and the dichotomous outcome case of

Sect. 10.7.1. Extended LCV (LCV^+) scores computed with multivariate normal likelihoods extended to address count/rate outcomes, using either matched-set-wise deletion as in Sect. 4.4.1 or measurement-wise deletion as in Sect. 4.13, are used to evaluate and compare models as part of the adaptive modeling process. LCV^+ scores for GEE-based models are computed with multivariate normal likelihoods while LCV and $QLCV^+$ scores for transition and general conditional models are computed with Poisson likelihoods for count/rate outcomes, and so these are not comparable. However, it is possible to compute LCV^+ scores for marginal models induced by transition and general conditional models, which can be compared to LCV^+ scores for GEE-based models. The formulation is essentially the same as the formulation of Sect. 14.7.3 for dichotomous discrete outcomes and so is not provided. It is also possible to compute extended penalized likelihood criteria (PLCs; see Sect. 2.10.1) adding the usual penalty factors to extended likelihoods giving the extended AIC (AIC^+), extended BIC (BIC^+), and extended TIC (TIC^+), assumed to be in larger is better form. These are alternatives to the quasi-likelihood information criterion (QIC) of Pan (2001), which extends readily to the count/rate outcome context from the continuous outcome context of Sect. 4.11.1. In contrast to QIC, the extended PLCs AIC^+, BIC^+, and TIC^+ are not based in part on results for independent correlations but are wholly based on the working correlation structure.

14.6   Adaptive GEE-Based Modeling of Post-Baseline Seizure Rates

For brevity, only constant dispersions models for seizure rates are considered in this section. Also all extended LCV (LCV^+) scores are based on $k = 5$ folds as for transition modeling of these data. The adaptive GEE-based additive model for seizure rate means in terms of visit and rate0 with order 1 autoregressive (AR1) correlation structure is based on the transform $rate0^{0.099}$ with an intercept and LCV^+ score 0.048238. The corresponding adaptive GEE-based model with exchangeable correlation (EC) structure is the model based on the transforms $rate0^{0.079}$ and $visit^{19}$ with an intercept and larger LCV^+ score 0.049804. Consequently, EC is the more appropriate correlation structure for these data and is used in subsequent analyses.

The adaptive GEE-based model in visit, rate0, int, and GCs is based on the two predictors: $rate0^{0.139}$ and $(visit^{-9} \cdot rate0^{-11})^{-0.798}$ with an intercept and improved LCV^+ score 0.050294. Consequently, GEE-based modeling leads to the conclusion that seizure rate means do not change distinctly with treatment as also held for constant dispersions transition models. However, the associated transition model induces a marginal model with LCV^+ score 0.051199, which is a distinct improvement over the associated GEE-based model with substantial PD in the LCV^+ scores of 1.77 %. In this case, transition modeling distinctly outperforms GEE-based modeling, suggesting that multivariate count/rate outcomes may be reasonable analyzed using only transition models without considering GEE-based marginal models. Moreover, the clock time to compute the above GEE-based marginal model is about 62.6 min in comparison to 18.2 min to compute the associated transition model or about 3.4 times as long.

14.7   Overview of Analyses of Post-Baseline Seizure Rates

1. For post-baseline seizure rates (Sect. 14.2), analyses use $k = 5$ folds (Sect. 14.4.1).
2. Models for post-baseline seizure rates based on constant dispersions with offsets are distinctly better than models based on constant dispersions without offsets, on unit dispersions without offsets, and on unit dispersions with offsets (this and the following results reported in Sect. 14.4.1). Using constant dispersions with offsets, mean post-baseline seizure rates are reasonably considered to change with the average of the up to four prior seizure rates, the baseline seizure rate, and visit, but not with treatment group.
3. Using constant dispersions with offsets and GEE-based marginal models, mean post-baseline seizure rates are reasonably considered to change with the baseline seizure rate and visit, but not with treatment group (this and the following results reported in Sect. 14.6). The marginal model induced by the associated constant dispersions transition model distinctly outperforms the GEE-based marginal model.
4. Using non-constant dispersions with offsets, mean post-baseline seizure rates are reasonably considered not to depend on treatment group (this and the following results reported in Sect. 14.4.2). However, dispersions do change distinctly with treatment group and are smaller when taking the drug progabide.

14.8   Chapter Summary

This chapter presents a series of analyses of the epileptic seizure data, addressing how seizure rates per week over four post-baseline clinic visits depends on visit, the baseline seizure rate, and treatment on progabide versus on a placebo for 59 epileptic patients using both adaptive transition models and adaptive marginal models with generalized estimating equations (GEE) parameter estimation. These analyses demonstrate adaptive Poisson regression modeling of multivariate count/rate outcomes using fractional polynomials, including how to model dispersions as well as means. The chapter has also provided formulations for these alternative regression models; for associated k-fold likelihood cross-validation (LCV) scores for unit dispersions transition models, extended quasi-likelihood cross-validation $(QLCV^{+})$ scores for non-unit dispersions transition models, pseudolikelihood cross-validation (PLCV) and extended PLCV (PLCV^+) scores for general conditional models of means and/or dispersions, and extended LCV (LCV^+) scores for GEE-based models of means and/or dispersions; and for residuals, standardized or Pearson residuals and scaled residuals.

The example analyses demonstrate assessing whether log-transformed means of a count/rate outcome are nonlinear in individual predictors, whether those relationships are better addressed with multiple predictors in combination, whether those relationships interact using geometric combinations (GCs), and whether there is a benefit to considering non-constant dispersions. The example analyses also demonstrate how to compare GEE-based marginal models to marginal models induced by transition models. The results of these analyses demonstrate the need to consider non-constant dispersions since taking progabide only affects dispersions for seizure rates not the means. These results also indicate that transition models for multivariate count/rate outcomes can induce marginal models that distinctly outperform associated GEE-based marginal models and in much less time. Thus, it seems reasonable not to consider GEE-based marginal models when analyzing multivariate count/rate discrete outcomes. Example residual analyses are not reported in this chapter for brevity. See Chap. 15 for a description of how to conduct analyses of multivariate count/rate outcomes in SAS.

References

Fitzmaurice, G. M., Laird, N. M., & Ware, J. H. (2011). *Applied longitudinal analysis* (2nd ed.). Hoboken, NJ: John Wiley & Sons.

Liang, K.-Y., & Zeger, S. L. (1986). Longitudinal data analysis using generalized linear models. *Biometrika, 73*, 13–22.

McCullagh, P., & Nelder, J. A. (1999). *Generalized linear models* (2nd ed.). Boca Raton, FL: Chapman & Hall/CRC.

Molenberghs, G., & Verbeke, G. (2006). *Models for discrete longitudinal data*. New York: Springer.

Pan, W. (2001). Akaike's information criterion in generalized estimating equations. *Biometrics, 57*, 120–125.

Thall, P. F., & Vail, S. C. (1990). Some covariance models for longitudinal count data with overdispersion. *Biometrics, 46*, 657–671.

Chapter 15
Adaptive Poisson Regression Modeling of Multivariate Count Outcomes in SAS

15.1 Chapter Overview

This chapter describes how to use the genreg macro for adaptive Poisson regression modeling of multivariate count outcomes, possibly converted to rates using offsets, as described in Chap. 14, and its generated output. See Supplementary Materials for a more complete description of the macro. See Stokes et al. (2012) for details on standard generalized estimating equations (GEE) modeling of multivariate count/rate outcomes in SAS. Familiarity with adaptive modeling in SAS of univariate count/rate outcomes as described in Chap. 13 and of transition and GEE-based modeling in SAS as described in Chaps. 5, 7, and 11 is assumed in this chapter. Section 15.2 describes the epileptic seizure data (see Sect. 14.2) used in the analyses of Chap. 14. Section 15.3 provides examples of transition modeling of seizure rates while Sect. 15.4 provides examples of GEE-based marginal modeling of seizure rates.

15.2 Loading in the Epileptic Seizures Data

Analyses are conducted in Chap. 14 of post-baseline seizure rates for 59 patients with epilepsy (see Sect. 14.2). Assume that these epileptic seizure data have been loaded into the default library (for example, by importing them from a spreadsheet file) in wide format (see Sect. 5.2) under the name seizures. An output title line, selected system options, labels for the variables, and formats for values of selected variables can be assigned as follows.

```
options nodate pageno=1 pagesize=53 linesize=76;
title1 "Epileptic Seizures Data";
proc format; value intfmt 0="Placebo" 1="Progabide"; run;
```

© Springer International Publishing Switzerland 2016
G.J. Knafl, K. Ding, *Adaptive Regression for Modeling Nonlinear Relationships*,
Statistics for Biology and Health, DOI 10.1007/978-3-319-33946-7_15

```
data seizures;
 set seizures;
 int=(treatment=1);
 rate0=count0/8;
 label id="Subject ID" int="Treatment Group" age="Age in Years"
       count0="Seizure Count in Prior 8 Weeks at Time 0"
       count1="Seizure Count in Prior 2 Weeks at Visit 1"
       count2="Seizure Count in Prior 2 Weeks at Visit 2"
       count3="Seizure Count in Prior 2 Weeks at Visit 3"
       count4="Seizure Count in Prior 2 Weeks at Visit 4"
       int="Progabide versus a Placebo"
       rate0="Seizure Rate per Week in Prior 8 Weeks at Time 0";
 format int intfmt.;
run;
```

Patient identifiers are stored in the variable id. Seizure count outcome measurements at visits 0–4 are stored in the variables count0–count4, respectively. The variable int indicates the treatment group with value 1 for patients on progabide and 0 for patients on a placebo. A format is created with PROC FORMAT for the values of the variable int and assigned with the format statement in the data step. The variable rate0 is loaded with baseline rates; the baseline period is 8 weeks long for all patients.

The following code converts the data to long format, storing it in the longseiz data set.

```
data longseiz;
 set seizures;
 array counts{5} count0-count4;
 do i=1 to 5;
  visit=i-1; count=counts{i};
  if i=1 then dltatime=8; else dltatime=2;
  output;
 end;
 label visit="Visit" count="Seizure Count"
       dltatime="Prior # of Weeks for Count";
 keep id int age visit rate0 count dltatime;
run;
data longseiz;
 set longseiz;
 xoffset=log(dltatime); voffset=log(dltatime);
 y=count; w=visit;
 label xoffset="Offset for Expectations"
       voffset="Offset for Dispersions"
       y="Seizure Count" w="Visit";
 run;
```

The variable count is created from count0 to count4. The variable visit is loaded with indexes from 0 to 4 for clinic visits. The variable dltatime is loaded with the length of associated periods in weeks. All post-baseline periods are 2 weeks long. This variable is used to create the offset variables xoffset and voffset for means and dispersions, respectively. Since these two variables have the same values, a single variable could have been used instead. A copy y of the outcome variable count and a copy w of the within-subject variable visit are created for use in shortening the length of names for dependence predictors in the code of Sect. 15.3. The postseiz data set containing only post-baseline data is created as follows.

```
data postseiz;
  set longseiz;
  if visit=0 then delete;
run;
```

The cutoff for a substantial percent decrease (PD) in the $QLCV^+$ and LCV^+ scores (see Sect. 4.4.2 for the formula) for the 236 post-baseline seizure rates per week is 0.81 %. Since there are no missing measurements, all these scores are computed with matched-set-wise deletion (Sect. 4.4.1; using the default setting "measdlte=n" of the genreg macro parameter measdlte).

15.3   Transition Modeling of Post-Baseline Seizure Rates

Assume that genreg has been loaded into SAS (see Supplementary Materials). An adaptive transition model for count can be generated as follows.

```
%genreg(modtype=poiss,datain=longseiz,yvar=count,
        xoffstvr=xoffset,voffstvr=voffset,conditnl=y,
        corrtype=IND,matchvar=id,withinvr=visit,
        winfst=1,foldcnt=5,expand=y,expxvars=pre_y_w_1_4,
        contract=y);
```

The parameter setting "modtype=poiss" requests a Poisson regression model. The datain parameter specifies the input data set, in this case the longseiz data set. The yvar parameter specifies the count outcome variable, in this case the variable count. The xoffstvr and voffstvr parameters specify the variables in the datain data set containing offset values for the means and dispersions, respectively. A conditional model is requested since "conditnl=y". This requires an independent correlation structure as requested with "corrtype=IND". It also requires that the matchvar and withinvr parameters have nonempty settings specifying, respectively, the variable whose unique values determine the matched sets, the variable id in this case, and the variable whose values indicate the different conditions under which the outcome variable has been measured, the variable visit in this case.

The parameter setting "foldcnt=5" (as justified in Sect. 14.4.1) requests that 5-fold QLCV$^+$ scores be computed for models and is used in all further analyses of the seizure rates. The parameter setting "expand=y" requests that the base model be expanded. The model for the means is expanded by adding in transforms of primary predictor variables listed in the setting for the expxvars parameter. The model for the dispersions is not changed since the expvvars macro parameter has its default empty setting. The parameter setting "contract=y" requests that the expanded model be contracted. In this case, the one dependence predictor pre_y_w_1_4 (called PRE(y,1,4) in Chap. 14) is considered in the expansion (see Sect. 5.4.1 for more on how dependence predictors are specified). Using the copies y and w shortens the names of these predictors. Alternate transition models can be generated by changing the expxvars list to depend on pre_y_w_1_3, pre_y_w_1_2, or pre_y_w_1_1 (called PRE(y,1,3), PRE(y,1,2), and PRE(y,1,1) in Chap. 14, respectively).

The winfst parameter specifies the first value of the withinvr variable to use in the analysis, in this case the value of 1 for that variable is the first to be considered. By default (with setting "winfst=."), the first value of that variable, in this case 0, is used. There is also a winlst parameter controlling the last value of the withinvr variable to use in the analysis. In this case, its default value ("winlst=.") is requested, meaning that the last value 4 of the withinvr variable is to be used in the analysis. Taken together, these settings of winfst and winlst request that the post-baseline seizure rates from visit 1 to 4 be modeled. The advantage of modeling the post-baseline outcome values from the longseiz data set over using the postseiz data set with baseline values deleted is that the baseline counts can be used in computing values for prior dependence predictors like pre_y_w_1_4. Since the baseline counts are not missing for any of the patients, there is always at least one prior outcome value available to use in computing all prior dependence predictors. That means that indicators of no prior outcome values for computing dependence predictors like pre_y_w_1_4 have all zero values and need not be considered in analyses. If a data set with baseline values deleted is used instead (as in the analyses of Chaps. 10 and 11), this is no longer the case and these indicators are needed, for example, pre_y_w_1_4_m is the missing indicator corresponding to pre_y_w_1_4. When non-zero offset variables are specified and the base variable (the variable y in this case) for a dependence predictor equals the outcome variable defined through the yvar macro parameter, the values for the dependence predictor is based on averages of the outcome variables divided by the exponent of the associated offset variable (defined with xoffstvr for means and voffstvr for dispersions). In this way, the dependence predictor is based on averages of associated rates rather than of the counts.

The default setting"measdlte=n" is requested so that generated QLCV$^+$ scores are based on matched-set-wise deletion with all measurements of a matched set assigned to the same fold (see Sect. 4.4.1). Measurement-wise deletion (see Sect. 4.13) with individual measurements assigned to folds instead can be requested with the setting "measdlte=y". For transition and general conditional models, partial measurement-wise deletion (Sect. 4.13) can be requested with the setting "measdlte=p".

The base model is generated first, in this case the model with constant means (since the default settings of "xintrcpt=y" and "xvars=" are used) with offsets, constant dispersions (since the default settings of "vintrcpt=y" and "vvars=" are used) with offsets, and $QLCV^+$ score 0.17268. This is expanded by adding in the single transform for the means: $pre\_y\_w\_1\_4^{0.05}$ with associated LCV score 0.31873. The contraction leaves the model unchanged and there is no need for a conditional transformation since there is only one transform in the model.

An adaptive model in $pre\_y\_w\_1\_4$, visit, rate0, int, and geometric combinations (GCs; see Sect. 4.5.4) can be generated as follows.

```
%genreg(modtype=poiss,datain=longseiz,yvar=count,
        xoffstvr=xoffset,voffstvr=voffset,conditnl=y,
        corrtype=IND,matchvar=id,withinvr=visit,
        winfst=1,foldcnt=5,expand=y,
        expxvars=pre_y_w_1_4 visit rate0 int,geomcmbn=y,
        contract=y);
```

The primary predictors for the expansion are set through the expxvars parameter. GCs are requested as part of this expansion with the "geomcmbn=y" setting. The default setting "geomcmbn=n" generates the associated additive model. The expansion adds six transforms to the base model: $pre\_y\_w\_1\_4^{0.05}$, $(pre\_y\_w\_1\_4^{-0.8} \cdot rate0^{1.5} \cdot visit^{-1})^{3.4}$, $int \cdot pre\_y\_w\_1\_4^{-0.7} \cdot visit^{-0.7} \cdot rate0^{-0.1}$, $(rate0^{-5} \cdot pre\_y\_w\_1\_4^{2.1} \cdot visit^{1.2})^2$, $visit^{11} \cdot pre\_y\_w\_1\_4^{-1.07}$, and $(rate0^{-3} \cdot pre\_y\_w\_1\_4^{-2})^{1.2}$ with $QLCV^+$ score 0.34274. This is contracted to the model based on the four transforms: $pre\_y\_w\_1\_4^{0.073}$, $(pre\_y\_w\_1\_4^{-0.8} \cdot rate0^{1.5} \cdot visit^{-1})^{3.27}$, $int \cdot pre\_y\_w\_1\_4^{-0.7} \cdot visit^{-0.7} \cdot rate0^{-0.1}$, and $(rate0^{-5} \cdot pre\_y\_w\_1\_4^{2.1} \cdot visit^{1.2})^{2.92}$ with an intercept and $QLCV^+$ score 0.33995 as also reported in Sect. 14.4.1.

Adaptive models for both the means and dispersions can be generated as follows. For example, the following code generates a model with both means and dispersions a function of the primary predictors: $pre\_y\_w\_1\_4$, visit, rate0, int, and GCs.

```
%genreg(modtype=poiss,datain=longseiz,yvar=count,
        xoffstvr=xoffset,voffstvr=voffset,conditnl=y,
        corrtype=IND,matchvar=id,withinvr=visit,
        winfst=1,foldcnt=5,expand=y,
        expxvars=pre_y_w_1_4 visit rate0 int,
        expxvars=pre_y_w_1_4 visit rate0 int,geomcmbn=y,
        contract=y);
```

The generated model for the means has the one transform: $PRE(y,1,4)^{0.056}$ with an intercept. The adaptively generated model for the dispersions is based on the four transforms: $PRE(y,1,4)^{0.3}$, $(visit^9 \cdot PRE(y,1,4))^{1.001}$, and $(visit^3 \cdot int \cdot PRE(y,1,4))^{1.1}$ without an intercept. The $QLCV^+$ score is 0.36552, which substantially improves on the associated constant dispersions model (see Sect. 14.4.2).

This latter adaptive model can be generated directly as follows.

```
%genreg(modtype=poiss,datain=longseiz,yvar=count,
        xoffstvr=xoffset,voffstvr=voffset,conditnl=y,
        corrtype=IND,matchvar=id,withinvr=visit,
        winfst=1,foldcnt=5,xvars=pre_y_w_1_4,
        xpowers=0.056,vvars=pre_y_w_1_4 rate0,
        vpowers=0.3 -0.09,
        vgcs=visit 9 pre_y_w_1_4 1 :
            visit 3 in. 1 pre_y_w_1_4 1,
        vgcpowrs=1.001 1.1);
```

The vgcs parameter is used to specify GCs for the dispersions with GCs separated by colons (:) and the vgcpowrs parameter to specify powers for transforming those GCs. For example, the GC $visit^9 \cdot pre\_y\_w\_1\_4$ is requested with "visit 9 pre_y_w_1_4 1". Since this is the first requested GC and 1.001 is the first power in the vgcpowrs list, together they request the transform $(visit^9 \cdot pre\_y\_w\_1\_4)^{1.001}$. The xgcs and xgcpowrs parameters are used in the same way to generate transformed GCs for means, but those are not needed in this case. Table 15.1 contains part of the output generated by this code. GCs generated for the means (dispersions) have names starting with "XGC_" ("VGC_") followed by an index number. Lists are provided describing each of the GCs using the SAS

Table 15.1 The adaptive model for post-baseline seizure rates in terms of the average of the up to four prior seizure rates (pre_y_w_1_4), clinic visit, the baseline seizure rate (rate0), the indicator for being on probagide (int), and geometric combinations in these four primary predictors

```
         geometric combination log dispersion variables:
              VGC_1 visit**(9)*pre_y_w_1_4
              VGC_2 visit**(3)*int*pre_y_w_1_4
...
```

base log expectation component

predictor	power	estimate
XINTRCPT	1	-15.5775
pre_y_w_1_4	0.056	15.602623

base log dispersion component

predictor	power	estimate
pre_y_w_1_4	0.3	1.586029
rate0	-0.09	-1.711018
VGC_1	1.001	-5.96E-7
VGC_2	1.1	-0.002186

...

mth root of quasi+ likelihood using deleted predictions: 0.3655243 operators "*" for multiplication and "**" for exponentiation. Powers used to transform these GCs and estimated slopes for those power transforms are also provided in the output.

15.4 Marginal GEE-Based Modeling of Post-Baseline Seizure Rates

An adaptive GEE-based model can be generated for post-baseline seizure rates in terms of visit, rate0, int, and GCs as follows.

```
%genreg(modtype=poiss,datain=postseiz,yvar=count,
        xoffstvr=xoffset,voffstvr=voffset,GEE=y,
        corrtype=EC,biasadj=y,matchvar=id,
        withinvr=visit,foldcnt=5,expand=y,
        expxvars=visit rate0 int,geomcmbn=y,
        contract=y);
```

The winfst and winlst parameters are only supported for conditional modeling (requested by "conditnl=y"), and so the postseiz data set needs to be used to be able to model only post-baseline values. If the longseiz data set is used instead, seizure rates for all five visits are analyzed. Only constant dispersions models are considered since the default settings "vintrcpt=y" and "expvvars=" (that is, the empty setting) are requested. The setting "GEE=y" requests a GEE parameter estimation (see Sect. 14.5). The default setting is "GEE=n", meaning use maximum likelihood parameter estimation, but that is only supported for marginal models with "modtype=norml". The corrtype parameter has the same meaning as for marginal models of continuous outcomes (see Sect. 5.3.1). Exchangeable correlations (EC) are requested in this case. The setting "biasadj=y" requests that correlation and dispersion estimates be bias-corrected (see Sect. 12.7.1) adjusting the number of measurements by subtracting the number of terms in the model for the means as is standard for GEE-based modeling. The default setting "biasadj=n" means compute those estimates without adjusting for bias, dividing instead by the unadjusted number of measurements. The other choices are "corrtype=AR1" for order 1 autoregressive correlations and "corrtype=UN" for unstructured correlations. For the AR1 case, the spatial parameter determines the type of autoregression. The default setting of "spatial=y" requests a spatial autoregression where the actual withinvr values are used in computing correlations while "spatial=n" requests a standard autoregression where the indexes for the withinvr values are used in computing correlations. These are only equivalent when the actual values are equally spaced.

The search starts at the constant means and dispersions model with extended LCV (LCV$^+$) score 0.025958. The expansion adds in the five transforms for the means: $\text{rate0}^{0.309}$, $\text{int} \cdot \text{visit}^5 \cdot \text{rate0}^{0.1}$, $\text{int} \cdot \text{rate0}^{-2} \cdot \text{visit}^{-0.3}$, visit^{18}, and $\text{visit}^{-9} \cdot \text{rate0}^{-11}$ with improved LCV^+ score 0.049973, and then the contraction removes three transforms leaving the model based on $\text{rate0}^{0.139}$ and $(\text{visit}^{-9} \cdot \text{rate0}^{-11})^{-0.798}$ with an intercept and further improved LCV^+ score 0.050294 as also reported in Sect. 14.6.

LCV^+ scores for GEE-based models of count/rate outcomes are computed with extended multivariate normal likelihoods while QLCV^+ scores for transition and PLCV^+ scores for general conditional models of those outcomes are computed with Poisson likelihoods, and so these two types of scores are not comparable. However, transition and general conditional models for count/rate outcomes induce marginal models (see Sect. 14.5), whose LCV^+ scores can be compared to those for GEE-based marginal models. The induced LCV^+ score for a transition and general conditional model is reported in the genreg output when requested with the setting "GEEscore=y".

15.5 Practice Exercises

15.1 Patients' ages are also available in the epileptic seizure data set, stored in the variable age. Assess the impact of also including age as a primary predictor for post-baseline seizure rates. Use $k = 5$ folds as justified in Sect. 14.4.1. First, generate the adaptive transition model for the post-baseline seizure rate means in pre_y_w_1_4, rate0, visit, int, age, and GCs with constant dispersions. How does this model depend on int? Does also considering age as a primary predictor provide a distinct improvement in predicting seizure rate means when dispersions are constant? Next, generate the adaptive transition model for the post-baseline seizure rate means and dispersions in pre_y_w_1_4, rate0, visit, int, age, and GCs. How does this model depend on int? Does also considering age as a primary predictor provide a distinct improvement in predicting seizure rate means and dispersions in combination in comparison to using constant dispersions modeling? Finally, generate the adaptive transition model for the post-baseline seizure rate means and dispersions in pre_y_w_1_4, rate0, visit, age, and GCs without int to assess the impact of int on seizure rates when age is also considered. Is this model a competitive alternative to the one based also on int as for analyses conducted without considering age? Or does consideration of age lead to the opposite conclusion that there is a substantial effect to int?

For Practice Exercises 15.2 and 15.3, use the aspartame study data available on the Internet (see Supplementary Materials). Aspartame is an artificial sweetener used as a sugar substitute. The data are in long format. There are 122 measurements for 27 subjects over weeks 1–5 with an average of 4.5 measurements per subject. The outcome variable for this data set is called headaches and contains counts of headaches within each week. The predictors to be considered are called week and int, the indicator for being on aspartame versus being on a placebo. The variable days contains the number of days of exposure for the associated week (not always the whole 7 days). For all models use offsets for means and dispersions set equal to the logs of days so that the Poisson regression models for headache counts are converted into models for headache rates per day. The load code for this data set creates the variables xoffset and voffset and loads them with these offset values. It also creates copies called y and w of headaches and week, respectively, for use in creating shorter names for dependence predictors.

15.2 For the aspartame data, use the adaptive additive transition model for the means of headache rates per day in pre_y_w_1_4 and pre_y_w_1_4_m as a benchmark analysis to set the number of folds for QLCV$^+$ scores. Use constant dispersions models in all analyses of this practice exercise. Next generate the adaptive model for the means in pre_y_w_1_4, pre_y_w_1_4_m, week, and GCs and assess whether consideration of week has a distinct effect on the means for headache rates. Finally generate the adaptive model for the means in pre_y_w_1_4, pre_y_w_1_4_m, week, int, and GCs and assess whether consideration of int has a distinct effect on the means for headache rates. Does being on aspartame have an effect on the means for headache rates per day compared to being on a placebo?

15.3 For the aspartame data, use the number of folds selected in Practice Exercise 15.2 for all analyses of this practice exercise. First generate the adaptive model for the means and dispersions in pre_y_w_1_4, pre_y_w_1_4_m, week, and GCs and assess whether consideration of week has a distinct effect on means and dispersions for headache rates. Next generate the adaptive model for the means and dispersions in pre_y_w_1_4, pre_y_w_1_4_m, week, int, and GCs and assess whether consideration of int has a distinct effect on means and dispersions for headache rates. Does being on aspartame have an effect on means and/or dispersions for headache rates per day compared to being on a placebo?

Reference

Stokes, M. E., Davis, C. S., & Koch, G. G. (2012). *Categorical data analysis using the SAS system* (3rd ed.). Cary, NC: SAS Institute.

Part IV
Alternative Nonparametric Regression Modeling

Chapter 16
Generalized Additive Modeling

16.1   Chapter Overview

This chapter formulates and demonstrates generalized additive models (GAMs) (Hastie and Tibshirani 1999) for means of continuous outcomes treated as independent and normally distributed with constant variances as in linear regression and for logits (log odds) of means of dichotomous outcomes with unit dispersions as in logistic regression. GAMs for these two cases are also compared to adaptive fractional polynomial models. PROC GAM, which supports generation of GAMs in SAS, currently supports GAMs for the logistic case only with unit dispersions, and so constant dispersion models are not considered for that case. Poisson regression analyses are not conducted in this chapter for brevity. See Chap. 17 for a description of how to conduct analyses like those described in this chapter in SAS.

GAMs provide an alternative to fractional polynomial models for modeling nonlinear relationships between univariate outcomes and predictors. Since GAMs are nonparametric regression alternatives to generalized linear models, they only address univariate outcomes and not multivariate outcomes. GAMs can be used in the regression context with univariate continuous outcomes as well as in other types of regression contexts like logistic regression with dichotomous discrete outcomes. GAMs can be generated in SAS using cubic splines (Ahlberg et al. 1967), local regression (loess) (Cleveland et al. 1988), or thin plate splines (Meinguet 1979). SAS macros are available (see Chap. 17) for computing GAMs and their likelihood cross-validation (LCV) scores.

Section 16.2 formulates GAMs for continuous outcomes. Section 16.3 formulates likelihood cross-validation (LCV) for GAMs. Section 16.4 formulates leave-one-out (LOO) least squares cross-validation (LSCV) and generalized cross-validation (GCV) (Wahba 1990) commonly used with GAMs. Sections 16.5–16.7 provided example analyses using GAMS of the death rate data analyzed in Chaps. 2, 3, 6, and 7 (see Sect. 2.2 for a description of these data). These data are a subset of a larger data set described and analyzed in Sect. 16.8. Section 16.9

G.J. Knafl, K. Ding, *Adaptive Regression for Modeling Nonlinear Relationships*,
Statistics for Biology and Health, DOI 10.1007/978-3-319-33946-7_16

formulates GAMs for dichotomous outcomes. Section 16.10 provides example analyses using GAMs of the dichotomous outcome of the fish mercury data analyzed in Chaps. 8 and 9 (see Sect. 8.2 for a description of these data). Sections 16.11 and 16.12 provide overviews of the results of analysis of death rates and dichotomous mercury levels, respectively. Formulations can be skipped to focus on analyses.

16.2   Formulation of GAMs for Univariate Continuous Outcomes

GAMs in the normal distribution case use a generalization of the multiple regression model of Sect. 2.17. For $s \in S = \{s : 1 \leq s \leq n\}$, decompose the $r \times 1$ vector $\mathbf{x}_s$ into $\mathbf{x}_s = (\mathbf{x}_s'^T, \mathbf{x}_s''^T)^T$ where $\mathbf{x}_s'$ has the r' entries x'_{sj} for $j' \in J' = \{j' : 1 \leq j' \leq r'\}$ and $\mathbf{x}_s''$ has the r'' entries x''_{sj} for $j'' \in J'' = \{j'' : 1 \leq j'' \leq r''\}$ where $r' + r'' = r$. Assume that $y_s = \mathbf{x}_s'^T \cdot \boldsymbol{\beta} + f(\mathbf{x}_s'') + e_s$ for an arbitrary function f. This model is parametric in the predictor vectors $\mathbf{x}_s'$ and nonparametric in the predictor vectors $\mathbf{x}_s''$. The first entry of $\mathbf{x}_s'$ satisfies $x'_{s1} = 1$ for $1 \leq s \leq n$ so that an intercept parameter β_1 is always included in the model. The function f decomposes into separate functions $f_{j''}$ for predicting the additive impact of each of the predictors x''_{sj}. These separate functions can be estimated with either the loess or cubic spline smoothing approaches. The effect of pairs of predictors can also be estimated using the thin plate spline smoothing approach (for the formulation for thin plate splines, see the documentation on PROC TPSPLINE in SAS Institute 2004).

Let $\mathbf{y}$ denote the $n \times 1$ vector of outcome values y_s. Under the cubic spline and loess approaches applied to the predictor values x''_{sj} for $1 \leq s \leq n$, the $n \times 1$ vector $\mathbf{f}_{j''}$ with entries $f_{j''}(x''_{sj})$ for $1 \leq s \leq n$ is estimated as a linear function $\mathbf{K}_{j''} \cdot \mathbf{y}$ for a $n \times n$ matrix $\mathbf{K}_{j''}$ with entries $K_{ss'j''}$. The matrices $\mathbf{K}_{j''}$ depend on smoothing parameters and possibly also on x''_{sj} and $\mathbf{y}$, but this dependence has been suppressed to simplify the notation. When symmetric, the matrices $\mathbf{K}_{j''}$ are analogous to hat matrices for regression models. For cubic spline GAMs, the matrices $\mathbf{K}_{j''}$ are symmetric, and so the associated degrees of freedom (DF) are defined as the trace $\text{tr}(\mathbf{K}_{j''}) = \sum_{1 \leq s \leq n} K_{ssj''}$ of $\mathbf{K}_{j''}$. For loess, associated DF values are defined as the trace $\text{tr}(\mathbf{K}_{j''}^T \cdot \mathbf{K}_{j''})$ since the matrices $\mathbf{K}_{j''}$ are not symmetric. Associated DF can be similarly defined for thin plate splines in terms of pairs of predictor values within the predictor vectors $\mathbf{x}_s''$. DF values represent effective numbers of slope parameters used by alternative smoothing approaches to estimate the effects of predictors. They are analogous to degrees for polynomial models and so can be compared to degrees for standard and fractional polynomial models. Note also that the matrices $\mathbf{K}_{j''}$ can be combined over $j'' \in J''$ together with a similar matrix $\mathbf{K}'$ for the parametric part of the model into the hat matrix $\mathbf{K}$ with entries $K_{ss'}$ generating predictions $\mathbf{K} \cdot \mathbf{y}$ of means for all the observations based on the complete model in terms of all predictor vectors $\mathbf{x}_s$ for $s \in S$.

Residuals are computed as $e_s(S) = y_s - {\mathbf{x}_s'}^T \cdot \boldsymbol{\beta}(S) - f(S)(\mathbf{x}_s'')$ for $s \in S$ where $f(S)$ denotes the estimate of the function f. LCV scores are then computed using deleted residuals $e_s(S \backslash F(h))$ for $s \in F(h)$ and $h \in H$ as defined in Sect. 2.5.3. However, the associated deleted estimates $f(S \backslash F(h))(\mathbf{x}_s'')$ are not always computable, in which case the LCV score is adjusted as described in Sect. 16.3.

16.3 Formulation of Likelihood Cross-Validation for GAMs

To compute LCV scores for GAMs, an adjustment is needed since predictions generated by PROC GAM can sometimes be missing when fold predictor values are outside the range of predictor values for the complement of that fold. Let $n(h)$ denote the number of observations in fold $F(h)$, $miss(h)$ the possibly empty set of observations in fold $F(h)$ with missing predictions, and $nmiss(h)$ the number of observations in $miss(h)$. Assuming $nmiss(h) < n(h)$, define LCV scores for GAMs as

$$LCV = \prod_{h \in H} L'(F(h); \boldsymbol{\theta}(S \backslash F(h)))^{\frac{1}{n}},$$

where $\log(L'(F(h); \boldsymbol{\theta})) = \log(L(F(h) \backslash miss(h); \boldsymbol{\theta})) \cdot n(h)/(n(h) - nmiss(h))$ and $\boldsymbol{\theta} = (\boldsymbol{\beta}, f)$ is the combination of the parameters and the nonparametric function underlying a given GAM. This is equivalent to replacing the log-likelihood terms for observations in fold $F(h)$ with missing predictions with the average of the log-likelihoods for the observations in fold $F(h)$ with non-missing predictions, and so is a common form of single imputation. In the normal distribution case, the deleted log likelihood for observation $(y_{s'}, \mathbf{x}_{s'})$ with $s' \in miss(h)$ is imputed as

$$-\frac{1}{2} \cdot \sum_{s \in F(h) \backslash miss(h)} \frac{(y_s - y(\mathbf{x}_s; S \backslash F(h)))^2}{(n(h) - nmiss(h)) \cdot \sigma^2(S \backslash F(h))} - \frac{1}{2} \cdot \log(\sigma^2(S \backslash F(h))) - \frac{1}{2} \cdot \log(2 \cdot \pi),$$

where $y(\mathbf{x}_s; S \backslash F(h))$ denotes the predicted value for an observation $(y_s, \mathbf{x}_s)$ from the observations with indexes in $S \backslash F(h)$. Thus, the imputed squared deleted error for $(y_{s'}, \mathbf{x}_{s'})$ is the average of the squared deleted errors for the observations in fold $F(h)$ with non-missing predictions. Consequently, predicted values for $(y_{s'}, \mathbf{x}_{s'})$ with $s' \in miss(h)$ are likely not to be as extreme as if they had been obtained by extrapolation of the predicted values for the observations with indexes in $S \backslash F(h)$, and so this imputation approach is likely to provide relatively favorable imputed LCV scores for

GAMs. This adjusted LCV score cannot be computed when one or more folds have all missing predictions (that is, nmiss(h) = n(h) for some h), but that will not often occur. If it does occur, reduce the number of folds until this is resolved.

16.4   Other Forms of Cross-Validation

A least squares form of leave-one-out (LOO) cross-validation (CV) is often used with GAMs (see eq. 3.10, Hastie and Tibshirani 1999) with least squares CV scores

$$ \text{LSCV} = \frac{1}{n} \sum_{1 \le s \le n} \left(e_s(S \backslash \{s\}) \right)^2 $$

for the normal distribution case. Smaller LSCV scores indicate better models. Using LSCV in the standard regression context is equivalent to using PRESS as defined in Sect. 2.5.1 since $\text{LSCV} = \text{PRESS}/n$ and so is similar to LOO LCV generalizing PRESS and LSCV to account for deleted variance estimates (as shown in Sect. 2.5.3). It can be shown that the LSCV score satisfies

$$ \text{LSCV} = \frac{1}{n} \sum_{1 \le s \le n} \left(\frac{e_s(S)}{1 - K_{ss}} \right)^2 $$

(eq. 3.19, Hastie and Tibshirani 1999) where K_{ss} are the diagonal entries of the hat matrix $\mathbf{K}$ as defined in Sect. 16.2. Generalized CV (GCV) uses the approximation to this LSCV score given by

$$ \text{GCV} = \frac{1}{n} \sum_{1 \le s \le n} \left(\frac{e_s(S)}{1 - \text{tr}(\mathbf{K})/n} \right)^2 , $$

replacing the diagonal entries K_{ss} by their average $\text{tr}(\mathbf{K})/n$. PROC GAM supports GCV selection of GAMs.

16.5   GAM Analyses of Deathrate as a Function
of the Nitric Oxide Pollution Index

Models can be generated in PROC GAM using non-integer degrees of freedom (DF) values, but analyses reported in this chapter are restricted to only integer valued DF. The DF for such cubic spline GAMs equal the requested integer values. The DF for such loess models, on the other hand, are non-integer values close to the requested DF. For cubic spline and loess GAMs, predictors are also included as linear terms in those predictors. This means that integer valued DF of at least 2 are required for cubic splines to avoid degenerate cases, but $\text{DF} = 1$ is a possible alternative for loess GAMs. Thin plate spline GAMs do not generate linear terms for predictors, but since they involve two predictors, they require integer valued DF of at least 2 (but requests for lower DF are changed by PROC GAM to DF = 2).

The GAM for deathrate as a function of NOindex generated with the cubic spline approach selected through GCV has DF = 7.03 (including a linear term in NOindex and DF = 6.03 for the nonparametric component in NOindex) with GCV = 2929.960. In contrast, the GAM generated with the loess approach selected through GCV has DF = 2.86 (including a linear term in NOindex and DF = 1.86 for the nonparametric component in NOindex) with smaller and so better GCV = 54.328. Predicted value curves for these two alternative GAMs are displayed in Fig. 16.1 (see Fig. 2.1 for a plot of the data). Both approaches generate similar predicted values for relatively small and relatively large NOindex values. In between, the cubic spline GAM is more highly influenced by variability in the data than the loess GAM due to its much larger DF, resulting in a much larger (worse) GCV score. However, both are highly influenced by the two observations with very large NOindex values (see the scatter plot of the data in Fig. 2.1).

Table 16.1 contains 5-fold (as justified in Sect. 2.8) LCV scores for GAMs for deathrate as a function of the singleton predictor NOindex based on both the cubic spline and loess approaches chosen either by GCV or with specified DF values ranging from 2 to 4 for cubic spline GAMs and from 1 to 4 for loess GAMs. All GAMs include a constant term not counted in reported DF values and a linear term counted in reported DF values, and so the associated nonparametric components are based on 1 less DF than reported in the table. Actual DF values for loess models are only close to the requested values: actual DF values (not reported in Table 16.1) for requested DF values of 1–4 are 1.30, 2.14, 3.03, and 3.75, respectively. Note that DF = 4 is an example where the actual DF is less than the requested integer DF. Actual DFs when DF = 1 is requested appear to be greater than 1 (as in this case) so that such choices are reasonable to consider. The loess model with DF = 2

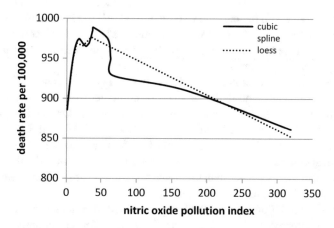

Fig. 16.1 Comparison of estimated mean death rate per 100,000 as a function of the nitric oxide pollution index for generalized additive models based on the cubic spline and loess approaches selected through generalized cross-validation

Table 16.1 Comparison of alternative generalized additive models to the adaptive fractional polynomial model for death rate per 100,000 as a function of the nitric oxide pollution index

Modeling approach	DF	5-fold LCV score	Percent decrease (%)[a]	Percent decrease (%)[b]	Percent decrease (%)[c]	Percent decrease (%)[d]
Cubic spline GAM	2	0.0039184	0.00		2.43	7.37
	3	0.0030058	23.29		25.16	28.95
	4	0.0020098	48.71		49.96	52.49
	7.03[e]	0.0019354	50.61		51.81	54.25
Loess GAM	1	0.0039407		1.88	1.88	6.85
	2	0.0040161		0.00	0.00	5.06
	2.86[e]	0.0039866		0.73	0.73	5.76
	3	0.0040119		0.10	0.10	5.16
	4	0.0036823		8.31	8.31	12.95
Adaptive	–	0.0042303				0.00

DF: degrees of freedom, GAM: generalized additive model, LCV: likelihood cross-validation
[a]Among all cubic spline models
[b]Among all loess models
[c]Among all cubic spline and loess models
[d]Among all cubic spline, loess, and adaptive models
[e]DF chosen through generalized cross-validation including 1 DF for the linear term

generates the best LCV score of 0.0040161 for all the GAMs of Table 16.1. Among all cubic spline GAMs, the model with DF = 2 generates the best LCV score of 0.0039184 and a percent decrease (PD) in the LCV scores of 2.43 % compared to the best loess model. This is an insubstantial PD since it is smaller than the cutoff of 3.15 % for the data (as reported in Chap. 2).

By default, PROC GAM uses the DF value of 4. The default DF = 4 cubic spline model has LCV score 0.0020098 with substantial PD of 48.71 % compared to the cubic spline model with the best LCV score of 0.0039184. The default DF = 4 loess model has LCV score 0.0036823 with substantial PD of 8.31 % compared to the loess model with the best LCV score of 0.0040161. Consequently, using the default DF value can generate substantially inferior models.

The loess model generated with GCV has DF = 2.86 and LCV score of 0.0039866 with insubstantial PD of 0.73 % compared to the best loess model with specified DF = 2, and so is a competitive alternative. On the other hand, the cubic spline GAM generated with GCV has DF = 7.03 and LCV score of 0.0019354 with very substantial PD of 50.61 % compared to the best cubic spline model with specified DF = 2. Thus, consideration of ranges of DF values is likely to generate better LCV scores than GCV and sometimes substantially better, and so GCV is not considered in subsequent analyses.

The LCV score 0.0040161 for the best overall GAM generates a substantial PD of 5.06 % compared to the LCV score 0.0042303 for the adaptive fractional polynomial model (see Sect. 2.8). Thus, adaptive fractional polynomial models provide a distinctly better depiction of the nonlinearity of deathrate in NOindex

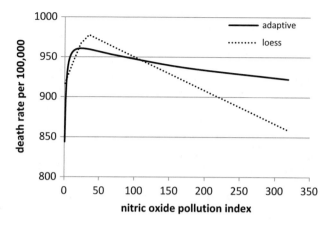

Fig. 16.2 Comparison of estimated mean death rate per 100,000 as a function of the nitric oxide pollution index for the adaptive fractional polynomial model and the best generalized additive model

than GAMs. Also, the generated adaptive model is based on two transforms without an intercept (as reported in Sect. 2.6) and so is less complex than the best GAM based on two DF plus an intercept. Figure 16.2 provides a comparison of estimated mean curves for these two models (see Fig. 2.1 for a plot of the data). Compared to the adaptive fractional polynomial model, the estimated mean deathrate for the best GAM starts out larger for low NOindex levels, is smaller for a while, then larger, and ends up much smaller for very large NOindex values. The GAM is more highly influenced by the few extreme observations with very large NOindex values (see Fig. 2.1) than the fractional polynomial model, thereby accounting for its substantially inferior LCV score.

16.6 GAM Analyses of Deathrate as a Function of Other Singleton Predictors

Table 16.2 contains a comparison of GAMs to adaptive models for deathrate in terms of the three singleton predictors NObnded (that is, min(NOindex,12), see Sect. 2.15), SO2index, and rain. The best LCV score for loess GAMs with DF ranging from 1 to 4 is generated at DF = 1 for all three predictors. The best LCV score for cubic spline GAMs with DF ranging from 2 to 4 is generated at DF = 4 for rain and at DF = 2 for the other two predictors. For NObnded, SO2index, and rain the loess approach generates the better LCV score than the cubic spline approach, as was also the case for NOindex as reported in Table 16.1. For NObnded and SO2index, adaptive models generate larger LCV scores than the GAMs, and substantially so for NObnded but not for SO2index. For rain, the best cubic spline GAM generates a larger LCV score than the adaptive model, but the PD for the

Table 16.2 Comparison of adaptive and generalized additive models for death rate per 100,000 as a function of singleton predictors

	5-fold LCV score			Percent decrease in LCV score for best GAM (%)	Percent decrease in LCV score for adaptive model (%)
		GAM			
Predictor	Adaptive model	Loess[a]	Cubic spline[b]		
NObnded	0.0042303	0.0040471	0.0040118	4.33	0.00
SO2index	0.0040239	0.0039902	0.0039730	0.84	0.00
rain	0.0044527	0.0045353	0.0045212	0.00	1.82

GAM: generalized additive model, LCV: likelihood cross-validation, NObnded: nitric oxide pollution index bounded at 12, SO2index: sulfur dioxide pollution index, rain: annual average precipitation
[a]Best LCV score for $DF = 1 - 4$ achieved at $DF = 1$ for all three predictors
[b]Best LCV score for $DF = 2 - 4$ achieved at $DF = 2$ for NObnded and SO2index and at $DF = 4$ for rain

adaptive model is insubstantial at 1.52 %. Moreover, that model is based on a single transform of rain without an intercept (as described in Sect. 2.16) while the cubic spline is based on $DF = 4$ plus an intercept, and so it is a parsimonious, competitive alternative.

16.7   GAM Analyses of Deathrate as a Function of Two Predictors

Table 16.3 contains a comparison of selected GAMs in NObnded and SO2index for alternate DF values based on the cubic spline approach alone, the loess approach alone, either the cubic spline or loess approaches, and the thin plate spline approach alone. The best model based on either the cubic spline or the loess approaches is the same as the best model based on the loess approach alone with $DF = 1$ for both predictors. GAMs based on combinations of cubic splines and loess are truly additive models compared to thin plate spline models which also account for possible interaction between NObnded and SO2index. The best thin plate spline model is generated for $DF = 2$ and has LCV score 0.0040743 while the best of the GAMs combining cubic spline and/or loess models for individual predictors has LCV score 0.0037297 with substantial PD of 8.46 %. The latter model avoids consideration of the complexity of interactions between predictors. This has the advantage of simplifying computations, but these results indicate that there will be situations where ignoring interactions can impose a substantial penalty. On the other hand, the GAM for NObnded by itself is the better of the two singleton predictor GAMs with LCV score 0.0040471 (Table 16.2) and insubstantial PD of 0.67 %. This indicates that NObnded by itself provides a competitive, parsimonious alternative and so explains essentially all of the effect of SO2index on death rate

Table 16.3 Comparison of generalized additive models for death rate per 100,000 as a function of the bounded nitric oxide pollution index and the sulfur dioxide pollution index in combination

Model type	Model	DF		5-fold LCV score	Percent decrease in LCV score (%)
		NObnded	SO2index		
Both cubic spline	cubic spline (NObnded) cubic spline(SO2index)[a]	2	2	0.0035018	14.05
Both loess	loess(NObnded) loess(SO2index)[b]	1	1	0.0037297	8.46
Cubic spline or loess	loess(NObnded) loess(SO2index)[c]	1	1	0.0037297	8.46
Thin plate spline	thin plate spline (NObnded, SO2index)[d]	2		0.0040743	0.00

DF: degrees of freedom, LCV: likelihood cross-validation, NObnded: nitric oxide pollution index bounded at 12, SO2index: sulfur dioxide pollution index
[a]With best LCV score for all nine cubic spline models in both NObnded and SO2index with DF $= 2 - 4$
[b]With best LCV score for all 16 loess models in both NObnded and SO2index with DF $= 1 - 4$
[c]With best LCV score for all 49 models in NObnded and SO2index, either as cubic spline with DF $= 2 - 4$ or loess with DF $= 1 - 4$
[d]With best LCV score for all three thin plate splines models in NObnded and SO2index with DF $= 2 - 4$

(as also concluded in Sect. 2.16 through adaptive analyses). For this reason, SO2index is not considered further in the analyses.

Table 16.4 contains a comparison of selected GAMs in NObnded and rain for alternate DF values based on the cubic spline approach alone, the loess approach alone, either the cubic spline or loess approaches, or the thin plate spline approach alone. The best model for all cases is based on loess models for both NObnded and rain, both with DF $= 1$, and has LCV score 0.0055341. The best thin plate spline model is generated for DF $= 2$ and has LCV score 0.0053103. The associated PD of 4.04 % is substantial, indicating that thin plate models can be distinctly inferior and suggesting that the effects of NObnded and rain on deathrate are truly additive and do not interact. The best GAM for rain by itself is the better of the two singleton predictor GAMs with LCV score 0.0045212 (Table 16.2) and substantial PD of 18.30 % compared to the best composite GAM of Table 16.4, indicating that rain and NObnded explain distinct aspects of deathrate not explained by the other (as also concluded in Sect. 2.16 through adaptive analyses). These analyses address both additive models and models addressing interactions (through thin plate splines). The analyses of the effects of NObnded and rain on deathrate of Chap. 2 only address the additive case since geometric combinations (GCs) are not introduced until Chap. 4. The adaptive model in NObnded, rain, and GCs between these two predictors is based on the single transform $(\text{rain}^{-0.2} \cdot \text{NObnded}^{-0.09})^{-0.59}$

Table 16.4 Comparison of generalized additive models for death rate per 100,000 as a function of the bounded nitric oxide pollution index and the average annual precipitation in combination

Model type	Model	DF		5-fold LCV score	Percent decrease in LCV score (%)
		NObnded	Rain		
Both cubic spline	cubic spline(NObnded) cubic spline(rain)[a]	2	2	0.0054271	1.93
Both loess	loess(NObnded) loess(rain)[b]	1	1	0.0055341	0.00
Cubic spline or loess	loess(NObnded) loess(rain)[c]	1	1	0.0055341	0.00
Thin plate spline	thin plate spline (NObnded,rain)[d]	2		0.0053103	4.04

DF: degrees of freedom, LCV: likelihood cross-validation, NObnded: nitric oxide pollution index bounded at 12, rain: average annual precipitation
[a]With best LCV score for all nine cubic spline models in both NObnded and rain with DF $= 2 - 4$
[b]With best LCV score for all 16 loess models in both NObnded and rain with DF $= 1 - 4$
[c]With best LCV score for all 49 models in NObnded and rain, either as cubic spline with DF $= 2 - 4$ or loess with DF $= 1 - 4$
[d]With best LCV score for all three thin plate splines models in NObnded and rain with DF $= 2 - 4$

without an intercept and LCV score 0.0057296. This provides a substantial improvement over the GAM with the best LCV score 0.0055341 in Table 16.4 with PD 3.41 %. The adaptive additive model (see Sect. 2.16) has LCV score 0.0056386 with insubstantial PD 1.59 % compared to the adaptive GC-based model, indicating as for GAMs that the effects of NObnded and rain are reasonably treated as additive. However, the additive model is based on two transforms without an intercept and so is more complex.

16.8 GAM Analyses of the Full Deathrate Data

There are a total of 15 predictor variables available in the full death rate data (Table 16.5). The predictor NOindex has been replaced by its bounded version NObnded as justified in Sect. 2.15. Because they are additive and so do not consider interactions, GAMs based on the cubic spline and/or loess smoothing approaches can reduce the complexity of models for how deathrate changes with large numbers of predictors as in this case. However, it is likely that not all of these predictors are needed to generate an effective model for mean deathrate. Moreover, the number of observations per predictor is only $60/15 = 4$, and so a model in all the predictors is likely to be a poor choice for these data. An approach is needed to identify which predictors to include in a composite model, which smoothing approach to use with that predictor, and what DF value to use with that smoothing approach.

Table 16.6 presents results for an approach for systematically including predictors into a composite GAM for deathrate. Predictors based on GAMs are added one at a time starting from the constant model. Among all predictors not currently in

Table 16.5 Complete set of predictors for deathrate per 100,000

Predictor	Description
educatn	Number of years of schooling for persons over 22
HCindex	Hydrocarbon pollution index
HHsize	Number of members per household
JANtemp	Average January temperature
JULtemp	Average July temperature
kitchens	Number of households with fully equipped kitchens
lowinc	Number of families with income less than $3000
moisture	Degree of atmospheric moisture
NObnded	Nitrous oxide pollution index bounded by 12
nonwhite	Size of non-White population
over65	Size of population older than 65
oworkers	Number of office workers
pop	Population per square mile
rain	Average annual precipitation in inches
SO2index	Sulfur dioxide pollution index

Table 16.6 Systematic inclusion of GAM predictors for deathrate per 100,000

Inclusion order	GAM term[a]	5-fold LCV score	Percent decrease in LCV score
1	loess(nonwhite,DF=1)	0.0049107	31.20
2	loess(rain,DF=1)	0.0055887	21.70
3	param(NObnded)	0.0066243	7.14
4	loess(JANtemp,DF=2)	0.0070116	1.72
5	param(SO2index)	0.0070922	0.59
6	param(HHsize)	0.0071340	0.00
7	param(oworkers)	0.0071181	0.22
8	param(pop)	0.0070122	1.71
9	param(lowinc)	0.0068106	4.53
10	loess(JULtemp,DF=2)	0.0067206	5.79
11	loess(HCindex,DF=1)	0.0065364	8.38
12	param(moisture)	0.0062490	12.40
13	param(over65)	0.0059502	16.60
14	param(kitchens)	0.0057244	19.80
15	loess(educatn,DF=1)	0.0038808	45.60

DF: degrees of freedom, GAM: generalized additive model, LCV: likelihood cross-validation
[a]See Table 16.5 for definitions of the predictors

the model, the next predictor added to the model is the one that maximizes the LCV score generated by adding one predictor at a time to the current model. For each predictor not yet included in the model, the parametric model as well as cubic spline GAMs with DF = 2 − 4 and loess GAMs with DF = 1 − 4 are considered. The best

LCV score of 0.0071340 is generated with the inclusion of six predictors (nonwhite, rain, NObnded, JANtemp, SO2index, and HHsize in that order) each either parametric or loess with $DF = 1$ or $DF = 2$ for a total $DF = 7$ plus an intercept. The LCV score decreases after that. As expected, models based on large numbers of predictors are ineffective for modeling the death rate data with only 60 observations. The simpler model with HHsize and SO2index removed generates LCV score of 0.0070116 and insubstantial PD of 1.72 %, and so is a competitive, parsimonious alternative to the full six predictor GAM, but the further removal of JANtemp generates a substantial PD of 7.14 %.

The adaptive modeling process used in Chap. 2 to analyze the limited deathrate data can also be used to generate an additive fractional polynomial model in power transforms of the predictors of Table 16.5. Since the models of Table 16.6 all have an intercept, the adaptive modeling process is restricted not to remove the intercept in the contraction step. The expanded model is based on the seven transforms: nonwhite, educatn$^{11.1}$, NObnded$^{-0.1}$, rain$^{-0.4}$, SO2index$^{1.9}$, lowinc^{-9}, and kitchens^{-19}. As in Table 16.6 up to step 6, the LCV score increases with each additional term to the value 0.0073736. Consequently, this is the appropriate adaptive model to compare to the best model of Table 16.6, which generates a substantial PD of 3.35 % compared to the adaptive expanded model. The contraction reduces this to the model based on the following five transforms: nonwhite$^{0.7}$, NObnded$^{-0.3}$, rain$^{-0.4}$, SO2index$^{1.9}$, and lowinc^{-7} and LCV score is 0.0072154. The associated model of Table 16.6 is the one based on the first four terms with LCV score 0.0070116. The PD in the LCV scores compared to the fully adaptive model is insubstantial at 2.82 %, but the GAM is not simpler involving $DF = 5$ plus an intercept compared to five terms with an intercept. Allowing the contraction to also remove the intercept, the generated model is based on the four transforms: nonwhite$^{0.5}$, educatn$^{10.1}$, NObnded$^{-0.1}$, and rain$^{0.05}$ without an intercept. The LCV score is 0.0070948, larger that the score for the reduced GAM and simpler. In this case, adaptive additive fractional polynomial modeling generates preferable models compared to generalized additive modeling and sometimes distinctly so.

16.9   Formulation of GAMs for Dichotomous Outcomes

Using the logistic regression notation of Sect. 8.3 and the GAM notation of Sect. 16.2, model the logits of the means as

$$\text{logit}(\mu_s) = \mathbf{x}_s'^{\,\text{T}} \cdot \boldsymbol{\beta} + f(\mathbf{x}_s'')$$

for $s \in S$. Estimates f(S) of the nonparametric function f can be generated with the cubic spline, loess, and thin plate spline approaches as for continuous outcomes. Estimates of the means satisfy

$$\mu_s(S) = \frac{\exp\left(\mathbf{x}_s'^{\,\mathrm{T}} \cdot \boldsymbol{\beta}(S) + f(S)(\mathbf{x}_s'')\right)}{1 + \exp\left(\mathbf{x}_s'^{\,\mathrm{T}} \cdot \boldsymbol{\beta}(S) + f(S)(\mathbf{x}_s'')\right)}.$$

These can be used to compute LCV scores using the adjustment of Sect. 16.3 for missing predictions. Residuals are computed as $e_s(S) = y_s - \mu_s(S)$. See Hastie and Tibshirani (1999) for details on generalizations of degrees of freedom (DF), least square cross-validation (LSCV), and generalized CV (GCV) to outcomes with distribution in the exponential family including the case of dichotomous discrete outcomes.

16.10   GAM Analyses of the Mercury Level Data

Among cubic spline GAMs for merchigh (a high mercury level over 1.0 ppm versus low; see Chap. 8) as a function of the weight of fish with $DF = 2 - 4$, the $DF = 2$ model generates the best LCV score of 0.54803 (using $k = 15$ folds as justified in Sect. 8.4). Among loess GAMs with $DF = 1 - 4$, the $DF = 3$ model generates the best LCV score of 0.54824. The best cubic spline GAM is a competitive alternative with insubstantial PD of 0.04 % (that is, lower than the cutoff of 1.13 % for the data as reported in Sect. 8.2). Moreover, it is simpler having $DF = 2$ compared to $DF = 3$ for the loess GAM, and so is preferable as a parsimonious, competitive alternative. On the other hand, the adaptive model for merchigh in weight is based on the single transform weight$^{-0.5}$ with an intercept (as do all adaptive models for merchigh reported in this section) with improved LCV score of 0.56081 (as reported in Sect. 8.4). The loess GAM in weight with the best LCV score for GAMs generates a substantial PD of 2.24 % and is more complex with $DF = 3$ plus an intercept (all GAMs have intercept). Consequently, the adaptive fractional polynomial model distinctly outperforms GAMs in this case.

Among cubic spline GAMs for merchigh as a function of the length of fish with $DF = 2 - 4$, the $DF = 3$ model generates the best LCV score 0.58795. Among loess GAMs with $DF = 1 - 4$, the $DF = 1$ model has the smaller LCV score of 0.56966 and substantial PD of 3.11 %. Consequently, the cubic spline model distinctly outperforms the loess model in this case. The adaptive fractional polynomial model for merchigh in length is based on the single transform length$^{0.5}$ and has LCV score of 0.59140 (as reported in Sect. 8.5). The PD for the cubic spline GAM is insubstantial at 0.58 %, but this GAM is more complicated than the adaptive model with $DF = 3$ compared to one power transform. Consequently, the adaptive fractional polynomial model is preferable to the best GAM in this case.

For modeling merchigh as a function of both weight and length, the best cubic spline GAM in both predictors with combinations of $DF = 2 - 4$ for each is achieved at $DF = 2$ for weight and $DF = 3$ for length with LCV score 0.60005. The best loess GAM in both predictors with combinations of $DF = 1 - 4$ for each is achieved at DF = 1 for weight and DF = 2 for length with improved LCV score 0.60103. Considering either cubic splines with DF = 2 − 4 or loess with DF = 1 − 4, the best GAM is the same as the best GAM with loess for both predictors. The adaptive additive model for merchigh in weight and length is based on the two transforms $length^{0.9}$ and $weight^{0.3}$ with LCV score of 0.60382 (as reported in Sect. 8.6). The best GAM has a lower LCV score but with an insubstantial PD of 0.46 %. However, it is more complex with DF = 3 compared to only two transforms for the adaptive model. The best thin plate spline GAM in both predictors over DF = 2 − 4 has DF = 4 and improved LCV score of 0.60637. The PD for the best prior GAM is insubstantial at 0.88 % and is simpler with DF = 3. The PD for the adaptive additive model is also insubstantial at 0.42 % and is based on only two transforms compared to DF = 4, and so the adaptive additive model is preferable to GAMs in this case as a parsimonious, competitive alternative. Furthermore, the adaptive model allowing for geometric combinations (GCs) in weight and length is based on three transforms plus an intercept with LCV score 0.61585 (as reported in Sect. 8.6). The PD for the thin plate spline model is substantial at 1.54 %. Consequently, adaptive models are more effective at identifying the effects of weight and length on merchigh.

16.11 Overview of Analyses of Death Rates

1. For deathrates (Sect. 2.2), analyses use k = 5 folds (Sect. 2.8).
2. The loess approach generates a better LCV score than the cubic spline approach for modeling NOindex but not distinctly better (this and the following results reported in Sect. 16.5). The cubic spline approach with DF based on GCV produces distinctly inferior results. Both the loess and cubic spline approaches with default DF setting of four produce distinctly inferior results. The adaptive model in NOindex distinctly outperforms GAMs based on either the loess approach with DF from 1 to 4 or the cubic spline approach with DF from 2 to 4.
3. The adaptive model in NObnded distinctly outperforms GAMs based on either the loess approach with DF from 1 to 4 or the cubic spline approach with DF from 2 to 4 (this and the following results reported in Sect. 16.6). The loess GAM in SO2index with DF = 1 is a competitive alternative to the associated adaptive model but is more complex (since it also includes an intercept while the adaptive model does not). The cubic spline GAM in rain with DF = 4 generates a better LCV score than the associated adaptive model but not substantially better and is much more complex.
4. The thin plate spline in NObnded and SO2index distinctly outperforms models in these two predictors using the loess approach with DF from 1 to 4 and/or the cubic spline approach with DF from 2 to 4 (this and the following results reported in Sect. 16.7). The thin plate spline in NObnded and rain is distinctly outperformed by the loess GAMs with DF = 1 for both of these predictors. The adaptive model based on NObnded, rain, and GCs distinctly outperforms this

GAM in NObnded and rain. The associated adaptive additive model generates a competitive LCV score but is more complex.

5. Considering all 15 predictors available in the full death rate data set, a model based on either the loess approach or as linear terms in six of these predictors for a total DF = 7 generates the best LCV score considering only GAMs and linear terms (this and the following results reported in Sect. 16.8). The model based on four of these predictors with DF = 5 is a parsimonious, competitive alternative. These first of these GAM-based models is distinctly outperformed by the associated adaptive model. The associated adaptive model is preferable to the second of these GAMs.

16.12   Overview of Analyses of Dichotomous Mercury Levels

1. For dichotomous mercury levels (Sect. 8.2), analyses use k = 15 folds (Sect. 8.4).
2. For models in weight, the loess approach generates a better LCV score than the cubic spline approach, but the cubic spline approach is a parsimonious, competitive alternative (this and the following results reported in Sect. 16.10). The adaptive model in weight distinctly outperforms both of these GAMs.
3. For models in length, the cubic spline approach distinctly outperforms the loess approach (this and the following results reported in Sect. 16.10). The adaptive model in length generates a better LCV score than the cubic spline GAM but not substantially better. However, the cubic spline GAM is more complex.
4. For models in weight and length, using the loess approach with DF from 1 to 4 and/or the cubic spline approach with DF from 2 to 4, the best choice is based on a loess GAM with DF = 1 for weight and a loess GAM with DF = 2 for length. The thin plate spline with DF = 4 generates a better score but the first GAM is a parsimonious, competitive alternative. The adaptive additive model in weight and length is a parsimonious, competitive alternative to the thin plate spline. The adaptive model in weight, length, and GCs distinctly outperforms the thin plate spline.

16.13   Chapter Summary

This chapter presents a series of analyses of the full death rate data using generalized additive models (GAMs), addressing how the continuous outcome deathrate per 100,000 depends on the 15 available predictors for 60 metropolitan statistical areas. It also presents analyses of the mercury level data using GAMs, addressing how the dichotomous outcome a high level of mercury over 1.0 ppm versus a lower level depends on the weight and length of 169 fish. These analyses demonstrate generalized additive modeling in these two important contexts.

The chapter also provides a formulation extending linear regression and logistic regression models to GAMs for univariate continuous and dichotomous outcomes, respectively. Likelihood cross-validation (LCV) scores are extended to be able to compare GAMs to adaptive models and to other GAMs. Other alternatives for conducting cross-validation are also defined including the leave-one-out (LOO) form of least squares cross-validation (LSCV) and generalized cross-validation (GCV) commonly used to evaluate GAMs. Adaptive fractional polynomials often generate better LCV scores than associated GAMs and sometimes substantially better scores. In all reported analyses, adaptive models are less complex than GAMs. They are also always preferable due to having either larger LCV scores or competitive scores generating insubstantial percent decreases using more parsimonious models. Other data sets may exist for which GAMs generate substantially better scores than adaptive models. The example analyses only considered relatively smooth GAMs with degrees of freedom (DF) at most 4. GAMs based on larger DF values may provide substantial improvements over adaptive models. However, the results of reported analyses indicate that consideration of only GAMs can sometimes produce either distinctly inferior results or more complex models than needed, and so it is important to consider adaptive fractional polynomial models in general to address nonlinearity. Other advantages of adaptive fractional polynomial modeling include the ability to compute odds ratio functions for dichotomous outcomes (see Sect. 8.3) and to model polytomous outcomes, multivariate outcomes, and variances/dispersions in combination with means. See Chap. 17 for details on conducting analyses in SAS like those presented in this chapter.

References

Ahlberg, J. H., Nilson, E. N., & Walsh, J. L. (1967). *The theory of splines and their applications.* New York: Academic.

Cleveland, W. S., Devlin, S. J., & Gross, E. (1988). Regression by local fitting. *Journal of Econometrics, 37*, 87–114.

Hastie, T. J., & Tibshirani, R. J. (1999). *Generalized additive models.* Boca Raton, FL: Chapman & Hall/CRC.

Meinguet, J. (1979). Multivariate interpolation at arbitrary points made simple. *Journal of Applied Mathematics and Physics (ZAMP), 30*, 292–304.

SAS Institute. (2004). *SAS/STAT 9.1 user's guide.* Cary, NC: SAS Institute.

Wahba, G. (1990). *Spline models for observational data.* Philadelphia: SIAM.

Chapter 17
Generalized Additive Modeling in SAS

17.1 Chapter Overview

This chapter provides a description of how to use PROC GAM for generating
generalized additive models (GAMs) (Hastie and Tibshirani 1999; SAS Institute
2004) for univariate continuous and dichotomous outcomes and available SAS
macros for computing their likelihood cross-validation (LCV) scores. Comparison
of GAMS to adaptive fractional polynomial models is also covered. Reported
output is produced using version 9.4. Sections 17.2–17.4 present code for modeling
the univariate continuous outcome death rate per 100,000 in terms of available
predictors (see Sects. 2.2 and 16.8) as well as models for predicting the univariate
dichotomous outcome a high mercury level in fish over 1.0 ppm versus a lower
level in terms of available predictors (see Sect. 8.2).

17.2 Invoking PROC GAM

A data set on death rates for $n = 60$ metropolitan statistical areas in the US is
analyzed in Chap. 16 as described in Sect. 16.8 (see Sect. 2.2 for description of the
part of these data analyzed in Chaps 2 and 3). Assuming this full data set has been
loaded into the SAS default library under the name fulldr, a GAM for deathrate as a
function of NOindex using the cubic spline (Ahlberg et al. 1967) approach with
$DF = 3$ and treating deathrate as normally (or Gaussian) distributed with identity
link function (PROC GAM only supports canonical link functions) can be requested
in SAS as follows.

```
proc gam data=fulldr;
  model deathrate=spline(NOindex,DF=3) / dist=gaussian;
run;
```

© Springer International Publishing Switzerland 2016   315
G.J. Knafl, K. Ding, *Adaptive Regression for Modeling Nonlinear Relationships*,
Statistics for Biology and Health, DOI 10.1007/978-3-319-33946-7_17

Table 17.1 Output generated by PROC GAM for the cubic spline generalized additive model for the death rate per 100,000 in the nitric oxide pollution index (NOindex) with three degrees of freedom

```
                        Regression Model Analysis
                          Parameter Estimates

                        Parameter       Standard
        Parameter       Estimate         Error      t Value     Pr > |t|

        Intercept       942.66509        8.35984     112.76      <.0001
        Linear(NOindex)  -0.10383        0.16320      -0.64      0.5272

                       Smoothing Model Analysis
                Fit Summary for Smoothing Components

                                                                      Num
                        Smoothing                                    Unique
        Component       Parameter         DF            GCV           Obs

     Spline(NOindex)    0.983984       2.000000    3381.769650        30
```

Part of the SAS output is displayed in Table 17.1. The model always includes an intercept term (the PROC GAM model statement does not currently support a "noint" option as do other SAS regression procedures). Note that a linear term in NOindex is included in the model while the associated DF for the nonparametric component in NOindex is $3 - 1 = 2$. A χ^2 test for a zero nonparametric component is also generated but not included in Table 17.1. A linear model in NOindex without a nonparametric NOindex component can be requested by changing "spline(NOindex,DF=3)" to "param(NOindex)".

The loess (Cleveland et al. 1988) approach with DF = 3 can be requested by changing "spline" to "loess" in the above code. Part of the SAS output is displayed in Table 17.2. Note that the actual DF = 3.029048 only rounds to the requested value of DF = 3 and is composed of DF = 1 for the linear term and DF = 2.029048 for the loess nonparametric component. Note also that a generalized cross-validation (GCV) (Wahba 1990) score is reported in Table 17.2 (and also in Table 17.1). The DF value can be chosen for that loess model through GCV using the following code.

```
proc gam data=fulldr;
 model deathrate=loess(NOindex) / dist=gaussian method=GCV;
run;
```

Table 17.2 Output generated by PROC GAM for the local regression (loess) generalized additive model for the death rate per 100,000 in the nitric oxide pollution index (NOindex) with three degrees of freedom

```
                      Regression Model Analysis
                        Parameter Estimates

                    Parameter         Standard
   Parameter        Estimate            Error     t Value    Pr > |t|

   Intercept        942.66509          7.92746     118.91     <.0001
   Linear(NOindex)   -0.10383          0.15476      -0.67     0.5050

                      Smoothing Model Analysis
                 Fit Summary for Smoothing Components

                                                               Num
                   Smoothing                                  Unique
   Component       Parameter          DF            GCV         Obs

Loess(NOindex)     0.708333        2.029048      54.616385       60
```

The option "method=GCV" in the PROC GAM model statement requests selection of the DF through GCV scores as defined in Sect. 16.4. In this case, the selected DF = 2.858578 (DF = 1 for the linear term and DF = 1.858578 for the loess nonparametric component). When "method=GCV" is requested in the model statement, the GCV request is ignored if a DF value is also provided for a predictor in that model statement. If neither a DF value nor method=GCV is provided in the model statement, the default value DF = 4 is used. Requesting a cubic spline with DF = 1 generates a degenerate model with an essentially zero DF for the nonparametric part of the model along with a warning message in the SAS log window that the DF is outside the appropriate range, and so should be avoided. On the other hand, the loess GAM with requested DF = 1 has actual DF = 1.30351 with DF = 1 for the linear term and DF = 0.30351 for the loess nonparametric component, and so a requested DF = 1 is an acceptable alternative for loess GAMs (however, since DF < 0.5 for the loess nonparametric component of the model, the p-value for the associated χ^2 test is not generated by PROC GAM).

17.3   Generating LCV Scores for GAMs

SAS PROC GAM does not currently support LCV as needed to compare GAMs to adaptive fractional polynomial models (or to other GAMs), and so a SAS macro called LCVGAM has been developed for computing LCV scores for GAMs. Assuming that this macro has been loaded (and in what follows, all the other macros to be described as well), the model for deathrate as a function of NOindex using the loess approach with DF = 3 and its 10-fold LCV score is generated as follows.

```
%LCVGAM(datain=fulldr,yvar=deathrate,disttype=gaussian,
        xvars=loess(NOindex,DF=3),foldcnt=5,scorefmt=9.7,
        procmod=y);
```

The datain, yvar, and foldcnt macro parameters have the same meanings as for the genreg macro (see Chap. 3). The xvars macro parameter has similar meaning as for genreg but with its setting a list of model terms allowed by PROC GAM. The above xvars setting requests a model in NOindex using the loess approach with DF set to 3. The setting "xvars=loess(NOindex)" requests the default value DF = 4. Changing to "xvars=spline(NOindex,DF=3)" requests a model in NOindex using the cubic spline approach with DF = 3. Changing to "xvars=param(NOindex)" requests a linear model in NOindex. The disttype macro parameter must be set to a valid value for the "dist=" option of the PROC GAM model statement. The setting "disttype=gaussian" (which is the default value) requests a model for the untransformed means (that is, using the identity link function) of the outcome variable under standard normality-based regression modeling as used to model continuous outcomes like deathrate. The scorefmt macro variable is used to specify the format for printing of the generated LCV score. It must be a valid SAS w.d format. In this case, the width w equals nine characters with decimal digits d equal to 7. The setting "procmod=y" requests that PROC GAM output be generated for the requested GAM. The LCV score for that model will also be outputted as long as "noprint=n", which is the default setting. In this case, the actual DF = 3.02905, rounding to the requested DF = 3, and the LCV score is 0.0040119 as also reported in Table 16.1.

The following code requests a loess model in NOindex with DF chosen through GCV. A DF value must not be included in the xvars setting. If it is, PROC GAM will ignore the "method=GCV" request. As reported in Table 16.1, the actual DF = 2.85858, rounding to DF = 2.86, and the LCV score is 0.0039866.

```
%LCVGAM(datain=fulldr,yvar=deathrate,disttype=gaussian,
        xvars=loess(NOindex),method=GCV,foldcnt=5,
        scorefmt=9.7, procmod=y);
```

Several other SAS macros have been developed to systematically invoke the LCVGAM macro to generate LCV scores for multiple GAMs. One of these is called multGAM1 and is used to generate models using one smoothing approach over ranges of DF values. The following code requests LCV scores for cubic spline GAMs of deathrate as a function of NOindex with DF = 2–4 as reported in Table 16.1.

Table 17.3 Output generated by multGAM1 for alternate cubic spline generalized additive models for the death rate per 100,000 in the nitric oxide pollution index (NOindex)

xvar1	Type for xvar1	DF for xvar1	10-fold LCV Score	Percent Decrease
NOindex	spline	2	0.0039184	0.00%
NOindex	spline	3	0.0030058	23.3%
NOindex	spline	4	0.0020098	48.7%

```
%multGAM1(datain=fulldr,yvar=death rate,disttype=gaussian,
         xvar1=NOindex,GAMtype=spline,DFfst=2,DFlst=4,
         foldcnt=5,scorefmt=9.7);
```

The datain, yvar, disttype, foldcnt, and scorefmt macro parameters have the same meaning as for LCVGAM. The xvar1 macro parameter should be set to the name of a single predictor, in this case NOindex. The type of smoothing approach to use with that predictor is set with the GAMtype macro parameter, in this case "spline" to request cubic splines (as also used by PROC GAM to denote cubic splines). DFfst and DFlst are set to the first and last DF values, respectively, to be generated by multGAM1, in this case DF = 2–4. The default value for DFfst is 1, but multGAM1 will automatically adjust a request for a cubic spline with DF = 1 to DF = 2, and so DFfst is not needed. Neither is "DFlst=4" since that is the default value for DFlst. The output generated by multGAM1 is displayed in Table 17.3. To generate the results for loess models reported in Table 16.1 change to "GAMtype=loess" and "DFfst=1" (or drop the DFfst setting since 1 is the default value).

17.4   Multiple Predictor GAMs

The GAM for deathrate as a function of NObnded and rain combining the best singleton predictor GAMs for NObnded and rain of Table 16.2 (that is, using the loess approach with DF = 1 for each of the predictors) is requested in SAS as follows.

```
proc gam data=fulldr;
  model deathrate=loess(NObnded,DF=1) loess(rain,DF=1)
                  / dist=gaussian;
run;
```

The LCV score of 0.0055341 (see Table 16.4) for this model can be generated as follows.

Table 17.4 Output generated by PROC GAM for the thin plate spline generalized additive model for the death rate per 100,000 in the nitric oxide pollution index bounded at 12 (NObnded) and rain with two degrees of freedom

```
                          Regression Model Analysis
                            Parameter Estimates


                        Parameter        Standard
          Parameter     Estimate          Error     t Value     Pr > |t|

          Intercept     940.31333        5.52863     170.08      <.0001

                          Smoothing Model Analysis
                    Fit Summary for Smoothing Components


                                                                          Num
                              Smoothing                                 Unique
   Component                  Parameter         DF          GCV            Obs

   Spline2(NObnded rain)        24233      2.000186   1930.473360           54
```

```
%LCVGAM(datain=fulldr,yvar=deathrate,disttype=gaussian,
        xvars=loess(NObnded,DF=1) loess(rain,DF=1),
        foldcnt=5,scorefmt=9.7);
```

Thin plate splines (Meinguet 1979) are denoted as "spline2" by PROC GAM, and so a thin plate spline in NObnded and rain with DF = 2 is requested as follows.

```
proc gam data=fulldr;
   model deathrate=spline2(NObnded,rain,DF=2) / dist=gaussian;
run;
```

Table 17.4 contains part of the generated output. Note that no linear terms are added to the model for thin plate splines as they are for cubic splines and loess. The LCV score of 0.0053103 (see Table 16.4) for this model can be generated as follows.

```
%LCVGAM(datain=fulldr,yvar=deathrate,disttype=gaussian,
        xvars=spline2(NObnded,rain,DF=2),foldcnt=5,
        scorefmt=9.7);
```

Composite cubic spline models for NObnded and rain with varying DF values can be generated using multGAM1 as follows.

```
%multGAM1(datain=fulldr,yvar=deathrate,disttype=gaussian,
         xvar1=NObnded,xvar2=rain,GAMtype=spline,
         foldcnt=5,scorefmt=9.7);
```

The default DF range of 1–4 is requested, but is adjusted to DF = 2–4 for cubic splines. All nine combinations of DF = 2–4 for each predictor are generated. The best score of 0.0054271 occurs with DF = 2 for both predictors and is reported in the first row of Table 16.4. Changing to "GAMtype=loess" generates the 16 combinations of loess models with DF = 1–4 for each predictor. The best score of 0.0055341 occurs with DF = 1 for both predictors and is reported in Table 16.4. Changing to "GAMtype=spline2" generates the three thin plate spline models with DF = 2–4. As for cubic splines, requests for DF = 1 with thin plate splines are changed to DF = 2 to avoid degenerate cases. The best thin plate spline score of 0.0053103 occurs with DF = 2 and is also reported in Table 16.4.

The third row of Table 16.4 involves combinations of both cubic splines with DF = 2–4 and loess with DF = 1–4, a total of 49 different models. These can be requested using the multGAM2 macro as follows.

```
%multGAM2(datain=fulldr,yvar=deathrate,disttype=gaussian,
         xvar1=NObnded,xvar2=rain,foldcnt=5,
         scorefmt=9.7);
```

The best cubic spline or loess term for one new predictor to add to a GAM based on other predictors is generated with the add1GAM macro. Include the loess term for nonwhite selected in the first step of Table 16.6 with alternative models in NObnded as follows.

```
%add1GAM(datain=fulldr,yvar=deathrate,disttype=gaussian,
         fxdxvars=loess(nonwhite,DF=1),xtraxvar=NObnded,
         foldcnt=5,scorefmt=9.7);
```

The fxdxvars macro parameter setting is a list of smoothing requests for individual predictors using the format required by PROC GAM. The xtraxvar macro parameter setting is the name of an extra predictor. It should not be included in the fxdxvars list. The default DFfst and DFlst values are requested, and so seven models will be considered including models with extra cubic spline terms in NObnded with DF = 2–4 and extra loess terms in NObnded with DF = 1–4, each combined with the loess DF = 1 term for nonwhite. The output is displayed in Table 17.5. The extra "spline(NObnded,DF=2)" term generates the best LCV score.

The addGAM macro is used to iteratively call the add1GAM macro to augment a fixed GAM as determined by the fxdxvars macro parameter with an additional predictor, one at a time from the list of predictors in the xtraxvars macro parameter setting. The following code augments the loess term for nonwhite as selected in the first step of Table 16.6 with each of the other 14 possible predictors.

Table 17.5 Output generated by add1GAM augmenting the loess DF = 1 term for the indicator for being non-White with alternate param, cubic spline, and loess terms for the nitric oxide pollution index bounded at 12 (NObnded)

Extra x Variable	GAM Type	DF	5-fold LCV Score	Percent Decrease
NObnded	spline	2	0.0052521	0.00%
NObnded	loess	1	0.0052449	0.14%
NObnded	spline	3	0.0052337	0.35%
NObnded	loess	3	0.0052283	0.45%
NObnded	param	- -	0.0052043	0.91%
NObnded	spline	4	0.0051968	1.05%
NObnded	loess	2	0.0051966	1.06%
NObnded	loess	4	0.0051561	1.83%

```
%addGAM(datain=fulldr,yvar=deathrate,disttype=gaussian,
        fxdxvars=loess(nonwhite,DF=1),
        xtraxvars=NObnded SO2index rain JANtemp JULtemp
                  over65 HHsize educatn kitchens pop
                  oworkers lowinc HCindex moisture,
        foldcnt=5,scorefmt=9.7);
```

The addition of the loess term in rain with DF = 1 generates the best LCV score of 0.0055887, and so is the result of the second step of Table 16.6. The complete results of Table 16.6 can be generated by the addGAMs macro as follows.

```
%addGAMs(datain=fulldr,yvar=deathrate,disttype=gaussian,
         fxdxvars=,
         xtraxvars=NObnded SO2index rain JANtemp JULtemp
                   over65 HHsize educatn kitchens pop
                   nonwhite oworkers lowinc HCindex moisture,
         foldcnt=5,scorefmt=9.7);
```

The addGAMs macro first calls the addGAM macro to find the best term in all of the 15 predictors of xtraxvars to add to the constant model as requested by the empty setting for fxdxvars. This term is added to the fxdxvars parameter setting and the associated variable removed from the xtraxvars list. Then addGAM is called with these revised parameter settings and the process continues until one term for each of the xtraxvars variables is added to the fxdxvars model.

17.5   GAMs for Dichotomous Outcomes

Analyses are conducted in Sect. 16.10 of categorized mercury levels for $n = 169$ largemouth bass caught in one of two rivers (Lumber and Wacamaw) in North Carolina (see Sect. 8.2 for a description of these data). Assuming that these mercury data have been loaded into the SAS default library under the name mercury, a GAM for merchigh (a high mercury level of over 1.0 ppm versus low) as a function of the weight of fish using the cubic spline approach with $DF = 3$ and treating merchigh as binomially distributed with logit link function can be requested in SAS as follows.

```
proc gam data=mercury;
  model merchigh(descending)=spline(weight,DF=3)
                 / dist= binomial;
run;
```

By default, PROC GAM models the first or lower value of a binomial outcome like merchigh, and so the higher value is then treated as the reference value. This is reversed in the above code by adding the descending option in parentheses after the name of the outcome. In this way, models are generated for the chance of high levels of mercury versus low levels as the reference value.

Part of the SAS output is displayed in Table 17.6. The link function used with "dist=binomial" is the canonical logit function. The note in the output is important to check for "dist=binomial" cases to correctly interpret predicted values. In this case, it indicates that the larger outcome value of 1 is modeled so that the lower value of 0 is the reference value. This is achieved in the above code with the descending option. Another alternative is to use the "event=last" option as in the following model statement.

```
model merchigh(event=last)=spline(weight,DF=3) / dist=binomial;
```

The output suggests that using "event=1" would also work, but that is only the case if the outcome variable merchigh has not been assigned a format. If the outcome variable is formatted, use the formatted value not the actual value. This issue is avoided by designating the outcome value as the last one. The rest of the output is similar to results for continuous outcomes except that estimates are for logit transforms of the means rather than identity transformed (that is, untransformed) means.

The 15-fold LCV score for this model is 0.54745 (reported LCV scores are based on 15-folds as justified in Sect. 8.4) and can be generated for the cubic spline GAM as follows, rounded to five decimal digits within seven character positions.

```
%LCVGAM(datain=mercury,yvar=merchigh,disttype=binomial,
        xvars=spline(weight,DF=3),foldcnt=15,scorefmt=7.5);
```

Table 17.6 Output generated by PROC GAM for the cubic spline generalized additive model for a high mercury level over 1.0 ppm (merchigh) in weight of the fish with three degrees of freedom

```
                        The GAM Procedure
                   Dependent Variable: merchigh
              Smoothing Model Component(s): spline(weight)

                    Summary of Input Data Set

              Number of Observations              169
              Number of Missing Observations        0
              Distribution                    Binomial
              Link Function                      Logit
...
NOTE: PROC GAM is modeling the probability that merchigh=1. One way to
      change this to model the probability that merchigh=0 is to specify
      the response variable option EVENT='0'.
...
                    Regression Model Analysis
                      Parameter Estimates

                    Parameter      Standard
      Parameter      Estimate        Error    t Value    Pr > |t|

      Intercept       -1.30191      0.30362     -4.29     <.0001
      Linear(weight)   1.08144      0.21974      4.92     <.0001

                    Smoothing Model Analysis
                Fit Summary for Smoothing Components

                                                                  Num
                     Smoothing                                   Unique
      Component      Parameter        DF          GCV             Obs

      Spline(weight)  0.999994     2.000000     5.768278          162
```

LCV scores for cubic spline GAMs of merchigh as a function of weight with DF = 2–4 can be generated as follows.

```
%multGAM1(datain=mercury,yvar=merchigh,disttype=binomial,
          xvar1=weight,GAMtype=spline,DFfst=2,DFlst=4,
          foldcnt=15,scorefmt=7.5);
```

As reported in Sect. 16.10, the best such LCV score is 0.54803 and is achieved at DF = 2. The multGAM1 macro can be used to generate LCV scores for GAMs of dichotomous outcomes in terms of singleton predictors similar to those generated for the continuous outcomes reported in Sect. 17.3. It can also be used to generate LCV scores for GAMs of dichotomous outcomes in terms of two predictors similar to those generated for the continuous outcomes reported in Sect. 17.4. For example,

LCV scores for thin plate spline GAMs in weight and length can be requested as follows.

```
%multGAM1(datain=mercury,yvar=merchigh,disttype=binomial,
         xvar1=weight,xvar2=length,GAMtype=spline2,
         DFfst=2,DFlst=4,foldcnt=15,scorefmt=7.5);
```

The DFfst and DFlst options request scores for the choices DF = 2–4. The initial DF value of 2 is requested using the DFfst macro parameter since DF = 1 is not appropriate for thin plate splines. However, it is not needed since multGAM1 skips requests for DF = 1 when "GAMtype=spline2" (and also "GAMtype=spline"). The multGAM2 macro (see Sect. 17.4) can also be used to generate GAMs for merchigh as a function of weight and length using combinations of cubic spline and loess terms similarly to GAMs for continuous outcomes. The add1GAM, addGAM, and addGAMs macros (see Sect. 17.4) can be used with dichotomous outcomes to generate multiple predictor GAMs.

The variable river, indicating the river in which the fish were caught, is demonstrated in Sect. 8.4 using adaptive fractional polynomial modeling to distinctly moderate the effect of weight on merchigh, leading to the question of how this variable can be incorporated into GAMs. One way is as a linear predictor using the term "param(river)". Use of the term "spline(river,DF=2)" generates an error message, and the model cannot be computed by PROC GAM. Hence, cubic spline GAMs in indicator variables should not be requested. The model with the term "loess(river,DF=1)" does not generate an error message and the model can be computed by PROC GAM. However, only the linear term is estimated while the loess nonparametric term of the model has a missing DF value. The LCV score for this model is the same as for the model in "param(river)", and so loess GAMs in indicator variables are degenerate and should also not be requested. On the other hand, the model with the term "spline2(river,weight,DF=2)" is not degenerate and this term is significant (P < 0.001). In standard regression analyses, a main effect to a moderator like river could also have an effect when its interaction with another variable like weight is included in the model, but the LCV score of 0.54469 for the thin plate GAM in river and weight without the term "param(river)" is the same as with it, indicating there is no need for a linear term in an indicator variable that is included in a thin plate term of the model. The multGAM1 macro can be used to identify the best DF for the thin plate GAM in river and weight. A search over DF = 2–4 identifies DF = 4 as the best choice with LCV score is 0.56025 while the loess GAM in weight with DF = 3 with the best LCV score for GAMs in weight alone is 0.54824 (see Sect. 16.10) with substantial PD of 2.14 %. Hence, a GAM analysis indicates that river distinctly moderates the effect of weight on merchigh as also holds for the adaptive analysis of Sect. 8.4. The adaptive moderation model in river and weight has LCV score 0.57192 (see Sect. 8.4), which is a substantial improvement over the best thin plate spline GAM with PD 2.04 % in the LCV scores. Moreover, it is simpler having two terms besides an intercept in comparison to the DF = 4 of the thin plate spline GAM plus an intercept.

17.6 Practice Exercises

17.1 Assess the effectiveness of the first two steps of the adaptive process for adding GAMs in individual predictors to a model described in Sect. 16.8. With k = 5 folds as justified in Sect. 2.8, use the multGAM2 macro to generate all possible combinations of loess and cubic splines GAMs in the first two predictors nonwhite and rain added to the model for deathrate (see Table 16.6). What model is generated by multGAM2? Is the Step 2 model of Table 16.6 either better than or a competitive alternative to the multGAM2 model, indicating that the first two steps of the adaptive process are effective? Or is the multGAM2 model distinctly better, indicating that the adaptive process is not effective and a more exhaustive search is required to effectively identify GAMs in two predictors?

17.2 Compare GAMs and adaptive fractional polynomial models for the two predictors NObnded and nonwhite of the death rate data. First, with k = 5 as justified in Sect. 2.8, use the multGAM2 macro to generate all possible combinations of loess and cubic splines GAMs in these two predictors with DF = 2–4 for spline terms and DF = 1–4 for loess terms. Next, generate the adaptive additive fractional polynomial model in these two predictors. Which of these two models is more preferable? Next, use the multGAM2 macro to generate thin plate splines in these two predictors with DF = 2–4. Does this improve on the results of multGAM2? Finally, generate the adaptive model in these two predictors and GCs. Does this improve on the adaptive additive fractional polynomial model? Compare the effectiveness of fractional polynomial models for identifying interaction effects between these two predictors through GCs to that of thin plate splines.

17.3 Assess moderation of the effect of length on merchigh by river using thin plate splines. With k = 15 folds as justified in Sect. 8.4, use the multGAM1 macro to generate thin plate spline GAMs in these two predictors with DF = 2–4. Compare this best thin plate spline GAM to the best GAM in length alone identified in Sect. 16.10. Does a GAM analysis indicate distinct moderation or not? Compare the better of these two latter GAMs to the adaptive fractional polynomial model in river, length, and geometric combinations identified in Sect. 8.5. Which model has the better LCV score? Is the other model a parsimonious, competitive alternative or not? Which of these models is the more preferable one?

For Practice Exercise 17.4, use the body fat data set available on the Internet (see Supplementary Materials). The outcome variable for this data set is called bodyfat and contains body fat values in gm/cm^3 for 252 men. The file contains several predictors. Practice Exercises 17.4 uses only three of these predictors, called weight, height, and BMI containing weights in pounds, heights in inches, and body mass index values in kg/cm^2, respectively.

17.4 Generate the spline GAMs for bodyfat in terms of BMI with DF = 2–4. Use the number of folds for this practice exercise determined as part of Practice Exercise 3.5. Then, generate the loess GAMs for bodyfat in terms of BMI with DF = 1–4. Do loess or spline GAMs generate a better model. Compare the better of these two types of GAMs to the adaptive model in BMI computed for Practice Exercise 3.5. Next, generate the thin plate spline GAM in weight and height and compare it to the GAM model in BMI.

For Practice Exercise 17.5, use the Titanic survival data available on the Internet (see Supplementary Materials). Data are available for 756 passengers with no missing data. The outcome variable for this data set is called survived and is the indicator for having survived the sinking of the Titanic. The predictors to be considered are age and the indicator fstclass for the passenger being in first class versus second or third class. The gender of the passenger is also available in the data set but is not used in the practice exercises.

17.5 Generate the spline GAMs for survived in terms of age with DF = 2–4. Use the number of folds determined as part of Practice Exercise 9.5. Then, generate the loess GAMs for survived in terms of age with DF = 1–4. Do loess or spline GAMs generate a better model. Compare the better of these two types of GAMs to the adaptive model in age computed for Practice Exercise 9.5. Next, generate the thin plate spline GAM in age and fstclass; compare it to the best GAM model in age.

References

Ahlberg, J. H., Nilson, E. N., & Walsh, J. L. (1967). *The theory of splines and their applications.* New York: Academic Press.

Cleveland, W. S., Devlin, S. J., & Gross, E. (1988). Regression by local fitting. *Journal of Econometrics, 37,* 87–114.

Hastie, T. J., & Tibshirani, R. J. (1999). *Generalized additive models.* Boca Raton, FL: Chapman & Hall/CRC.

SAS Institute. (2004). *SAS/STAT 9.1 user's guide.* Cary, NC: SAS Institute.

Meinguet, J. (1979). Multivariate interpolation at arbitrary points made simple. *Journal of Applied Mathematics and Physics (ZAMP), 30,* 292–304.

Wahba, G. (1990). *Spline models for observational data.* Philadelphia: SIAM.

Chapter 18
Multivariate Adaptive Regression Spline Modeling

18.1 Chapter Overview

This chapter demonstrates multivariate adaptive regression splines (MARS) (Friedman 1991) for modeling means of continuous outcomes treated as independent and normally distributed with constant variances as in linear regression and of logits (log odds) of means of dichotomous outcomes with unit dispersions as in logistic regression. MARS models for these two cases are compared to adaptive fractional polynomial models. Poisson regression is not considered for brevity. See Chap. 19 for a description of how to conduct analyses like those described in this chapter using SAS.

MARS models provide an alternative to fractional polynomial models for modeling nonlinear relationships between univariate outcomes and predictors. Since MARS models are nonparametric regression alternatives to standard generalized linear models, they only address univariate outcomes and not multivariate outcomes (the "multivariate" in the abbreviation MARS refers to the fact that the models can be based on multiple variables but does not mean the outcome is multivariate as that term has been used elsewhere in this book). MARS models can be used in the regression context with univariate continuous outcomes as well as in other types of regression contexts like logistic regression with dichotomous discrete outcomes. Support for MARS models is provided in SAS through PROC ADAPTIVEREG (starting with version 9.4). A SAS macro called MARSmodl is available (see Chap. 19) for generating a data set containing the splines for a MARS model that can be inputted to the genreg macro to compute its likelihood cross-validation (LCV) score or to adaptively power transform its splines.

Section 18.2 describes MARS modeling. Section 18.3 provides example MARS analyses of the death rate data analyzed in Chaps. 2, 3, 16 and 17 (see Sects. 2.2 and 16.8 for a description of these data). Section 18.4 provides example MARS analyses of the dichotomous outcome of the fish mercury data analyzed in Chaps. 8, 9, 16 and 17 (see Sect. 8.2 for a description of these data). Sections 18.5–18.6 provide

© Springer International Publishing Switzerland 2016
G.J. Knafl, K. Ding, *Adaptive Regression for Modeling Nonlinear Relationships*,
Statistics for Biology and Health, DOI 10.1007/978-3-319-33946-7_18

overviews of the results of MARS analyses of death rates and dichotomous mercury levels, respectively.

18.2 Description of MARS Modeling

Only an informal description of the MARS modeling process is provided here; see Friedman (1991) or the SAS version 9.4 documentation for the formulation. MARS modeling first generates a maximal set of splines. Then, a forward selection process selects a subset of this maximal set by systematically adding in splines to the model. Finally a backward selection process systematically removes splines from the forward selection model to obtain the final subset determining the MARS model. Forward selection and backward selection serve similar purposes to the expansion and contraction phases of the adaptive modeling process: first to grow the model and then to prune it back to an effective model.

When a primary predictor u is a categorical variable, its associated basic splines are indicator variables for subsets of the observed values for u. When a primary predictor u is continuous, its associated basic splines have the forms $f(u) = \max(u - u_0, 0)$ and $f'(u) = \max(u_0 - u, 0)$ where u_0 is an observed value for u called a knot. Note that $f(u)$ is zero for $u \leq u_0$ and linear for $u \geq u_0$ while $f'(u)$ is zero for $u \geq u_0$ and linear for $u \leq u_0$. Interactions between these basic splines are considered as part of the default MARS modeling process, but this process can be constrained to be additive in its primary predictors. General MARS models can contain interactions of arbitrary order. By default, PROC ADAPTIVEREG supports only pairwise interactions, but this can be changed using the "maxorder=" option on the model statement. PROC ADAPTIVEREG only supports nonzero intercept models; the model statement does not have a "noint" option.

Parameters of MARS models can be estimated using maximum likelihood estimation, but an alternate approach is used by PROC ADAPTIVEREG to speed up processing. See Buja et al. (1991) or the SAS version 9.4 documentation for details. Splines based on continuous predictors are linear when nonzero but models based on power transforms of these splines can be generated using adaptive modeling.

18.3 MARS Analyses of Death Rates

18.3.1 MARS Analyses Based on NObnded

The MARS model for deathrate (the death rate per 100,000) as a function of NObnded (the nitric oxide pollution index bounded to be no more than 12 as justified in Sect. 2.15) is generated using the pairs of splines for NObnded at the 10 knots 5, 7, 9, 11, 10, 6, 4, 8, 3, and 2 (generated in that order), a total of 20 splines. The forward selection model is based on 11 of these splines and is reduced by backward elimination to the single spline max(NObnded $-$ 2, 0). Its 5-fold (as justified in Sect. 2.8) LCV score is 0.0041056. The corresponding adaptive model has larger LCV score 0.0041968 (as reported in Sect. 2.15), but the percent decrease (PD) for the MARS model is insubstantial at 2.17 % (that is, smaller than the cutoff of 3.15 % as reported in Sect. 2.7). However, the adaptive model is simpler with one transform and no intercept compared to the MARS model with one spline and an intercept.

The adaptive modeling process using the spline of the MARS model is based on the transform max(NObnded $-$ 2, 0)$^{0.3}$ with an intercept. Its LCV score is 0.0042039 and the untransformed MARS model has insubstantial PD 2.34 %. Consequently, there is not a substantial benefit in this case to considering power transformed splines. The adaptive model in NObnded has a lower LCV score and insubstantial PD 0.17 %, is simpler, and so is preferable.

18.3.2 MARS Analyses Based on Rain

The MARS model for deathrate as a function of rain (the annual average precipitation in inches) is generated using the pairs of splines for rain at the four knots 34, 31, 44, and 39 (generated in that order), a total of eight splines. The forward selection model is based on five of these splines and is reduced by backward elimination to the single spline max(34 $-$ rain, 0). Its LCV score is 0.0043796. The corresponding adaptive model has larger LCV score 0.0044527 (as reported in Sect. 2.16), but the PD for the MARS model is insubstantial at 1.64 %. However, the adaptive model is simpler with one transform and no intercept compared to the MARS model with one spline and an intercept.

The adaptive modeling process using the spline of the MARS model is based on the transform max(34 $-$ rain, 0)$^{0.7}$ with an intercept. Its LCV score is 0.0044095 and the untransformed MARS model has insubstantial PD 0.68 %. Consequently, there is not a substantial benefit in this case to considering power transformed splines. Also, the adaptive model has a better LCV score and is simpler than the adaptive MARS model.

18.3.3 MARS Analyses Based on NObnded and Rain

The MARS model for death rate as an additive function of NObnded and rain is generated using the pairs of splines for NObnded at the eight knots 4, 8, 7, 11, 6, 10, 2, and 5 and the pairs of splines for rain at the two knots 33 and 38, a total of 20 splines. The forward selection model is based on 12 of these splines and is reduced by backward elimination to the four splines max(33 $-$ rain, 0), max(4 $-$ NObnded, 0), max(rain $-$ 38, 0), and max(NObnded $-$ 7, 0). Its LCV score is 0.0052894. The corresponding adaptive additive model has larger LCV score 0.0056386 (as reported in Sect. 2.16), which is a substantial improvement over the MARS model with PD 6.19 %. Moreover, the adaptive model is simpler with two transforms and no intercept compared to the MARS model with four splines and an intercept.

The adaptive modeling process using the splines of the additive MARS model is based on the two transforms $\max(33 - \text{rain}, 0)^{0.8}$ and $\max(\text{NObnded} - 7, 0)^{0.1}$ with an intercept. Its LCV score is 0.0054876 and the untransformed MARS model has substantial PD 3.61 %. Consequently, there is a substantial benefit in this case to considering power transformed splines. Furthermore, the PD compared to the corresponding adaptive model is now insubstantial at 2.68 %, but the adaptive model is simpler.

The MARS model in NObnded and rain allowing for interactions is based on five pairwise spline interactions and has improved LCV score 0.0056596. However, the adaptive additive model is a parsimonious, competitive alternative with insubstantial PD 0.37 %.

18.3.4 MARS Analyses Based on the Full Set of Available Predictors

The MARS model for deathrate as an additive function of the 15 predictors of Table 16.5 is based on the four splines $\max(\text{nonwhite} - 4.7, 0)$, $\max(\text{educatn} - 10.7, 0)$, $\max(10 - \text{NObnded}, 0)$, and $\max(35 - \text{rain}, 0)$. Its LCV score is 0.0071189. The corresponding adaptive additive model has larger LCV score 0.0072154 (as reported in Sect. 16.8), but the PD for the MARS model is insubstantial at 1.34 %. However, it is not simpler since it is based on four splines with an intercept while the adaptive additive model is based on five transforms without an intercept.

The adaptive additive MARS model using the splines of the additive MARS model is based on the four transforms $\max(\text{nonwhite} - 4.7, 0)^{0.7}$, $\max(\text{educatn} - 10.7, 0)^{2.1}$, $\max(10 - \text{NObnded}, 0)$, and $\max(35 - \text{rain}, 0)^{0.6}$ with an intercept. The LCV score is 0.0074000 and the untransformed additive MARS model has substantial PD 3.80 %. Consequently, there is a substantial benefit in this case to considering power transformed splines. The PD for the adaptive additive model compared to the corresponding adaptive additive MARS model is insubstantial at 2.49 % but it is not simpler.

18.4 MARS Analyses of the Mercury Level Data

As in Chaps. 8 and 9, all models of this section are constrained to include an intercept.

18.4.1   MARS Analyses Based on Weight of Fish

The MARS model for merchigh (the indicator for having a high mercury level >1 ppm) as a function of the weight of the fish is generated using the pairs of splines for weight at the ten knots 0.869, 2.541, 0.977, 0.844, 2.709, 0.6, 0.498, 0.38, 0.656, and 0.308 (generated in that order), a total of 20 splines. The forward selection model is based on 11 of these splines and is reduced by backward elimination to the two splines max(weight $- 0.6$, 0) and max(weight $- 0.498$, 0). Its 15-fold (as justified in Sect. 8.4) LCV score is 0.56281. The corresponding adaptive model has smaller LCV score 0.56081 (as reported in Sect. 8.4), but the PD is insubstantial at 0.36 % (that is, smaller than the cutoff of 1.13 % as reported in Sect. 8.2). Moreover, the adaptive model is simpler with one transform and an intercept compared to the MARS model with two splines and an intercept.

The adaptive modeling process using the splines of the MARS model is based on the transform max(weight $- 0.498$, 0)$^{0.27}$ with an intercept. Its LCV score is 0.56565 and the untransformed MARS model has insubstantial PD 0.50 %. Consequently, there is not a substantial benefit in this case to considering power transformed splines, but the adaptive MARS model is simpler. The adaptive model in weight has a lower LCV score but with insubstantial PD 0.86 %, but it is also based on one transform and an intercept so that the adaptive MARS model is preferable. Figure 18.1 provides a comparison of the estimated probability for a high mercury level >1.0 ppm under the adaptive MARS and adaptive models. The benefit for the adaptive MARS model is in treating the probability to be constant for small weights less than or equal to 0.498 kg (or essentially 0.5 kg).

18.4.2   MARS Analyses Based on Length of Fish

The MARS model for merchigh as a function of the length of the fish is generated using the pairs of splines for length at the ten knots 37.4, 45.4, 34.9, 36.2, 33.3, 43.4, 28.5, 29.5, 30.5, and 50 (generated in that order), a total of 20 splines. The forward selection model is based on 11 of these splines and is reduced by backward elimination to the three splines max(length $- 45.4$, 0), max(length $- 34.9$, 0), and max(length $- 36.2$, 0). Its LCV score is 0.60701. The corresponding adaptive model has smaller LCV score 0.59144 (as reported in Sect. 8.5) with substantial PD 2.57 %. The adaptive modeling process using the splines of the MARS model is based on the transforms max(length $- 45.4$, 0)^4 and max(length $- 34.9$, 0)$^{0.12}$ with an intercept. Its LCV score is 0.60816 and the untransformed MARS model has insubstantial PD 0.19 %. Consequently, there is not a substantial benefit in this case to considering power transformed splines. However, the adaptive MARS model is simpler based on two transforms plus an intercept compared to three splines plus an intercept.

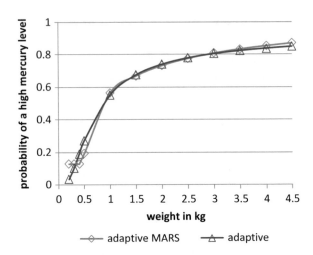

Fig. 18.1 Estimated probability of a high mercury level over 1.0 ppm as a function of weight of fish under the adaptive MARS model compared to the adaptive model

Figure 18.2 provides a comparison of the estimated probability for a high mercury level >1.0 ppm under the adaptive MARS and adaptive models. Under the adaptive MARS model, the estimated probability of a high mercury level > 1 ppm is constant up to 34.9 cm, increases nonlinearly from there to 45.4 cm, then close to linearly from there up to 55 cm after which it is constant at 1. In contrast, the estimated probability curve for the adaptive model is smoother, which is not as effective in this case.

18.4.3   MARS Analyses Based on Weight and Length of Fish

The MARS model for merchigh as an additive function of weight and length of the fish is generated using the pairs of splines for weight at the six knots 0.503, 0.362, 0.573, 0.313, 0.937, and 0.647 and the pairs of splines for rain at the four knots 37, 45.2, 36, and 31.7, a total of 20 splines. The forward selection model is based on 12 of these splines and is reduced by backward elimination to the six splines max(weight − 0.503, 0), max(length − 45.2, 0), max(weight − 0.362, 0), max(weight − 0.313, 0), max(length − 36, 0), and max(length − 31.7, 0). Its LCV score is 0.62140. The corresponding adaptive additive model has smaller LCV score 0.60382 (as reported in Sect. 8.6) with substantial PD 2.83 %. Consequently, in this case, the MARS model distinctly outperforms the adaptive model.

The adaptive Model using the splines of the additive MARS model is based on the four transforms max(length − 31.7, 0)$^{0.7}$, max(weight − 0.362, 0)$^{0.61}$, max(length − 45.2, 0)^4, and max(weight − 0.503, 0)$^{0.4}$ with an intercept. Its LCV score is 0.62259. The untransformed MARS model has insubstantial PD 0.19 %, but it is more complex, based on six splines with an intercept compared to four transforms plus an intercept.

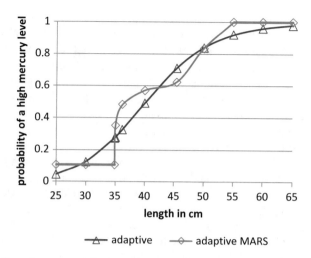

Fig. 18.2 Estimated probability of a high mercury level over 1.0 ppm as a function of length of fish under the adaptive MARS model compared to the adaptive model

The MARS model in weight and length allowing for interactions is based on 15 terms with five involving splines and the other ten pairwise interactions of splines. Its LCV score is the very low value 0.00027, indicating that this model seriously overfits the data. A standard spline analysis in this case suggests that the log odds for merchigh are reasonably considered to be additive in weigh and length of the fish. In contrast, the adaptive analysis of Sect. 8.6 indicates that the model considering geometric combinations (GCs) in weight and length provides a distinct improvement over the adaptive additive model. Moreover, this model has LCV score 0.61585 with insubstantial PD of 1.08 % compared to the adaptive additive MARS model with the best score for MARS models and is simpler, based on three transforms plus an intercept compared to four transforms plus an intercept. Consequently, in this case adaptive modeling generates a parsimonious, competitive alternative to MARS modeling as long as both additive models and models considering interactions or GCs are considered.

18.5   Overview of MARS Analyses of Death Rates

1. For death rates (Sect. 2.2), analyses use k = 5 folds (Sect. 2.8).
2. The adaptive model in NObnded generates a larger LCV score than the MARS model in NObnded (this and the following results reported in Sect. 18.3.1). The PD for the MARS model is insubstantial but the adaptive model is simpler. The adaptive MARS model generates a larger LCV score than the MARS model. The PD for the MARS model is insubstantial. The adaptive MARS model generates a larger LCV score than the adaptive model. The PD for the adaptive model is insubstantial and the adaptive model is simpler.

3. The adaptive model in rain generates a larger LCV score than the MARS model
   in rain (this and the following results reported in Sect. 18.3.2). The PD for the
   MARS model is insubstantial but the adaptive model is simpler. The adaptive
   MARS model generates a larger LCV score than the MARS model. The PD for
   the MARS model is insubstantial. The adaptive MARS model generates a larger
   LCV score than the adaptive model. The PD for the adaptive model is insubstantial and the adaptive model is simpler.
4. The adaptive additive model in NObnded and rain generates a larger LCV score
   than the additive MARS model in NObnded and rain (this and the following
   results reported in Sect. 18.3.3). The PD for the additive MARS model is
   substantial. The adaptive additive MARS model generates a larger LCV score
   than the additive MARS model. The PD for the additive MARS model is
   substantial and the adaptive additive MARS model is simpler. The adaptive
   additive model generates a larger LCV score than the adaptive additive MARS
   model. The PD for the adaptive additive MARS model is insubstantial but the
   adaptive additive model is simpler. The MARS model allowing for interactions
   generates a larger LCV score than the adaptive model. The PD for the adaptive
   additive model is insubstantial and the model is simpler.
5. The adaptive additive model in the predictors of Table 16.5 generates a larger
   LCV score than the additive MARS model in those predictors (this and the
   following results reported in Sect. 18.3.4). The PD for the additive MARS model
   is insubstantial but the model is not simpler. The adaptive additive MARS model
   generates a larger LCV score than the additive MARS model. The PD for the
   additive MARS model is substantial. The adaptive additive model generates a
   smaller LCV score than the adaptive additive MARS model. The PD for the
   adaptive additive model is insubstantial but the model is not simpler.

18.6   Overview of MARS Analyses of Dichotomous
Mercury Levels

1. For dichotomous mercury levels (Sect. 8.2), analyses use $k = 15$ folds
   (Sect. 8.4).
2. The MARS model in weight generates a larger LCV score than the adaptive
   model in weight (this and the following results reported in Sect. 18.4.1). The PD
   for the adaptive model is insubstantial and the model is simpler. The adaptive
   MARS model generates a larger LCV score than the MARS model. The PD for
   the MARS model is insubstantial but the adaptive MARS model is simpler. The
   adaptive MARS model generates a larger LCV score than the adaptive model.
   The PD for the adaptive model is insubstantial but both models have the same
   number of terms. Figure 18.1 provides a comparison of estimated probabilities
   for the adaptive and adaptive MARS models. See Sect. 19.5 for an analysis of the
   combined effect of weight and the river in which the fish were caught.

3. The MARS model in length generates a larger LCV score than the adaptive model in length (this and the following results reported in Sect. 18.4.2). The PD for the adaptive model is substantial. The adaptive MARS model generates a larger LCV score than the MARS model. The PD for the MARS model is insubstantial but the adaptive MARS model is simpler. Figure 18.2 provides a comparison of estimated probabilities for the adaptive and adaptive MARS models.

4. The adaptive MARS model in weight and length generates a larger LCV score than the adaptive additive model in weight and length (this and the following results reported in Sect. 18.4.3). The PD for the adaptive additive model is substantial. The adaptive additive MARS model generates a larger LCV score than the additive MARS model. The PD for the additive MARS model is insubstantial but the adaptive additive MARS model is simpler. The MARS model allowing for interactions generates a very small LCV score. The adaptive model in weight, length, and GCs generates a smaller LCV score than the adaptive additive MARS model but with insubstantial PD and fewer terms.

18.7   Chapter Summary

This chapter presents a series of analyses of the full death rate data using multivariate adaptive regression splines (MARS), addressing how the continuous outcome death rate per 100,000 depends on the 15 available predictors for 60 metropolitan statistical areas. It also presents analyses of the mercury level data using MARS, addressing how the dichotomous outcome a high level of mercury over 1.0 ppm versus a lower level depends on the weight and length of 169 fish. These analyses demonstrate MARS in these two important contexts.

Comparisons are also conducted of MARS modeling to adaptive fractional polynomial modeling. An example is provided where adaptive additive modeling distinctly outperforms additive MARS modeling. However, adaptive adjustment in that case improved the MARS model to be a competitive alternative. An example is also provided where additive MARS modeling distinctly outperforms adaptive additive modeling and adaptively adjusting the MARS model provides further improvements. However, consideration of interactions generated a very poor MARS model while consideration of geometric combinations improved the adaptive additive model to be a competitive alternative. Adaptively adjusting a MARS model usually improves the LCV score and sometimes distinctly so while reducing the number of terms in the model. Adaptive models usually have fewer or the same number of terms than adaptive MARS models with competitive or better LCV scores. The exceptions correspond to situations where a less smooth alternative is required as in Fig. 18.2. See Chap. 19 for details on conducting analyses in SAS like those presented in this chapter.

References

Buja, A., Duffy, D., Hastie, T., & Tibshirani, R. (1991). Discussion: Multivariate adaptive regression splines. *Annals of Statistics, 19*, 93–99.

Friedman, J. H. (1991). Multivariate adaptive regression splines. *Annals of Statistics, 19*, 1–67.

Chapter 19
Multivariate Adaptive Regression Spline Modeling in SAS

19.1 Chapter Overview

This chapter provides a description of how to use PROC ADAPTIVEREG for generating multivariate adaptive regression splines (MARS) models (Friedman 1991) for univariate continuous and dichotomous outcomes and SAS macros for computing their likelihood cross-validation (LCV) scores. Comparison of MARS models to adaptive fractional polynomial models is also covered as well as adaptively transforming MARS models. PROC ADAPTIVEREG requires SAS version 9.4 or later. Sections 19.2, 19.3 and 19.4 present code for modeling the univariate continuous outcome death rate per 100,000 in terms of available predictors (see Sects. 2.2 and 16.8). Section 19.5 presents code for modeling the univariate dichotomous outcome a high mercury level in fish over 1.0 ppm versus a lower level in terms of available predictors (see Sect. 8.2).

19.2 Invoking PROC ADAPTIVEREG

A data set on death rates for $n = 60$ metropolitan statistical areas in the US is analyzed in Chap. 18 as described in Sect. 16.8 (also see Sect. 2.2 for description of the part of these data analyzed in Chaps 2, 3, 6 and 7). Assuming this full data set has been loaded into the SAS default library under the name fulldr, a MARS model for deathrate as a function of NObnded (the nitric oxide pollution index bounded by 12; Sect. 2.15) treating deathrate as normally distributed with identity link function can be requested in SAS as follows.

```
proc adaptivereg data=fulldr details=bases;
  model deathrate=NObnded / dist=normal link=identity;
run;
```

© Springer International Publishing Switzerland 2016
G.J. Knafl, K. Ding, *Adaptive Regression for Modeling Nonlinear Relationships*,
Statistics for Biology and Health, DOI 10.1007/978-3-319-33946-7_19

The normal distribution is requested with the "dist=normal" option on the model statement but this is not needed since it is the default distribution for continuous outcome variables. The canonical identity link function is requested with the "link=identity" option but this is not needed since it is the default link function for the normal distribution. Part of the SAS output is displayed in Table 19.1. Spline predictors are given names with prefix "Basis" plus an index number. The model

Table 19.1 Output generated by PROC ADAPTIVEREG for the MARS model for the death rate per 100,000 as a function of the bounded nitric oxide pollution index (NObnded)

```
                      Basis Information

       Name          Transformation

       Basis0        1
       Basis1        Basis0*MAX(NObnded -              5,0)
       Basis2        Basis0*MAX(         5 - NObnded,0)
       Basis3        Basis0*MAX(NObnded -              7,0)
       Basis4        Basis0*MAX(         7 - NObnded,0)
       Basis5        Basis0*MAX(NObnded -              9,0)
       Basis6        Basis0*MAX(         9 - NObnded,0)
       Basis7        Basis0*MAX(NObnded -             11,0)
       Basis8        Basis0*MAX(        11 - NObnded,0)
       Basis9        Basis0*MAX(NObnded -             10,0)
       Basis10       Basis0*MAX(        10 - NObnded,0)
       Basis11       Basis0*MAX(NObnded -              6,0)
       Basis12       Basis0*MAX(         6 - NObnded,0)
       Basis13       Basis0*MAX(NObnded -              4,0)
       Basis14       Basis0*MAX(         4 - NObnded,0)
       Basis15       Basis0*MAX(NObnded -              8,0)
       Basis16       Basis0*MAX(         8 - NObnded,0)
       Basis17       Basis0*MAX(NObnded -              3,0)
       Basis18       Basis0*MAX(         3 - NObnded,0)
       Basis19       Basis0*MAX(NObnded -              2,0)
       Basis20       Basis0*MAX(         2 - NObnded,0)


   Regression Spline Model after Backward Selection

   Name       Coefficient     Parent    Variable        Knot

   Basis0        897.17                  Intercept
   Basis19       6.8657        Basis0    NObnded      2.0000
```

always includes an intercept term (the PROC ADAPTIVEREG model statement does not currently support a "noint" option as do other SAS regression procedures) denoted as "Basis0". The "detail=bases" option on the model statement requests a description of the full set of basis splines. Note that these are created in pairs of the form $f(u) = max(u - u_0, \ 0)$ and $f'(u) = max(u_0 - u, \ 0)$ where in this case $u = NObnded$ and u_0 is a knot equal to an observed NObnded value. Ten pairs of splines are generated for knots at the observed NObnded values of 5, 7, 9, 11, 10, 6, 4, 8, 3, and 2 in that order. The combination of forward and backward elimination applied to these 20 splines generates the MARS model based on the single spline $Basis19 = max(NObnded - 2, 0)$. To find out which splines are generated by the forward selection process change the details option on the model statement to "details=(bases fwdparams)". In this case, the forward selection model is based on the intercept Basis0 and the 11 splines Basis1, Basis2, Basis3, Basis5, Basis7, Basis9, Basis11, Basis13, Basis15, Basis17, and Basis19.

PROC ADAPTIVEREG supports a class statement that serves a similar purpose to the class statement of PROC GLM. Splines for predictors in the model statement also listed in the class statement are based on indicators for subsets of that predictor's values (an example is provided in Sect. 19.5).

19.3 Generating LCV Scores for MARS Models

PROC ADAPTIVEREG does not currently support LCV for comparing MARS models to each other and to adaptive fractional polynomial models. Consequently, a SAS macro called MARSmodl has been developed for generating data sets containing the spline predictors for a given MARS model. Assuming that this macro has been loaded (and also the genreg macro), the spline predictors for the MARS model for deathrate as a function of NObnded are generated in the data set data1 as follows.

```
%MARSmodl(datain=fulldr,dataout=data1,yvar=deathrate,
        xvars=NObnded);
```

The datain, yvar, and xvars macro parameters have the same meanings as for the genreg macro (see Chap. 3). The MARSmodl macro has a modtype parameter with the same meaning as for the genreg macro, but that is not needed here since the default setting is "modtype=norml" as is also the case for the genreg macro. The dataout macro parameter names the data set that is generated with the variables of the datain data set along with all the MARS spline predictors with names Basis1 to Basis20 as generated for this MARS model. The MARSmodl macro also generates the global macro parameter bwdlist containing the list of names of the spline predictors generated by the MARS backward selection process, in this case, its value is "Basis19". By default, the MARSmodl macro generates the output for

PROC ADAPTIVEREG, but this can be turned off with the setting "noMARSprnt=y".

The 5-fold (as justified in Sect. 2.8) LCV score for this MARS model can be generated as follows.

```
%genreg(datain=data1,yvar=deathrate,xvars=&bwdlist,
        foldcnt=5);
```

The LCV score is 0.0041056 as is also reported in Sect. 18.3.1. Note that this only works because the MARSmodl macro has previously been executed to generate the data1 data set containing the splines for the backward selection model and the bwdlist macro parameter with the list of names for that backward selection model. If the data1 data set has not been changed but the MARSmodl macro has most recently been executed for a different model, the above model can be generated by changing the xvars macro parameter setting in the above code to "xvars=basis19".

An adaptively transformed MARS model for deathrate as a function of NObnded can be generated as follows.

```
%genreg(datain=data1,yvar=deathrate,foldcnt=5,expand=y,
        expxvars=&bwdlist,contract=y);
```

In this case, the expanded model is based on Basis19$^{0.3}$ with an intercept and LCV score 0.0042039. The contraction leaves the model unchanged as does the conditional transformation (Sect. 3.3).

The 5-fold LCV score for the MARS model for deathrate as function of rain can be generated as follows.

```
%MARSmodl(datain=fulldr,dataout=data2,yvar=deathrate,
          xvars=rain);
%genreg(datain=data2,yvar= deathrate,xvars=&bwdlist,
        foldcnt=5);
```

19.4   Multiple Predictor MARS Models

The MARS model for deathrate as an additive function of NObnded and rain is directly requested in SAS as follows.

```
proc adaptivereg data=fulldr details=bases;
  model deathrate=NObnded rain
        / dist=normal link=identity additive;
run;
```

The additive option is needed in the model statement to generate an additive model. Without it, a model with individual predictor splines and pairwise interaction splines is generated. The first and third pairs of splines are based on the predictor rain and knots at values 33 and 38 in that order. The remaining eight pairs of splines are based on the predictor NObnded and knots at values 4, 9, 7, 11, 6, 10, 2, and 5 in that order. The LCV score for this model can be generated as follows.

```
%MARSmodl(datain=fulldr,dataout=data3,yvar=deathrate,
        xvars=NObnded rain, additive=y);
%genreg(datain=data3,yvar=deathrate,xvars=&bwdlist,
        foldcnt=5);
```

The setting "additive=y" requests an additive model in NObnded and rain. The following code generates the MARS model for NObnded and rain allowing for interactions and its LCV score.

```
%MARSmodl(datain=fulldr,dataout=data4,yvar=deathrate,
        xvars=NObnded rain);
%genreg(datain=data4,yvar=deathrate,xvars=&bwdlist,
        foldcnt=5);
```

The default setting of "additive=n" is requested in the above code to generate a MARS model with pairwise spline interactions. Table 19.2 contains some of the PROC ADAPTIVEREG output for this above MARS model. A pair of splines for rain with knot at the value 33 is generated first, then a pair of splines for NObnded with knot at the value 4. This is followed by interactions of Basis3 = max(NObnded −4, 0) with the pair of splines for rain with knot at value 38, interactions of Basis2 = max(33−rain, 0) with the three pairs of splines for NObnded with knots at 5, 11, and 2 in that order, interactions of Basis4 = max(4−NObnded, 0) with the pairs of splines for rain with knot at 39, a pair of splines for NObnded with knots at values 10 and 7 as well as finally a pair of splines for NObnded with knot at 6. The backward selection model is based on the five pairwise interaction splines: Basis5 = Basis3*max(rain−38, 0), Basis6 = Basis3*max(38−rain, 0), Basis7 = Basis2*max(NObnded−5, 0), Basis9 = Basis2*max(NObnded−11, 0), and Basis14 = Basis4*max(39−rain, 0). The LCV score is 0.0056596 as also reported in Sect. 18.3.3.

19.5 MARS Models for Dichotomous Outcomes

Analyses are conducted in Sect. 18.4 of the dichotomous mercury level outcome for $n = 169$ largemouth bass caught in one of two rivers (Lumber and Wacamaw) in North Carolina (see Sect. 8.2 for a description of these data). Assuming that the mercury data have been loaded into the SAS default library under the name

Table 19.2 Output generated by PROC ADAPTIVEREG for the MARS model for the death rate per 100,000 as a function of the nitric oxide pollution index (NObnded) and the annual average precipitation (rain) allowing for spline interactions

```
                    Basis Information

   Name          Transformation

   Basis0        1
   Basis1        Basis0*MAX(rain -          33,0)
   Basis2        Basis0*MAX(       33 - rain,0)
   Basis3        Basis0*MAX(NObnded -          4,0)
   Basis4        Basis0*MAX(        4 - NObnded,0)
   Basis5        Basis3*MAX(rain -          38,0)
   Basis6        Basis3*MAX(       38 - rain,0)
   Basis7        Basis2*MAX(NObnded -          5,0)
   Basis8        Basis2*MAX(        5 - NObnded,0)
   Basis9        Basis2*MAX(NObnded -         11,0)
   Basis10       Basis2*MAX(       11 - NObnded,0)
   Basis11       Basis2*MAX(NObnded -          2,0)
   Basis12       Basis2*MAX(        2 - NObnded,0)
   Basis13       Basis4*MAX(rain -          39,0)
   Basis14       Basis4*MAX(       39 - rain,0)
   Basis15       Basis0*MAX(NObnded -         10,0)
   Basis16       Basis0*MAX(       10 - NObnded,0)
   Basis17       Basis0*MAX(NObnded -          7,0)
   Basis18       Basis0*MAX(        7 - NObnded,0)
   Basis19       Basis0*MAX(NObnded -          6,0)
   Basis20       Basis0*MAX(        6 - NObnded,0)


        Regression Spline Model after Backward Selection

 Name        Coefficient    Parent    Variable       Knot

 Basis0        924.91                 Intercept
 Basis5        1.2677       Basis3    rain          38.0000
 Basis6        1.7791       Basis3    rain          38.0000
 Basis7       -4.3302       Basis2    NObnded        5.0000
 Basis9        8.7180       Basis2    NObnded       11.0000
 Basis14      -3.3360       Basis4    rain          39.0000
```

mercury, a MARS model for merchigh (the indicator for a high mercury level of over 1.0 ppm versus low) as a function of the weight of fish and treating merchigh as binomially distributed with logit link function can be requested in SAS as follows.

```
proc adaptivereg data=mercury details=bases;
  model merchigh(descending)=weight / dist=binomial link=logit;
run;
```

By default, PROC ADAPTIVEREG models the first or lower value of a binomial outcome like merchigh, and so the higher value is then treated as the reference value. This is reversed in the above code by adding the descending option in parentheses after the name of the outcome. In this way, models are generated for the chance of high levels of mercury versus low levels as the reference value. The option "link=logit" is not needed since that is the default link function for the "dist=binomial" option. The LCV score for this model can be generated as follows.

```
%MARSmodl(datain=mercury,dataout=data5,yvar=merchigh,
          xvars=weight);
%genreg(datain=data5,modtype=logis,yvar=merchigh,
         xvars=&bwdlist,foldcnt=15);
```

By default, MARSmodl generates a MARS model for dichotomous outcomes in descending order. Ascending order can be requested with the setting "descend=n". The generated LCV score is 0.56281 as reported in Sect. 18.4.1.

The variable river, indicating the river in which the fish were caught, is available in the mercury data set. A MARS model in weight and river, treating river as a classification variable and allowing for spline interactions can be generated as follows.

```
proc adaptivereg data=mercury details=bases;
  class river;
  model merchigh(descending)=weight river / dist=binomial link=logit;
run;
```

Part of the output generated by this code is displayed in Table 19.3. For classification variables like river, pairs of splines are generated for the variable having a subset of its values or not having those values. Since river has only two values, only one pair of splines is needed. Note that PROC ADAPTIVEREG uses the formatted values for river so that the pair of splines satisfy Basis3=(river=0:Lumber) and Basis4=NOT(river=0:Lumber). However, these are used only once interacting with the spline Basis1 = max(weight−0.869, 0).

Table 19.3 Output generated by PROC ADAPTIVEREG for the MARS model for a high mercury level > 1 ppm versus lower as a function of the weight of the fish and the river in which they were caught treated as a classification variable

```
                    Probability modeled is merchigh='1:high'.
...

                             Basis Information

         Name                   Transformation

         Basis0                 1
         Basis1                 Basis0*MAX(weight -        0.869,0)
         Basis2                 Basis0*MAX(      0.869 - weight,0)
         Basis3                 Basis1*(river = 0:Lumber)
         Basis4                 Basis1*NOT(river = 0:Lumber)
         Basis5                 Basis0*MAX(weight -        0.977,0)
         Basis6                 Basis0*MAX(      0.977 - weight,0)
         Basis7                 Basis0*MAX(weight -        0.844,0)
         Basis8                 Basis0*MAX(      0.844 - weight,0)
         Basis9                 Basis0*MAX(weight -         1.71,0)
         Basis10                Basis0*MAX(       1.71 - weight,0)
         Basis11                Basis0*MAX(weight -          0.6,0)
         Basis12                Basis0*MAX(        0.6 - weight,0)
         Basis13                Basis0*MAX(weight -        0.498,0)
         Basis14                Basis0*MAX(      0.498 - weight,0)
         Basis15                Basis0*MAX(weight -         0.38,0)
         Basis16                Basis0*MAX(       0.38 - weight,0)
         Basis17                Basis0*MAX(weight -        0.656,0)
         Basis18                Basis0*MAX(      0.656 - weight,0)
         Basis19                Basis0*MAX(weight -        0.308,0)
         Basis20                Basis0*MAX(      0.308 - weight,0)


            Regression Spline Model after Backward Selection

Name      Coefficient      Parent      Variable      Knot      Levels

Basis0      -2.9187                     Intercept
Basis3      -1.6099        Basis1       river                    0
Basis11     -171.43        Basis0       weight       0.6000
Basis13      185.19        Basis0       weight       0.4980
Basis15     -126.17        Basis0       weight       0.3800
Basis17      63.4805       Basis0       weight       0.6560
Basis19      50.7817       Basis0       weight       0.3080
```

An LCV score for this model can be computed as follows.

```
%MARSmodl(datain=mercury,dataout=data6,yvar=merchigh,
          xvars=weight river,classvrs=river, modtype=logis);
%genreg(datain=data6,modtype=logis,yvar=deathrate,
          xvars=&bwdlist, foldcnt=15);
```

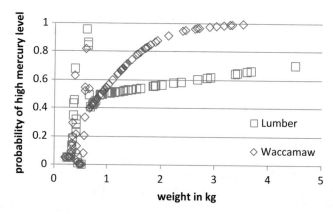

Fig. 19.1 Estimated probabilities for a high mercury level >1 ppm at unique weight values for the Lumber and Waccamaw Rivers generated by the MARS model allowing for spline interactions

The classvrs macro parameter of the MARSmodl macro specifies which of the xvars variables are to be treated as classification variables. The generated LCV score is 0.57883, which is a substantial improvement over the MARS model in weight alone with substantial PD 2.77 % (that is, greater than the cutoff of 1.13 % as reported in Sect. 8.2).

An LCV score for the additive MARS model in weight and river can be generated as follows.

```
%MARSmodl(datain=mercury,dataout=data7,yvar=merchigh,
          xvars=weight river,classvrs=river,
          modtype=logis,additive=y);
%genreg(datain=data7,modtype=logis,yvar=deathrate,
        xvars=&bwdlist,foldcnt=15);
```

The generated MARS model is based on splines for weight only and not on splines for river and is the same model as generated without consideration of river. Hence, the generated LCV score is also 0.56281 with substantial PD 2.77 % compared to the model allowing for interactions. Consequently, MARS modeling leads to the conclusion that river distinctly moderates the effect of weight on merchigh. This conclusion is also reached in Sect. 8.4 using adaptive modeling. However, the LCV score for that moderation model is 0.57192 with substantial PD 1.19 %, and so is outperformed by the MARS model.

Figure 19.1 displays estimated probabilities for a high mercury level > 1 ppm at unique weight values for the Lumber and Waccamaw Rivers generated by the MARS model allowing for spline interactions. For low weights, estimated probabilities are highly variable ranging from close to 0 to close to 1. However for weight values exceeding 0.869 kg, the estimated probabilities follow regular increasing patterns with the probabilities for the Waccamaw River increasing with increasing weights to a distinctly higher level than for the Lumber River. This model suggests that prediction of mercury levels is not reliable at relatively low weights for fish in either river.

19.6   Practice Exercises

19.1 In Sect. 18.8.3, the MARS model for deathrate in NObnded and rain allowing for interactions is addressed, but not the associated adaptive MARS model. Using $k = 5$ folds as justified in Sect. 2.8, regenerate the MARS model in NObnded and rain allowing for interactions. Then generate the associated adaptive MARS model. Compare this adaptive MARS model to the associated MARS model. Does consideration of transforms of interaction splines generate a distinct improvement or not?

19.2 Using the death rate data and $k = 5$ as justified in Sect. 2.8, generate the additive MARS model for deathrate in terms of NObnded, SO2index, and rain. Does this model depend on SO2index or not? Compare it to the additive MARS model for deathrate in terms of only NObnded and rain of Sect. 18.3.3. Next generate the adaptive additive MARS model for deathrate in terms of NObnded, SO2index, and rain. Does consideration of power transformations of splines provide a substantial improvement over using untransformed splines? Does the adaptive MARS model in these three predictors substantially improve on the adaptive MARS model generated using only NObnded and rain described in Sect. 18.3.3? Compare the adaptive additive MARS model in NObnded, SO2index, and rain to the adaptive additive model in these three predictors generated as part of Practice Exercise 3.3. Is the conclusion of any additive benefit to consideration of SO2index also controlling for additive effects to NObnded and rain the same when based on adaptive MARS models and on adaptive models?

19.3 Assess moderation of the effect of length on merchigh by river using MARS modeling. With $k = 15$ folds as justified in Sect. 8.4, generate the MARS model for merchigh in length and river allowing for interactions. Treat river as a classification variable. Compare this model to the MARS model in length of Sect. 18.4.2. Is there a substantial interaction effect between length and river and/or a substantial main effect to river using MARS modeling? Or is there no distinct river effect after controlling for length as reported for adaptive models in Sect. 8.5?

For Practice Exercise 19.4, use the body fat data set available on the Internet (see Supplementary Materials). The outcome variable for this data set is called bodyfat and contains body fat values in gm/cm^3 for 252 men. The file contains several predictors. Practice Exercises 19.4 uses only three of these predictors, called weight, height, and BMI containing weights in pounds, heights in inches, and body mass index values in kg/cm^2, respectively.

19.4 Generate the MARS model for bodyfat in terms of BMI. Use the number of folds determined as part of Practice Exercise 3.5. Compare this to the adaptive model in BMI computed for Practice Exercise 3.5. Next, generate the adaptive MARS model using the splines of the MARS model for BMI and compare it to that MARS model. Next, generate the MARS model in weight and height allowing for interactions and compare it to the MARS model in BMI. Finally, generate the adaptive MARS model in weight and height allowing for interactions and compare it to the adaptive MARS model in BMI.

For Practice Exercise 19.5, use the Titanic survival data available on the Internet (see Supplementary Materials). Data are available for 756 passengers with no missing data. The outcome variable for this data set is called survived and is the indicator for having survived the sinking of the Titanic. The predictors to be considered are age and the indicator fstclass for the passenger being in first class versus second or third class. The gender of the passenger is also available in the data set but is not used in the practice exercises.

19.5 Generate the MARS model for survived in terms of age. Use the number of folds determined as part of Practice Exercise 9.5. Compare this to the adaptive model in age computed for Practice Exercise 9.5. Next, generate the adaptive MARS model using the splines of the MARS model for age and compare it to that MARS model. Next, generate the MARS model for survived in terms of age and fstclass allowing for interactions. Compare this to the MARS model based on only age. Finally, generate the adaptive MARS model in age and fstclass allowing for interactions and compare it to the MARS model in age and fstclass allowing for interactions.

Reference

Friedman, J. H. (1991). Multivariate adaptive regression splines. *Annals of Statistics, 19*, 1–67.

Part V
The Adaptive Regression Modeling Process

Chapter 20
Adaptive Regression Modeling Formulation

20.1 Chapter Overview

This chapter provides a general formulation for adaptive regression modeling of nonlinear relationships. Since formulations for special cases have been provided earlier, only overviews are presented in Sect. 20.2 for alternative types of regression models and in Sect. 20.3 for alternate cross-validation scoring approaches. Section 20.4 then presents a detailed formulation for the adaptive regression modeling process used by the genreg macro, which has only been generally described earlier.

20.2 Overview of General Regression Modeling Formulation

Formulations for regression modeling of continuous outcomes have been provided in Chaps. 2 and 4. Sections 2.3 and 2.17 address regression modeling of means for univariate continuous outcomes using univariate normal likelihoods. This is extended to modeling of variances along with means in Sect. 2.19.1. These formulations are further extended for multivariate continuous outcomes using multivariate normal likelihoods to marginal modeling of means using maximum likelihood (ML) parameter estimation in Sect. 4.3 and generalized estimating equations (GEE) parameter estimation in Sect. 4.11.1 as well as modeling of variances along with means in Sect. 4.15.1. Section 4.7 provides a formulation for transition modeling of means of multivariate continuous outcomes expressing multivariate normal likelihoods as products of univariate conditional normal likelihoods, or equivalently in terms of dependence predictors computed from prior outcome measurements. Section 4.9 generalizes transition modeling of multivariate continuous outcomes to general conditional modeling using pseudolikelihoods defined as products of univariate conditional normal likelihoods, or equivalently in terms of dependence

© Springer International Publishing Switzerland 2016
G.J. Knafl, K. Ding, *Adaptive Regression for Modeling Nonlinear Relationships*,
Statistics for Biology and Health, DOI 10.1007/978-3-319-33946-7_20

predictors computed from prior and/or subsequent outcome measurements. The extension to transition and general conditional modeling of variances along with means for multivariate continuous outcomes is similar to the extension in Sect. 2.19.1 for univariate continuous outcomes (as also noted in Sect. 4.15.1).

Formulations for regression modeling of discrete outcomes, either dichotomous and polytomous, have been provided in Chaps. 8–10. Section 8.3 addresses logistic regression modeling of means for univariate dichotomous outcomes using Bernoulli likelihoods and Sect. 8.13.1 extends this to modeling of means and dispersions using associated extended quasi-likelihoods. The extension to binomial likelihoods for grouped data is addressed in Sect. 9.5. Section 8.7 addresses logistic regression modeling of means for univariate polytomous outcomes using categorical likelihoods and Sect. 8.13.2 extends this to modeling of means and dispersions using associated extended quasi-likelihoods. The extension to multinomial likelihoods for grouped data is addressed in Sect. 9.9. Nominal polytomous outcomes can be modeled using multinomial regression based on generalized logits (Sect. 8.7.1). Ordinal polytomous outcomes can be modeled using ordinal regression based on cumulative logits and proportional odds (Sect. 8.7.2) or using multinomial regression. Section 10.3 provides a formulation for general conditional modeling, including transition modeling as a special case, of multivariate dichotomous outcomes using pseudolikelihoods defined as products of univariate conditional Bernoulli likelihoods for modeling of means (Sect. 10.3.1) and also extended quasi-pseudolikelihoods for modeling dispersions along with means (Sect. 10.3.2). The extension to grouped multivariate dichotomous outcomes using binomial pseudolikelihoods and binomial extended quasi-pseudolikelihoods is similar to the extension in Sect. 9.5 for univariate dichotomous outcomes (and so a detailed formulation is not provided). Initial groups of measurements are computed in the same way as for the univariate case but then partitioned into actual groups of measurements with the same values of the variable specified by the withinvr macro parameter. The extension of conditional modeling of means and dispersions of multivariate polytomous outcomes using pseudolikelihoods defined as products of univariate conditional categorical likelihoods and associated extended quasi-pseudolikelihoods is addressed in Sect. 10.5. The extension to grouped multivariate polytomous outcomes using multinomial pseudolikelihoods and multinomial extended quasi-pseudolikelihoods is similar to the extension in Sect. 9.9 for univariate polytomous outcomes (and so a detailed formulation is not provided). Section 10.7 addresses marginal generalized estimating equations (GEE) modeling of means and dispersions for multivariate dichotomous (Sect. 10.7.1) and polytomous (Sect. 10.7.2) outcomes.

Formulations for modeling of count outcomes, possibly adjusted to rate outcomes using offsets, have been provided in Chaps. 12 and 14. Section 12.3.1 addresses Poisson regression modeling of means for univariate count/rate outcomes using Poisson likelihoods and Sect. 12.3.2 extends this to modeling of means and dispersions using associated extended quasi-likelihoods. Section 14.3 provides a formulation for general conditional modeling, including transition modeling as a special case, of multivariate count/rate outcomes using pseudolikelihoods defined as products of univariate conditional Poisson likelihoods for modeling of means (Sect. 14.3.1) and also extended quasi-pseudolikelihoods for modeling dispersions along with means (Sect. 14.3.2). Section 14.5 addresses marginal generalized estimating equations (GEE) modeling of means and dispersions for multivariate count/rate outcomes.

The normal, Bernoulli, and Poisson distributions are members of the exponential family of distributions. Modeling of means for univariate outcomes having any other distribution in this family, for example, the gamma distribution, is formulated similarly to the normal, Bernoulli, and Poisson cases, but with the likelihoods appropriately adjusted. Extensions to modeling of dispersions along with means for univariate outcomes having one of these other distributions is similar to the extension for the Bernoulli and Poisson cases, but extended quasi-likelihoods are computed with different deviance functions (see McCullagh and Nelder 1999). For example, the deviance function for the gamma distribution is $d(y; \mu) = 2 \cdot (-\log(y/\mu) + (y - \mu)/\mu)$. Transition and general conditional modeling of means and dispersions for multivariate outcomes with each of its univariate component outcome variables having a common distribution in the exponential family are formulated similarly to the Bernoulli and Poisson cases but with pseudolikelihoods and extended quasi-pseudolikelihoods appropriately adjusted. Marginal GEE modeling of means and dispersions for such multivariate outcomes is formulated similarly to the Bernoulli and Poisson cases. The variance function $V(\mu)$ for the mean-value parameter μ needs to be adjusted. For example, the variance function for the gamma distribution satisfies $V(\mu) = \mu^2$.

20.3 Overview of Model Selection Approaches

20.3.1 Using Cross-Validation Based on Likelihood or Likelihood-Like Functions

Likelihood cross-validation (LCV) scores are defined in Sect. 2.5.3. The k-fold approach partitions the data into disjoint subsets called folds, computes the likelihood for each fold from the data in that fold and parameters estimated using the data in the other folds, and combines these deleted likelihoods into a score with larger values indicating better models. The leave-one-out (LOO) approach assigns each observation to its own fold.

LCV scores are used to evaluate and compare models for univariate continuous outcomes using normal likelihoods in Chaps. 2, 3, 6, 7 and 16–19, for multivariate continuous outcomes using marginal multivariate normal likelihoods in Chaps. 4–7, univariate dichotomous outcomes using Bernoulli likelihoods in Chaps. 8, 9 and 16–19 as well as grouped binomial likelihoods in Chap. 9, univariate polytomous outcomes using categorical likelihoods in Chaps. 8 and 9 as well as grouped multinomial likelihoods in Chap. 9, and univariate count/rate outcomes using

Poisson likelihoods in Chaps. 12 and 13. Extended quasi-likelihood cross-validation ($QLCV^+$) scores are defined in Sect. 8.13 for modeling dispersions along with means of dichotomous (Sect. 8.13.1) and polytomous (Sect. 8.13.2) outcomes using associated deviance functions. $QLCV^+$ scores for modeling dispersions along with means of count/rate outcomes are addressed in Sect. 12.3.2. For the discrete outcome cases, the deviance function is equivalent to the associated likelihood and so LCV scores for unit dispersion models can be compared to $QLCV^+$ scores for non-unit dispersions models for the same data. In general, including the count/rate outcome case, the deviance function equals the likelihood plus a term constant in the model parameters, and so maximizing the deviance function with constant dispersions generates the same estimates of the parameters for the means as maximum likelihood estimation of those parameters under unit dispersions. The constant equals zero for dichotomous and polytomous outcomes, but not in general. Pseudolikelihood cross-validation (PLCV) scores for evaluating and comparing general conditional models of means and variances for multivariate continuous outcomes are defined in Sect. 4.9.1 using univariate conditional normal likelihoods. This is extended to models for means of dichotomous outcomes in Sect. 10.3.1, of polytomous outcomes in Sect. 10.5, and of count/rate outcomes in Sect. 14.3.1. Extended PLCV ($PLCV^+$) scores for models of dispersions along with means of dichotomous outcomes are addressed in Sect. 10.3.2, of polytomous outcomes in Sect. 10.5, and of count/rate outcomes in Sect. 14.3.2. Extended quasi-pseudolikelihoods and associated $PLCV^+$ scores are computed using extended conditional quasi-likelihoods for outcome measurements conditioned on subsets of other measurements. Transition models are the special case when the other measurements are subsets of the prior measurements. $PLCV/PLCV^+$ scores for transition models equal their $LCV/QLCV^+$ scores. Extended LCV scores (LCV^+) are defined in terms of multivariate normal likelihoods extended to address marginal GEE models for means and dispersions of dichotomous and polytomous outcomes in Sect. 10.7 and of count/rate outcomes in Sect. 14.5.

For marginal multivariate cases, LCV and LCV^+ scores can be based on matched-set-wise deletion (Sect. 4.4.1) with all measurements for a matched set randomly assigned to the same fold or on measurement-wise deletion (Sect. 4.13) with measurements of each matched set randomly assigned to possibly different folds. For conditional multivariate cases, PLCV and $PLCV^+$ scores can be based on matched-set-wise deletion, measurement-wise deletion, or partial measurement-wise deletion. Measurement-wise deletion, in this case, requires that conditional predictors based on averages of other measurements be recomputed for the data in the complement of each fold while matched-set-wise deletion uses conditional predictors computed for the complete data. Partial measurement-wise deletion is intermediate between these two other alternatives with measurements of each matched set randomly assigned to possibly different folds, but with conditional predictors computed from the complete data to reduce the computations.

Cross-validation scores can be computed in any context with parameter estimation computed by maximizing likelihoods or likelihood-like functions (e.g. extended quasi-likelihoods). LCV and PLCV scores can be computed in any context with parameter estimates based on maximizing likelihoods and pseudolikelihoods, respectively. $QLCV^+$ and $PLCV^+$ scores can be computed in any context with outcomes having a common distribution in the exponential family using the associated deviance function $d(y;\mu)$. LCV^+ scores can be computed for multivariate outcomes with each univariate component outcome having distribution in the exponential family using the associated variance function $V(\mu)$. As an example, Knafl et al. (2010) use LCV scores to evaluate and compare models for means for univariate count outcomes with unit dispersions based on Poisson likelihoods and $QLCV^+$ scores for both means and dispersions of univariate count outcomes based on Poisson extended quasi-likelihoods. They also evaluate and compare cluster analysis models using LCV scores based on likelihoods for multivariate normal mixture distributions. Knafl and Grey (2007) evaluate and compare exploratory and confirmatory factor analysis models using LCV scores based on factor-analytic multivariate normal likelihoods.

20.3.2   Alternate Model Selection Approaches

Least square cross-validation (LSCV) scores are often used for model selection, for example in the linear regression context (see Sect. 2.5.3) and in the generalized additive modeling context (see Sect. 16.4). A simplified form of LSCV called generalized cross-validation is also used in the latter context (Sect. 16.4), but can have problems (Sect. 16.5). Penalized likelihood criteria (PLCs) are commonly used as well, including among others the Akaike information criterion (AIC), the Bayesian information criterion (BIC), and the Takeuchi information criterion (TIC) (Sect. 2.10.1). These are usually formulated so that smaller scores indicate better models. PLCs can be used to control the adaptive modeling process (as described in Sect. 20.4) but need first to be adjusted so that larger scores indicate better models (as defined in Sect. 2.10.1). However, their use in adaptive modeling can have problems (Sects. 2.10.2 and 4.8.4). In the logistic regression context, the proportion of correct deleted predictions (PCDP) can be used as an alternative for controlling the adaptive modeling process for both dichotomous and polytomous discrete outcomes, but its use in adaptive modeling can have problems (Sects. 8.12.2 and 8.12.3).

In the case of modeling multivariate outcomes, the computation of likelihoods can be too complex for likelihood-based parameter estimation and model selection to be practical in general. Consequently, GEE techniques have been developed that circumvent the need to compute likelihoods. For that reason, the quasi-likelihood criterion (QIC) has been formulated (Sect. 4.11) with the "likelihood" part of the score based on the independent-data case and only the penalty factor accounting for dependence. However, the use of the QIC score in model selection can have problems (Sects. 4.11.3 and 11.4). Not being able to compute a likelihood function also complicates adaptive modeling since it requires a cross-validation score based on a likelihood-like function. However, LCV^+ scores based on extended multivariate normal likelihoods can be used to control the adaptive modeling process for such outcomes (as justified in Sect. 10.7.1) that fully accounts for the dependence. The extended likelihood in these cases can also be penalized to obtain extended PLCs that also fully account for the dependence (Sect. 10.7.1).

20.4   The Adaptive Modeling Process

This section describes the heuristic search process used by the genreg macro to generate adaptive models. The process is controlled by rules indicating how much of a percent decrease (PD) or percent increase (PI) in the cross-validation (CV) scores can be tolerated at each of the steps of the process. CV scores of any kind can be used as long as larger values indicate better models, including LCV, $QLCV^+$, PLCV, $PLCV^+$, and LCV^+ scores as well as adjusted penalized likelihood criteria including adjusted versions of AIC, BIC, and TIC (see Sect. 2.10.1) penalizing true likelihoods, adjusted versions of their extensions AIC^+, BIC^+, and TIC^+ (see Sect. 10.7.1) penalizing extended likelihoods, and adjusted versions for other extensions penalizing extended quasi-likelihoods, pseudolikelihoods, or extended quasi-pseudolikelihoods (not addressed elsewhere but readily formulated). The proportion of correct deleted predictions (PCDP; see Sect. 8.12.1) can also be used in the logistic regression context.

20.4.1   Conditional Predictors

For an outcome variable y multiply measured over conditions $c \in C$, let u be a variable with values changing with the conditions c, either the outcome variable y itself or some condition-varying predictor variable. Transition and general conditional models use dependence predictors for the current value of y computed from averages of subsets of the values for u. The prior predictors PRE(u,i,j) and associated missing indicators PRE(u,i,j,$\varnothing$) for integers $0 \leq i \leq j$ are used in transition models (and defined in Sect. 4.7). Subsequent predictors POST(u,i,j) and combined prior and subsequent predictors OTHER(u,i,j) along with associated missing indicators POST(u,i,j,$\varnothing$) and OTHER(u,i,j,$\varnothing$) are used in general conditional models (and defined in Sect. 4.9.1) possibly with prior predictors. When u = y, these predictors specify the dependence of each outcome measurement on subsets of the other outcome measurements, and so i should then be positive to avoid using the current outcome measurement. For condition-varying variables $u \neq y$, the option i = 0 can be used to model the current outcome measurement in terms of averages of the current as well as prior and/or subsequent values of u. Conditional models commonly use sums based on the other outcome values (e.g., Liang and Zeger 1989), but these are not comparable when the observed conditions sets C(s) for the matched sets s vary with s∈S. Using averages accounts for possible missing outcome measurements, which can happen even when the available outcome measurements C(s) is the full set C for all matched sets s∈S in cases with CV scores computed using measurement-wise deletion (Sect. 4.13). Conditional models sometimes include predictors based on sums of products of other outcome measurements (e.g., Eq. (2.2) of Liang and Zeger 1989). These are not directly supported by the genreg macro, but geometric combinations based on products of power transformations of the variables PRE(y,i,j), POST(y,i,j), and OTHER(y,i,j) can be included in models to achieve similar effects.

20.4.2   Power Transforms

Power transforms u^p of primary predictors u, either dependence or non-dependence, are not always well-defined for all real valued powers p. To avoid this, power transforms are defined as f(u,p) with value u^p when u > 0, 0 when u = 0, and $\cos(\pi \cdot p) \cdot |u|^p$ when u < 0 where |u| is the absolute value of u and 0^p is set to 0 even for negative powers p < 0 (see Sect. 4.6.1). The limit of f(u,p) as p → 0 depends on the other predictors in the model. For example, for u > 0, if the constant predictor $u^0 = 1$ (with associated intercept parameter) is not in the model, f(u,p) converges to 1 as p → 0. Otherwise, it converges to log(u) (see Sect. 2.13.2). To avoid having to decide which case holds during the adaptive modeling process, powers are restricted away from zero. Also, to avoid overly complex models, powers are rounded to a fixed number of digits. Any number of digits can be used, but four digits are recommended and then powers p are restricted away from 0 so that $|p| \geq 0.0001$. This value is controlled by the pwrround macro parameter with default value 0.0001. Note that when u > 0 and the model includes an intercept term, models based on u^p with p = ±0.0001 approximate the model based on log(u).

20.4.3   Selecting a Power for a Primary Predictor

Let M_0 denote a base model consisting of a set of power transforms for modeling the means and another set for modeling the variances/dispersions with each set possibly empty but not both. Let u be a possible primary predictor. If u is constant, two valued, or a three valued indicator with values −1, 0, and 1 or some fixed positive multiple of this, power transformation of u has no effect on the model and so the power p is set to 1 in such cases. Otherwise, let $CV(M_0, u, p)$ denote the CV score (of type determined by the setting of the macro parameter scretype) for the base model M_0 adjusted to include $f(u,p)$ in its set of predictors for modeling the means. The starting power p_0 is chosen as the power generating the best score $CV(M_0, u, p)$ in a grid search over a fixed set of powers. A grid search over powers $p = -3, -2.5, \cdots, -0.5, 0.5, \cdots, 2.5, 3$ has proven to be effective in practice while limiting the computations and is recommended. The case $p = 0$ is purposely skipped as discussed in Sect. 20.4.2. The values in the grid search are controlled by the expwrfst, expwrlst, and expwrstp (for first, last, and step for powers used to start the power search) macro parameters with default values -3, 3, and 0.5, respectively. The exskip0 macro parameter with default value y means skip the 0 power in this grid search. The choice exskip0=n is not recommended.

Given the current power p_i and the current change in power Δ_i, with $\Delta_0 = 1$ as set through the exdelpwr (for expansion power delta) macro parameter with default value 1, if

$$CV(M_0, u, p_i - \Delta_i) \geq CV(M_0, u, p_i + \Delta_i),$$

set the direction $d_i = -1$. Otherwise, set the direction $d_i = 1$. Vary the multiple $m_{i'}$, starting from $i' = 0$, by increments of 1 (i.e., $m_{i'+1} = m_{i'} + 1$ with $m_0 = 1$) until

$$CV\big(M_0, u, p_i + (m_{i'} - 1) \cdot d_i \cdot \Delta_i\big) < CV\big(M_0, u, p_i + m_{i'} \cdot d_i \cdot \Delta_i\big)$$
$$\geq CV\big(M_0, u, p_i + (m_{i'} + 1) \cdot d_i \cdot \Delta_i\big). \quad (20.1)$$

When $\Delta_i = 1$, the alternative multiples $m_{i'}$ may be unbounded, but for $\Delta_i < 1$, it is only necessary to search through $m_{i'} < 10$. Also, only continue the search as long as there is a distinct $PI > \tau_1 \cdot 100\,\%$ in the CV scores for the multiple $m_{i'}$ compared to the previous multiple $m_{i'} - 1$. Besides reducing the computations, this can sometimes avoid the generation of powers with very large absolute values when $\Delta_i = 1$. At the stopping value for $m_{i'}$, if there is a distinct $PD < \tau_2 \cdot 100\,\%$ for the smallest of the three CV scores of Eq. (20.1) compared to the largest of those scores, continue the search with $p_{i+1} = p_i + m_{i'} \cdot d_i \cdot \Delta_i$ and $\Delta_{i+1} = \Delta_i / 10$. Otherwise, stop the search and the selected model is the base model M_0 with its set of predictors for the means augmented with the power transform $f(u, p^+(u))$ where $p^+(u) = p_i + m_{i'} \cdot d_i \cdot \Delta_i$. The search also stops when the next value of Δ_i is smaller than the power rounding value given by the setting of the pwrround macro parameter.

The recommended settings are $\tau_1 = 0.0001$ and $\tau_2 = 0.005$. The value of τ_1 is assigned with the tracctol (for transform accept tolerance) macro parameter with default value 0.0001. By default, the value of τ_1 is adjusted with the total number of measurements $m(SC)$ (using the notation of Sect. 4.3) as described in Sect. 20.4.8. This is controlled by the trstptst (for transformation stopping test; that is, based on a CV ratio test, see Sect. 4.4.2) macro parameter with default setting "trsptst=y", meaning to adjust all transformation-related tolerance parameters. The setting "trstptst=n" means to use assigned values of all transformation-related tolerance parameters without adjustment. This is not recommended. Adjusting for the number of measurements has been found to generate more effective models. The value of τ_2 is assigned with the trgrdtol (for transformation grid tolerance) macro parameter with default value 0.005. Its value is also adjusted with the total number of measurements m(SC) when "trstptst $=$ y".

20.4.4   Adjusting the Transforms of a Base Model

Let M_0 denote a base model consisting of some set of power transforms for the means and another set for the variances/dispersions with each set possibly empty but not both. The power transforms of this model can be adjusted to improve the CV score through the following process.

For each transform $f(u,p)$ for the means of the current base model M_i, let M_i' denote the model M_i with $f(u,p)$ removed and use the process of Sect. 20.4.3 to add to the set of transforms of M_i' for the means a power transform of u. Start this search with p_0 set equal to the current power p for u in M_i (rather than using the grid search of Sect. 20.4.3) to generate a new power transform $f(u,p^+(u,p))$. Also conduct similar searches for each transform $f(u,p)$ for the variances/dispersions. Let u_{max} denote the primary predictor for either the means or the variances/dispersions whose adjustment generates the best CV score, i.e.

$$CV\left(M_i',u_{max},p^+(u_{max},p)\right) = \max\left\{CV\left(M_i',u,p^+(u,p)\right) : f(u,p)\,a\,predictor\,of\,M_i\right\}.$$

If there is a distinct PI $> \tau_3 \cdot 100\,\%$ for the model M_{i+1} given by M_i with the power for u_{max} adjusted to $p^+(u_{max},p)$ compared to the model M_i, change the base model to M_{i+1}. Otherwise, stop the search and select the current base model M_i as the transform-adjusted model for M_0. At each stage of this process, if the PI in CV scores for the current base model M_i with one of its transform $f(u,p)$ adjusted compared to M_i is distinct, that is, if PI $> \tau_4 \cdot 100\,\%$, keep it under consideration for further adjustment. Otherwise, drop the transform $f(u,p)$ from future consideration for adjustment. This can reduce the computations.

Recommended settings are $\tau_3 = 0.001$ and $\tau_4 = 0.0001$. The value of τ_3 is assigned with the trstptol (for transformation stop tolerance) macro parameter with default value 0.001 while the value of τ_4 is assigned with the trkeptol (for transformation keep tolerance) macro parameter with default value 0.0001. When "trstptst $=$ y", these transformation-related tolerance values are adjusted with the total number of measurements m(SC) (along with the values of τ_1 and τ_2 of Sect. 20.4.3).

20.4.5   Expanding a Base Model

Let M_0 denote a base model. Let U' be a set of primary predictors for modeling the means and U'' a set of primary predictors for modeling the variances/dispersions with each set possibly empty but not both. M_0 can be expanded to include transforms $f(u,p)$ of the predictors u of either U' or U'' through the following process.

For each primary predictor $u \in U'$ for the means, use the power selection process of Sect. 20.4.3 to add to the currently expanded model M_i a power transform $f(u, p^+(u))$ for the means. Also, for each primary predictor $u \in U''$ for the variances/dispersions, use the power selection process of Sect. 20.4.3 to add to the currently expanded model M_i a power transform $f(u, p^+(u))$ for the variances/dispersions. Let u_{max} denote the primary predictor for either the means or the variances/dispersions whose adjustment generates the best CV score, i.e.

$$CV(M_i, u_{max}, p^+(u_{max})) = \max\Big\{ CV(M_i, u, p^+(u)) \; : \; u \in U' \text{ or } u \in U'' \Big\}.$$

Let M_{i+1} be the model M_i with $f(u_{max}, p^+(u_{max}))$ added to its predictors for the means if $u_{max} \in U'$ and to its predictors for the variances/dispersions if $u_{max} \in U''$. If $u_{max} \in U'$ and there is a distinct PD $< \tau_{5x} \cdot 100\,\%$ for M_{i+1} compared to the prior expanded model with the largest CV score, then stop expanding the means. If $u_{max} \in U''$ and there is a distinct PD $< \tau_{5v} \cdot 100\,\%$ for M_{i+1} compared to the prior expanded model with the largest CV score, then stop expanding the variances/dispersions. Continue with M_{i+1} as the current expanded model until the expansion of the means and variance/dispersions have both been stopped.

At each stage of this process, if there is a distinct PD $< \tau_6 \cdot 100\,\%$ in CV scores for model M_i expanded to include the transform $f(u, p^+(u))$ compared to the prior expanded model with the largest CV score, drop the primary predictor u from future consideration for expanding the model. This adjustment can reduce the computations. Also, if the current expanded model M_i includes one or more other transforms of the predictor u for modeling the means (variances/dispersions), then drop u from future consideration for modeling the means (variances/dispersions) if the addition of its next transform for modeling the means (variances/dispersions) generates a distinct PD $< \tau_7 \cdot 100\,\%$ for the model M_i expanded to include the transform $f(u, p^+(u))$ compared to the prior expanded model with the largest CV score.

The values of the stopping tolerances τ_{5x} and τ_{5v} decrease with the number of non-unit transforms used to model the means and the variances/dispersions, respectively. This reduces the number of ineffective transforms in the model. If there are no non-unit transforms in the base model for the means (variances/dispersions), the initial value for $\tau_{5x}(\tau_{5v})$ is the value τ_5; otherwise the initial value for $\tau_{5x}(\tau_{5v})$ is τ_5 minus $\Delta\tau_5$ times the number of non-unit transforms in the base model for the means (variances/dispersions). As each transform is added to the model for the means (variances/dispersions), $\tau_{5x}(\tau_{5v})$ is decreased by $\Delta\tau_5$. Note that τ_{5x} and τ_{5v} can become negative. When they are positive, transforms can be added to the model that decrease the CV score; when negative, transforms need to increase the CV score to be added to the model. A single expansion stopping tolerance for the mean and variance/dispersion components of the model in combination is not used since that can result in stopping the expansion before one of these components has been effectively expanded in comparison to expanding each component separately.

Recommended settings are $\tau_5 = 0.05$, $\Delta\tau_5 = 0.01$, $\tau_6 = 0.05$, and $\tau_7 = 0.001$. The value of τ_5 is assigned with the exstptol (for expansion stop tolerance) macro parameter with default value 0.05. The value of $\Delta\tau_5$ is assigned with the exstpdel (for expansion stop delta) macro parameter with default value 0.01. The value of τ_6 is assigned with the exdrptol (for expansion drop tolerance) macro parameter with default value 0.05. The value of τ_7 is assigned with the mlttrtol (for multiple transform tolerance) macro parameter with default value 0.001. When invoked as part of the expansion, the power selection process of Sect. 20.4.3 uses different macro parameters to set its tolerances. The value of τ_1 is assigned with the exacctol (for expansion accept tolerance) macro parameter with default value 0.0001 and the value of τ_2 is assigned with the exgrdtol (for expansion grid tolerance) macro parameter with default value 0.005. These are the same default values as for the associated macro parameters tracctol and trgrdtol, but in general the settings for the tolerance parameters τ_1 and τ_2 can be different when set directly by the transform adjustment process of Sect. 20.4.4 or indirectly by the expansion process. When exstptst (for expansion stop test) has its default setting "exstptst=y", all of the expansion-related tolerance settings (as determined by exstptol, exstpdel, exdrptol, mlttrtol, exacctol, and exgrdtol) are adjusted with the total number of measurements m(SC) (as described in Sect. 20.4.8).

20.4.6   Considering Geometric Combinations

The expansion process of Sect. 20.4.5 only considers transforms of individual primary predictors separate from the other primary predictors, but not interactions between multiple primary predictors. One way to allow for interaction terms is to include products of predictors in the sets U' and U''. For example, if u_1 and u_2 are two distinct primary predictors, the interaction term $u_3 = u_1 \cdot u_2$ can be added as a primary predictor. However, the expansion process of Sect. 20.4.5 then only considers transforms $f(u_3, p)$ using a common power p for both u_1 and u_2. This is reasonable if one of u_1 or u_2 is an indicator variable and so unaffected by power transformation. In the general case, though, the more general transform $f(u_1, p_1, u_2, p_2) = f(u_1, p_1) \cdot f(u_2, p_2)$ might be a more effective predictor. The expansion process of Sect. 20.4.5 can be adjusted to consider such geometric combinations (GCs) as follows.

For each $u' \in U'$, let $f_0 = f(u', p^+(u'))$ be the transform selected as part of the power selection process of Sect. 20.4.3 invoked as part of the expansion process of Sect. 20.4.5 as the best transform of u' to add next to the means for the current expanded model M_i (the same process is also used for each $u'' \in U''$). Let $U_0 = U' \backslash \{u'\}$. The predictor u' is not considered since it generates the first term of the GC. Note that predictors are considered for use in GCs even if they have been dropped from consideration as predictors by themselves as part of the expansion process of Sect. 20.4.5. Even if a predictor cannot improve the model by itself, it might still generate an effective GC term to complement other predictors.

Starting at $i' = 0$, for each $u \in U_{i'}$ use a power selection process similar to that of Sect. 20.4.3 to find the best GC $f^+(u) = f_{i'} \cdot f(u, p^+(u))$ to include in the model for the means in place of $f_{i'}$ determined by transforms of u with associated score $CV(u)$. For simplicity, the search for each u is started at the initial power $p_0 = 1$ rather than choosing this power through a grid search (as is done in the expansion process of Sect. 20.4.5). This search for a power for u is controlled using an accept tolerance parameter τ_8 analogous to τ_1 and a grid tolerance τ_9 analogous to τ_2. If there is a distinct PD $< \tau_{10} \cdot 100$ % for the model with $f_{i'}$ changed to $f^+(u)$ for some $u \in U_{i'}$, then drop u from future consideration for inclusion in the current GC (i.e., remove u from $U_{i'+1}$ as defined below). Let $u_{i'+1}$ denote the primary predictor generating the GC resulting in the best CV score for $u \in U_{i'}$, that is,

$$CV(u_{i'+1}) = \max\{CV(u) : u \in U_{i'}\}.$$

Let $M_{i'+1}$ be the model $M_{i'}$ with $f_{i'}$ changed to $f_{i'+1} = f^+(u_{i'+1})$. If there is a distinct PD $< \tau_{11} \cdot 100$ % for the model based on $f_{i'+1}$ compared to the model based on $f_{i'}$, stop the search and select the current GC $f^+ = f_{i'}$ generating the current model $M^+ = M_{i'}$. Otherwise continue the process using $f_{i'+1}$ and $U_{i'+1} = U_j \backslash \{u_{i'+1}\}$.

The recommended settings for τ_8 and τ_9 are the same as for τ_1 and τ_2, that is, 0.0001 and 0.005. The other recommended settings are $\tau_{10} = 0.0001$ and $\tau_{11} = 0.001$. The value of τ_8 is assigned with the cmacctol (for combination accept tolerance) macro parameter with default value 0.0001. The value of τ_9 is assigned with the cmgrdtol (for combination grid tolerance) macro parameter with default value 0.005. The value of τ_{10} is assigned with the cmdrptol (for combination drop tolerance) macro parameter with default value 0.0001. The value of τ_{11} is assigned with the cmstptol (for combination stop tolerance) macro parameter with default value 0.001. When cmstptst (for combination stop test) has its default value "y", all four of these combination-related tolerance values are adjusted with the total number of measurements $m(SC)$ (as described in Sect. 20.4.8). By default, powers p used in GCs are restricted away from 0 so that $|p| \geq 0.0001$. This value is controlled by the wgtround macro parameter with default value 0.0001 (with the same effect for controlling powers in GCs as the pwrround macro parameter has for controlling power transforms).

Now with $u'' = f^+$, apply the power selection process of Sect. 20.4.3, but with initial power $p_0 = 1$, to select the power transform $f(u'', p^+(u''))$ to replace f^+ in M^+ with CV score $CV(u'')$. If $CV(u'') \leq CV(u)$, that is, if the CV score generated by the transformed GC generated from the power transform $f(u, p^+(u))$ of u does not improve on the CV score for $f(u, p^+(u))$, use $f(u, p^+(u))$ instead in the expansion search of Sect. 20.4.5. Also, If $CV(u'')$ does not improve on the best overall CV score generated in prior iterations of the expansion process of Sect. 20.4.5, also use $f(u, p^+(u))$ in the search of Sect. 20.4.5. Otherwise, replace $f(u, p^+(u))$ by $f(u'', p^+(u''))$ in the expansion search of Sect. 20.4.5. These latter adjustments mean only consider inclusion of the more complex GCs in models when they provide improvements to the overall model.

20.4.7 Contracting a Base Model

Power transforms of primary predictors generating reduced CV scores can be added to the model in the expansion as long as the reduction is tolerable (as measured by τ_{5x} and τ_{5v}). These transforms may become more effective if other previously included transforms are removed from the model. In any case, there is a need to consider contracted models with some of the expanded terms removed and the others possibly retransformed.

Let M_0 denote a base model consisting of a set of power transforms of primary predictors and/or of GCs for modeling the means and a set for modeling the variances/dispersions with each set possibly empty but not both. It can be contracted by removing transforms and adjusting the remaining transforms with the following process.

For each transform f for either the means or the variances/dispersions of the current base model M_i, let $M_i{}'(f)$ denote the model M_i with f removed. Use the transformation process of Sect. 20.4.4 to adjust the transforms of $M_i{}'(f)$ into the model $M_i{}''(f)$. Transforms f can be power transforms of primary predictors as generated in Sect. 20.4.3 or power transforms of GCs as generated in Sect. 20.4.6. While the terms comprising the GCs can have different powers, whole GCs are retransformed, not individual GC terms separately. Let f_{max} be the transform of M_i whose removal generates the best CV score among all the transforms of M_i, that is,

$$CV\left(M_i{}''(f_{max})\right) = \max\left\{CV\left(M_i{}''(f)\right) : f \text{ a transform of } M_i\right\}.$$

If there is a distinct PD $< \tau_{13} \cdot 100\%$ for the model $M_{i+1} = M_i{}''(f_{max})$ compared to the model M_i, stop the search and select the current base model M_i as the contracted model for M_0. Otherwise, change the base model to M_{i+1} and continue the process. At each stage i, if there is a distinct PD $< \tau_{14} \cdot 100\%$ in CV scores for the model $M_i{}''(f)$ compared to the prior model M_i, drop the transform f from future consideration for removal. The inclusion of this transform provides a strong enough benefit at the current stage of the contraction that it is unlikely to be removed at later stages. However, its power might be changed at later stages.

By default, the contraction for the means (variance/dispersions) also stops when there is only one remaining term in the model for the means (variance/dispersions). This can be overridden to consider removal of this term creating a zero model for the possibly transformed means (log transformed variances/dispersions) using the setting "cnxzero=y" ("cnvzero=y"). However, this is unlikely to be beneficial except when using "cnvzero=y" with a dichotomous or polytomous outcome, thereby creating a unit dispersions model.

Recommended settings are $\tau_{13} = 0.02$ and $\tau_{14} = 0.1$. The value of τ_{13} is assigned with the cnstptol (for contraction stop tolerance) macro parameter with default value 0.02 while the value of τ_{14} is assigned with the cndrptol (for contraction drop tolerance) macro parameter with default value 0.1. When "cnstptst=y", these contraction-related tolerance values are adjusted with the total number of measurements m(SC) as described in Sect. 20.4.8.

20.4.8   Tolerance Parameter Settings

Settings have been recommended in Sects. 20.4.3–20.4.7 for the tolerance parameters $\tau_1 - \tau_{14}$ and $\Delta\tau_5$ that control the adaptive model selection process. The settings of these parameters usually need to be adjusted with the number of measurements m(SC) for the process to be effective. For example, when the contraction stopping tolerance τ_{13} is too large, the contraction continues for too long and valuable transforms are removed from the model. On the other hand, when it is too small, the contraction stops too soon and ineffective transforms are retained in the model. The contraction stopping tolerance τ_{13} is set using a CV ratio test (see Sect. 4.4.2) with τ_{13} set to

$$\tau_{13}(m(SC)) = 1 - e^{-\delta(95\%, DF)/(2 \cdot m(SC))},$$

where $\delta(95\%, DF)$ is the 95th percentile of the χ^2 distribution with DF degrees of freedom (see the formula for computing the cutoff for a substantial percent decrease (PD) of Sect. 4.4.2). For multinomial regression models, DF is set to one less than the number of unique outcome values since that is the number of regression coefficient parameters removed when one transform is removed from the model for the means. In all other cases, DF = 1. When m(SC) is close to 95 and DF = 1, $\tau_{13}(m(SC))$ is close to the recommended setting of 0.02 for τ_{13}; hence the need to adjust the value of τ_{13} with m(SC). The other tolerances are adjusted similarly, but proportionally to account for their recommended value. For example, the expansion stopping tolerance τ_5 is set to

$$\tau_5(m(SC)) = 0.05 \cdot \tau_{13}(m(SC))/0.02$$

adjusting the recommended value 0.05 of the expansion stopping tolerance τ_5 by an amount proportional to the adjustment for the contraction stopping tolerance τ_{13}

from its recommended value of 0.02. If the recommended value of a tolerance parameter is changed using the associated macro parameter (e.g., exstptol for the expansion stopping tolerance or cnstptol for the contraction stopping tolerance), that value is used in place of the recommended value in these computations.

These adjustments occur for contraction (transformation, expansion, combination) tolerances when "cnstptst=y" ("trstptst=y", "exstptst=y", "cmstptst=y"). If the settings for any of these tolerances are changed from their default recommended values, those values are adjusted rather than the recommended values. When "cnstptst=n" ("trstpst=n", "exstpst=n", "cmstpst=y"), the settings for the contraction (transformation, expansion, combination) tolerances are used without adjustment. This is not recommended since it does not adjust for the number of measurements.

20.4.9   The Complete Adaptive Model Selection Process

The standard adaptive model selection process is as follows. Starting from a base model M, use the expansion process of Sect. 20.4.5 to generate the expanded model M′ (assuming "expand=y"). Then use the contraction process of Sect. 20.4.7, starting from the expanded model M′, to generate the contracted model M″ (assuming "contract=y"). If any terms are removed in the contraction, then the contracted model M″ is the selected adaptive model. If the contraction leaves the expanded model unchanged and if there might be a benefit to adjusting powers of the expanded model (that is, it has at least one power transform of a non-indicator predictor followed by at least one other transform possibly of an indicator predictor), use the transformation process of Sect. 20.4.4 to adjust the powers of the uncontracted expanded model M′ generating the model M‴ (assuming "condtrns=y"). In this case, M‴ is the final model. Otherwise, the final model is the uncontracted expanded model M′. The base model M can be arbitrary, but by default it is a constant model with constant means (assuming "xintrcpt=y" and "xvars=") and constant variances/dispersions (assuming "vintrcpt=y" and "vvars=").

A variety of adjustments to this standard process are possible. By default, "geomcmbn=n", and so the GC-generating adjustments of Sect. 20.4.6 are not considered in the expansion and additive models are generated. By default, the number of power transforms in GCs is arbitrary, but can be limited to a maximum number using the maxterms macro parameter. For example, the setting "maxterms=2" restricts to pairwise GCs, which can be more readily comprehended. The expansion process of Sect. 20.4.5 is adjusted to account for GCs when "geomcmbn=y".

Expansion steps can be restricted to models for only the means or for only the variances/dispersions (using an empty setting for one of the expxvars and expvvars macro parameters). The model for the means can be expanded before expanding the model for the variances/dispersions or in the other order. The order of the expansion

is controlled by the expordr macro parameter. The default setting "expordr=."
means to expand both the models for the means and the variances/dispersions in
combination. Setting "expordr=xv" means first expand the model for the means
("x") and then expand the model for the variances/dispersions ("v"). This order can
be reversed using "expordr=vx". The contraction order can be similarly controlled
using the contord macro parameter as can the transformation order using the
trnsordr macro parameter, but transformations as part of the contraction process
use the order determined by contordr not by trnsordr.

Terms in the base model can be held fixed so they are not removed in the
contraction. For example, "nocnxbas=y" means do not contract any of the terms
of the base model for the means and "nocnvbas=y" has the same effect on the base
model for the variances/dispersions. Linear models in the primary predictors can be
generated by (1) restricting the expansion to consider only unit powers $p = 1$ using
the "exptrans=n" and "multtrns=n" settings, meaning do not transform the primary
predictors in the expansion and do not allow multiple transforms of the same
primary predictor; (2) restricting the contraction not to adjust those powers using
the "cnretrns=n" setting, meaning do not retransform the powers of any transforms during the contraction, and (3) turning off the conditional transformation
using "condtrns=n", which would otherwise be executed if the contraction does
not change the expanded model. Models can also be expanded without being
contracted, using "expand=y" and "contract=n", or contracted without being
expanded, using "expand=n" and "contract=y". Transformation of the expanded
model can be requested with "trnsform=y". The transformed expanded model is
then the base model for the contraction, but this is unnecessary due to transformations generated as part of the contraction and conditional transformation processes.

20.4.10 Computing Transforms

SAS conducts its computations in double precision. However, the values of
power transforms of primary predictors can have more digits than can be
correctly represented in double precision. Moreover, they can be very large.
To avoid such irregularities, transformed values x are adjusted as follows. Rewrite
x as $x = \text{sign}(x) \cdot a \cdot 10^d$ where $0 \le a \le 1$ and $\text{sign}(x)$ is the usual sign
function with values -1, 0, and 1. Let a' equal a rounded to δ digits. Replace x by
$x' = \text{sign}(x) \cdot \min(a', b) \cdot 10^d$ in the associated design matrix for a bound b as
defined later. The recommended setting for the number δ of rounding digits is
12 and is set using the desgnrnd (for design matrix entry rounding) macro parameter
with default value "1e−12". The upper bound b is used to guarantee that the
transformed value is not too large. Its recommended setting is "1e12" and is set
using the mxtrnval (for maximum transform value) macro parameter with default
value "1e12".

Bounding transform values can have an effect on generated estimates. For
example, Sect. 4.15.4 reports on models for means and dispersions of strength

measurements from the exercise data of Sect. 4.12. Figure 4.6 displays post-baseline estimates for means generated by the best adaptive model for subjects in the increasing number of repetitions group. The transform $(\text{incrwgts} \cdot \text{time}^{-1} \cdot \text{PRE}(y,1)^{-11})^{-1.1}$ accounts for how much of a change there is for subjects in the increasing weights group. Since this transform is not constant in time and $\text{PRE}(y,1)$, it seems surprising that a constant change in the means of about 0.02 is reported in Sect. 4.15.4 for post-baseline times. However, the smallest values for post-baseline time and $\text{PRE}(y,1)$ are 2 and 74 so that the smallest value for $(\text{time}^{-1} \cdot \text{PRE}(y,1)^{-11})^{-1.1} = \text{time}^{1.1} \cdot \text{PRE}(y,1)^{12.1}$ is 8.89e22. Consequently, all the values for this transform exceed the upper bound "b=1e12", and so they are changed to b, resulting in the reported constant change.

20.4.11   Avoiding Redundant Transforms

Transforms f(u,p) are considered for adjusting a base model as part of the power selection process of Sect. 20.4.3, invoked as part of a request for the expansion process of Sect. 20.4.5 (when "expand=y" and "exptrans=y"). These can be transforms of either primary predictors or of GCs (when "geomcmbn=y"). Transforms are also considered as part of a request for the transformation process of Sect. 20.4.4, either indirectly as part of the contraction process of Sect. 20.4.7 (when "contract=y" and "cnretrns=y") or directly through a conditional (when "condtrns=y") or unconditional (when "trnsform=y") transformation request. When GCs are requested, GCs of the form $f_{i'} \cdot f(u, p(u))$ are also considered for adjusting a base model augmented with a previously generated GC $f_{i'}$ as part of the associated power selection process (see Sect. 20.4.6) within the expansion process. These newly generated transforms can be redundant in the sense that they are essentially equivalent to a linear combination of transforms already in the base model. The power selection processes of Sects. 20.4.3 and 20.4.4 are adjusted to drop such redundant transforms from consideration for adjusting the base model as follows.

   Let D be a $n \times (p + 1)$ design matrix for the means or variances/dispersions with the $(p + 1)$th transform added to a base model determined by the first p columns of D that has already been checked to have no redundant transforms. Let D' be the design matrix D with its columns reordered so that columns $D'[, k]$ (using the submatrix notation of SAS PROC IML; SAS Institute 2008) of D' for $1 \leq k \leq p+1$ have their maximum absolute values $\max_k = \max\{|D'[i, k]| : 1 \leq i \leq n\}$ in increasing order, i.e., $\max_1 \leq \max_2 \leq \cdots \leq \max_{p+1}$. Let D'' denote the design matrix with columns $D''[, k] = D'[, k]/\max_k$ (assuming $\max_k \neq 0$ for all k or that there are no identically zero columns in D). The transform used to generate the $(p + 1)$th column of D is considered to be redundant and skipped in the associated power selection process if the kth column of the matrix D'' is close to a linear combination of the prior $k-1$ columns of D'' for some k in the range $2 \le k \le p+1$. This latter condition holds when

$$d_k = D''[,k]` \cdot (I - X_k \cdot (X_k'X_k)^{-1} \cdot X_k`) \cdot D''[,k] < \varepsilon,$$

where $X_k = D''[,1:k]$, that is, the submatrix consisting of the first k columns of D'', I the $n \times n$ identity matrix, and the back quote ($`$) denotes the transpose operator (as for SAS PROC IML; previously denoted by a superscript "T"). The sweep function of SAS PROC IML is used to compute d_k. The recommended value for the redundancy tolerance ε is 0.00001, which is set using the eqtrntol (for equal transform tolerance) macro parameter with default value 0.00001.

Reordering of the columns of D guarantees that transforms are considered redundant no matter what order they are included in the design matrix. When models are generated adaptively, their transforms are included in design matrices in the order determined by the base model and the expansion. The contraction can remove some of these transforms and transformation can adjust the powers, but the order of the remaining transforms is not changed. When the transforms of an adaptively generated model are generated directly, transforms of primary predictors are generated first followed by transforms of GCs. Without reordering in the computation of d_k, an adaptive model can be generated that is considered not to have redundant transforms during the adaptive modeling process but considered to have redundant transforms when generated directly; reordering avoids this. The columns of D' are bounded by max_k to avoid floating point overflow when computing d_k.

References

Knafl, G. J., Delucchi, K. L., Bova, C. A., Fennie, K. P., & Williams, A. B. (2010). Chapter 1: A systematic approach for analyzing electronically monitored adherence data. In B. Ekwall & M. Cronquist (Eds.), *Micro electro mechanical systems (MEMS) technology, fabrication processes and applications* (pp. 1–66). Hauppauge, NY: Nova Science Publishers. Retrieved from https://www.novapublishers.com/catalog/product_info.php?products_id=19133

Knafl, G. J., & Grey, M. (2007). Factor analysis model evaluation through likelihood cross-validation. *Statistical Methods in Medical Research, 16*, 77–102.

Liang, K.-Y., & Zeger, S. L. (1989). A class of logistic regression models for multivariate binary time series. *Journal of the American Statistical Association, 84*, 447–451.

McCullagh, P., & Nelder, J. A. (1999). *Generalized linear models* (2nd ed.). Boca Raton, FL: Chapman & Hall/CRC.

SAS Institute. (2008). *SAS/IML 9.2 user's guide*. Cary, NC: SAS Institute.

Index

C
Conditional
  model of continuous outcomes, 83–86
  model of count outcomes, 276–279
  model of dichotomous outcomes, 215–218
  model of polytomous outcomes, 223, 224
  predictors, 75, 77, 78, 84, 85, 95, 356, 358, 359
  transformation, 46–48, 117, 126, 367, 368
Contraction, 6, 7, 33, 47, 50, 53, 55, 56, 59, 60, 99, 117, 122, 126, 127, 129, 189, 193, 204–206, 208, 209, 219–221, 226, 242, 243, 246, 247, 270, 291, 294, 310, 330, 365–368
Cross-validation, 14, 16, 17
  extended likelihood (LCV$^+$), 227–234, 282–283, 357, 358
  extended pseudolikelihood (PLCV$^+$), 217, 218, 223, 224, 278–279
  extended quasi-likelihood (QLCV$^+$), 178, 257–258, 355–357
  generalized, 302, 310, 311, 357, 358
  k-fold, 15–17, 355–357
  least square (LSCV), 16, 17, 302, 357, 358
  leave-one-out (LOO), 16, 17, 302, 355–357
  likelihood (LCV), 16, 17, 67, 94, 95, 256–258, 301, 355–357
  likelihood ratio test, 18, 68, 69
  power-adjusted likelihood, 134–136
  PRESS, 15
  pseudolikelihood (PLCV), 84, 85, 215, 216, 277–278, 355–357

D
Degree of freedom, 12, 13, 300, 301
Deletion
  matched-set-wise, 67
  measurement-wise, 94, 95
Deviance, 178, 217, 218, 257–258, 278–279, 353–355
Dispersion modeling, 178, 185, 205, 217, 218, 256–258, 278–279

E
Expansion, 6, 27, 47, 48, 50, 54–57, 113, 116, 117, 126, 127, 129, 164, 189, 206, 208, 220, 226, 242, 244, 246, 267, 269, 273, 290, 291, 293, 330, 360, 362–370

F
Fractional polynomials, 4, 5, 13, 14, 25, 27, 28
  degree 2, 29
  limits of, 30

G
Generalized additive models
  for continuous outcomes, 300, 301
  for dichotomous outcomes, 310, 311
Generalized estimating equations (GEE)
  of multivariate continuous outcomes, 87–91
  of multivariate count outcomes, 282–283
  of multivariate dichotomous/polytomous outcomes, 227–234

© Springer International Publishing Switzerland 2016
G.J. Knafl, K. Ding, *Adaptive Regression for Modeling Nonlinear Relationships*,
Statistics for Biology and Health, DOI 10.1007/978-3-319-33946-7

Printed in the United States
By Bookmasters